DRUG-INDUCED DYSFUNCTION IN PSYCHIATRY

DRUG-INDUCED DYSFUNCTION IN PSYCHIATRY

Edited by
Matcheri S. Keshavan, M.D.
Western Psychiatric Institute and Clinic
University of Pittsburgh
Pittsburgh, Pennsylvania

John S. Kennedy, M.D.
Department of Psychiatry, Neurology, and Psychology
Case Western Reserve University
Cleveland, Ohio

●HEMISPHERE PUBLISHING CORPORATION
A member of the Taylor & Francis Group

New York   Washington   Philadelphia   London

DRUG-INDUCED DYSFUNCTION IN PSYCHIATRY

Copyright © 1992 by Hemisphere Publishing Corporation. All rights reserved. Printed in the United States of America. Except as permitted under the United States Copyright Act of 1976, no part of this publication may be reproduced or distributed in any form or by any means, or stored in a data base or retrieval system, without the prior written permission of the publisher.

1 2 3 4 5 6 7 8 9   B R B R   9 8 7 6 5 4 3 2 1

This book was set in Times Roman by Hemisphere Publishing Corporation. The editors were Deena Williams Newman and Michele Nix; the production supervisor was Peggy M. Rote; and the typesetter was Sandra Watts. Cover design by Kathleen A. Ernst.
Printing and binding by Braun-Brumfield, Inc.

A CIP catalog record for this book is available from the British Library.

Library of Congress Cataloging-in-Publication Data

Drug-induced dysfunction in psychiatry / edited by Matcheri S.
   Keshavan, John S. Kennedy.
      p.   cm.
   Includes bibliographical references and index.
   1. Psychopharmacology.   2. Psychotropic drugs—Side effects.
3. Psychotropic Drugs—adverse effects.   I. Keshavan, Matcheri S.
II. Kennedy, John S.
   [DNLM: 1. Psychopharmacology.   2. Psychoses, Substance-Induced.
WW 220 D794]
RC483.D72   1992
615'.78—dc20
DNLM/DLC
for Library of Congress   91-20848
ISBN 0-89116-961-X   CIP

From inability to let well alone,

From too much zeal for the new and contempt for what is old;

From putting knowledge before wisdom, science before art, and cleverness before common sense

From treating the patients as cases, and from making the cure of the disease more grievous than the endurance of the same,

Good lord, deliver us.

Prayer of Sir Robert Hutchinson

Contents

III
DRUG-INDUCED SYSTEMIC SYNDROMES

Foreword

"A sort of popgun pharmacy hitting now the malady and again the patient, himself not knowing which"

This quotation from Osler refers to the physician whose treatment choice can give rise to adverse drug reactions. The problem raised by Osler more than 100 years ago is of even greater concern today. These concerns about medication are even greater in psychiatric patients where an interaction of adverse effects and underlying psychiatric disorders can further contribute to the patient's distress and complicate the clinical picture. The interaction can also distort the underlying course of the psychiatric disorder and the interpretation of the therapeutic response. For example, when a benzodiazepine is withdrawn from a patient with anxiety, the withdrawal symptoms may falsely suggest an increase or a recurrence of the underlying psychopathology.

These concerns about medication are of special relevance in the psychiatric population, but are even greater in two subgroups of this population, the elderly and those with dementia. To compound this, drug interactions contribute another grave area of adverse reactions. Thus, every time a physician adds another medication to that already being taken, he or she runs the risk of developing a novel combination with unsuspected effects.

The magnitude of this problem can be illustrated by data from the Boston Collaborative Drug Surveillance Program. In a 1973 report on 11,526 patients monitored with 103,770 drug exposures, the adverse reactions rate was 28.1% (Miller RR. Drug surveillance utilizing epidemiologic methods: A report from the Boston Collaborative Drug Surveillance Program. (1973). *American Journal of Hospital Pharmacy, 30*, 584–592).

Very little available material covers the topics addressed in this volume. *Drug-Induced Dysfunction in Psychiatry* is a comprehensive reference source for this field and thus merits the attention of all potential prescribers and consumers. The editors of this volume are both broadly trained in psychiatry and clinical psychopharmacology; they have put together contributions of their own and of other experienced colleagues, both in the United States and abroad, to prepare this volume. The various contributors provide practicing clinicians with information on the iatrogenic complications encountered in psychiatric practice and an understanding of the relevant basic and clinical research data. Their mission would be well served if practicing clinicians will turn to this book as a ready reference when their patients develop adverse effects during psychiatric treatment.

Samuel Gershon, M.D.
Professor of Psychiatry
Vice-President for Research
University of Pittsburgh Medical Center

Contributors

GERARD ADDONIZIO, M.D., Associate Professor of Clinical Psychiatry, The New York Hospital-Cornell Medical Center, Westchester Division, 21 Bloomingdale Road, White Plains, New York 10605

CHITTARANJAN ANDRADE, M.D., Assistant Professor of Psychiatry, National Institute of Mental Health & Neurosciences, Bangalore, India 560029

JULES ANGST, M.D., Psychiatric University Hospital, Research Department, P.O. Box 68, CH-8027, Zurich, Switzerland

RICHARD BALON, M.D., Assistant Professor of Psychiatry, Wayne State University, Lafayette Clinic, 951 East LaFayette, Detroit, Michigan 48207

K. N. ROY CHENGAPPA, M.D., F.R.C.P.(c), M.R.C.Psych, Assistant Professor of Psychiatry, University of Pittsburgh School of Medicine, Department of Psychiatry, Western Psychiatric Institute and Clinic, 3811 O'Hara Street, Pittsburgh, Pennsylvania 15213

JOHN R. DeQUARDO, M.D., Departmental Chief Resident, University of Michigan, Department of Psychiatry, 1500 East Michigan Center Drive, Ann Arbor, Michigan 48109-0704

VIKTORIA ERHARDT, M.D., Resident, University of Chicago, Department of Psychiatry, 5841 South Maryland Avenue, Chicago, Illinois 60637

PATRICK FLYNN, M.D., F.R.C.P.(c), Professor of Psychiatry, Victoria General Hospital, Department of Psychiatry, 1278 Tower Road, Halifax, Nova Scotia, Canada, B3H 2Y9

B. N. GANGADHAR, M.D., Associate Professor of Psychiatry, National Institute of Mental Health & Neurosciences, Bangalore, India, 560029

ROHAN GANGULI, M.D., Associate Professor of Psychiatry and Pathology, University of Pittsburgh School of Medicine, Department of Psychiatry, Western Psychiatric Institute and Clinic, 3811 O'Hara Street, Pittsburgh, Pennsylvania 15213

A. JAMES GIANNINI, M.D., Clinical Professor of Psychiatry, Ohio State University, P.O. Box 2169, Youngstown, Ohio 44504

MAURICE B. GOLDMAN, M.D., Assistant Professor of Psychiatry, University of Chicago Medical Center, 5841 South Maryland, Box 411, Chicago, Illinois 60637

R. KRISHNA KAMBHAMPATI, M.D., Assistant Professor of Psychiatry, University of Pittsburgh School of Medicine, Department of Psychiatry, Western Psychiatric Institute and Clinic, 3811 O'Hara Street, Pittsburgh, Pennsylvania 15213

SHITIJ KAPUR, M.D., Resident in Psychiatry, University of Pittsburgh School of Medicine, Department of Psychiatry, Western Psychiatric Institute and Clinic, 3811 O'Hara Street, Pittsburgh, Pennsylvania 15213

JOHN S. KENNEDY, M.D., F.R.C.P.(c), Assistant Professor of Psychiatry, Neurology and Psychology, University Hospitals of Cleveland and Case Western Reserve University, 2074 Abington Road, Cleveland, Ohio 44106

JOHN KENNY, Ph.D., Assistant Professor of Psychiatry, Department of Psychiatry, University Hospitals of Cleveland, 2074 Abington Road, Cleveland, Ohio 44106

ASHA KESHAVAN, M.D., Resident in Psychiatry, University of Pittsburgh School of Medicine, Department of Psychiatry, Western Psychiatric Institute and Clinic, 3811 O'Hara Street, Pittsburgh, Pennsylvania 15213

MATCHERI S. KESHAVAN, M.D., F.R.C.P.(c), M.R.C.Psych, Associate Professor of Psychiatry, University of Pittsburgh School of Medicine, Department of Psychiatry, Western Psychiatric Institute and Clinic, 3811 O'Hara Street, Pittsburgh, Pennsylvania 15213

JAMES B. LOHR, M.D., Assistant Professor of Psychiatry, University of California, San Diego, VA Medical Center San Diego, 3350 LaJolla Village Drive, San Diego, California 92161

JOSEPH P. McEVOY, M.D., Associate Professor of Psychiatry, Duke University Medical Center, John Umstead Hospital, Butner, North Carolina 27509

VISHWAJIT L. NIMGAONKAR, M.D., Ph.D., M.R.C.Psych, Assistant Professor of Psychiatry, University of Pittsburgh School of Medicine, Department of Psychiatry, Western Psychiatric Institute and Clinic, 3811 O'Hara Street, Pittsburgh, Pennsylvania 15213

KATHLEEN A. PAJER, M.D., M.P.H., Assistant Professor of Psychiatry and Epidemiology, School of Medicine, Department of Psychiatry, University of Pittsburgh, Western Psychiatric Institute and Clinic, 3811 O'Hara Street, Pittsburgh, Pennsylvania 15213

ROBERT POHL, M.D., Associate Professor of Psychiatry, Wayne State University, Lafayette Clinic, 951 East LaFayette, Detroit, Michigan 48207

RUDRA PRAKASH, M.D., Assistant Professor of Psychiatry, Department of Psychiatry, Vanderbilt University Medical Center, 21st Avenue South, Nashville, Tennessee 37232

MICHAEL D. RANCURELLO, M.D., Assistant Professor of Psychiatry, University of Pittsburgh School of Medicine, Department of Psychiatry, Western Psychiatric Institute and Clinic, 3811 O'Hara Street, Pittsburgh, Pennsylvania 15213

SANDRA STEINGARD, M.D., Assistant Professor of Psychiatry, University of Pittsburgh School of Medicine, Department of Psychiatry, Western Psychiatric Institute and Clinic, 3811 O'Hara Street, Pittsburgh, Pennsylvania 15213

RAJIV TANDON, M.D., Director, Schizophrenia Program, Department of Psychiatry, University of Michigan, 1500 E. Medical Center Drive, Ann Arbor, Michigan 48109-0704

BRIAN K. TOONE, M.R.C.P., M.R.C.Psych, Consultant Psychiatrist, King's College Hospital, Denmark Hill, DeCrespigny Park, London SE5 United Kingdom

GARY VALLANO, M.D., University of Pittsburgh School of Medicine, Department of Psychiatry, Western Psychiatric Institute and Clinic, 3811 O'Hara Street, Pittsburgh, Pennsylvania 15213

G. SCOTT WATERMAN, M.D., University of Pittsburgh School of Medicine, Department of Psychiatry, Western Psychiatric Institute and Clinic, 3811 O'Hara Street, Pittsburgh, Pennsylvania 15213

ROBERT M. WETTSTEIN, M.D., Assistant Professor of Psychiatry, University of Pittsburgh School of Medicine, Department of Psychiatry, Western Psychiatric Institute and Clinic, 3811 O'Hara Street, Pittsburgh, Pennsylvania 15213

KASHINATH G. YADALAM, M.D., Associate Professor of Psychiatry, Director, Neuropsychiatric Clinic, Medical College of Pennsylvania, Philadelphia, Pennsylvania 19129

VIKRAM K. YERAGANI, M.D., F.R.C.P.(c), Associate Professor of Psychiatry, Wayne State University, Lafayette Clinic, 951 East LaFayette, Detroit, Michigan 48207

Preface

An inescapable fact in medicine is that any drug that has an *effect* on illness, also has the potential to demonstrate *adverse effects*. It is therefore critical for the physician to be aware of the risks involved in his or her therapeutic strategies, and together with the patient weigh the potential benefits for healing versus the potential for harm to be caused by the treatment.

This book represents an application of this quintessential principle to the practice of clinical psychopharmacology, a field that has made rapid strides over the past three decades. Physicians now have an increasing variety of biological treatments for psychiatric ailments. At the same time, more is being learned about their adverse effects. Few volumes exist in the psychopharmacological literature specifically addressing this area.

In preparing this book we have classified drug-induced reactions into a disorder or syndrome-oriented approach in the belief that this is the most useful format for the practicing clinician. The book is organized into three sections. The first deals with general principles of therapeutics focusing on how to avoid or deal with adverse drug effects. The second section includes chapters on adverse neuropsychiatric effects of drugs used in psychiatry. The third section has chapters on non-neurological syndromes related to psychotherapeutic drug use. Each chapter, where appropriate, has been organized such that the pathophysiology, clinical features, diagnosis, treatment, and prevention of the given disorder are discussed. We have attempted to emphasize practical clinical diagnosis and management, and have discussed aspects of basic pharmacology where clinically relevant.

This volume is not designed to be another textbook of psychopharmacology, but to be a supplement to the study of psychopharmacotherapeutics. Within limits of a single text, we have focused our collective efforts on problems we believe are most important for the patient to be informed about, and for the physician to recognize early and, if possible, prevent. In this process we may have overlooked some problems the reader might consider significant; if so we would appreciate being informed of these so they may be included in a later edition. We hope this book will be useful for psychiatrists, psychiatric residents, nonpsychiatric physicians, and other health care professionals involved in the care of the mentally ill.

We are grateful to Christine Johnson for her tireless secretarial and editorial assistance. She also singlehandedly handled all the correspondence and telephone calls needed for the preparation of this book. Thanks are due to Ann McDaniels for her secretarial help during the early stages and to Linda Koerbel for administrative assistance. Dr. Lida Prypchan helped check the references and thoughtfully reviewed and critiqued individual chapters. We also wish to express our gratitude to Dr. Ashoka Prasad who helped formulate the original plan of this book, as well as Drs. Samuel Gershon, Renee Kubacka, David Kupfer, Phillip Resnick, Nina Schooler, Paul Soloff, and Loren Roth for their constructive criticism and advice.

Last, but most importantly, we are grateful to our many teachers who inspired us to undertake this work, and to our families, particularly Nina Engelhardt and Asha Keshavan, and our children who tolerated our late working hours, supported us, and provided assistance in many aspects of preparation of the book.

Matcheri S. Keshavan, M.D., F.R.C.P.(c), M.R.C.Psych
John S. Kennedy, M.D., F.R.C.P.(c)

I

GENERAL PRINCIPLES

This section reviews the general principles underlying the rational use of psychotherapeutic drugs. The pharmacoepidemiology of adverse drug reactions, their common mechanisms, and the fundamental principles of their diagnosis, prevention, and management are discussed at the beginning of this section. Next, the legal aspects of psychopharmacological practice and the guidelines of how to avoid malpractice liability are discussed. This is followed by drug-drug interactions in psychiatry; specific drug interactions of clinical significance are discussed, and guidelines as to how the perils of polypharmacy may be avoided are provided. An overview of psychotropic drug overdose is also offered, along with principles of management of individual psychotropic drug toxicity.

This book intends to serve a wide ranging population seen by the psychiatrist; the text includes a review of the implications of psychotherapeutic drug use for the unborn child (i.e., teratogenicity), childhood and adolescence, the elderly, and pharmacodynamic changes unique to the extremes of age and their relevance to rational psychotherapeutic drug use.

1

Principles of Drug Therapy in Psychiatry

How to do the Least Harm

Matcheri S. Keshavan

All drugs have multiple effects. In clinical medicine, only a limited number of such effects is identified for each drug as the primary goal(s) of treatment. All the other effects of the drug are called *side effects*, some of which may be trivial and inconsequential, and some of which may be significant and *adverse effects*. The categorization of what is a beneficial and what is a side effect is therefore made arbitrarily in the clinical context.

No drug is completely free of adverse effects, even when used as per standard modes of administration. When used inexpertly, they may occur more often. An adverse drug reaction refers to consequences of drug use, including "administration of the wrong drug (or drugs) in the wrong dosage (form, amount, route, or interval) at the wrong time and for the wrong disease" (Melmon, 1971). Adverse reactions can result from any single "wrong." This chapter describes the frequency of adverse effects, their mechanisms, approaches to identification, management, and prevention.

EPIDEMIOLOGY

How common are adverse drug effects? It is quite difficult to assess the incidence of drug-induced disease. The reported incidences vary depending on the methods of screening, the standard of medical practice, and the population being studied. Cause-effect relationships are often difficult to prove or disprove. In hospital medical and pediatric services about 2–5% of admissions result from one or another drug-induced syndrome (Woods & Oates, 1987). Among patients hospitalized on a general medical service, the incidence may be as high as 10%. About one third of patients have at least one adverse drug reaction during hospitalization (Borda, Slone, & Jick, 1968). The incidence increases in very ill patients, those treated with many drugs, in the elderly, and in those with multiple diseases. Prescription errors are frequently the cause of significant adverse drug reactions; a recent study reported 3.13 errors for every 1,000 orders in a teaching hospital (Lesar et al., 1990). The highest rate of prescribing errors occurred during afternoon hours when the majority of orders are being written. This may be related to the higher risk of prescriber fatigue among junior physicians (Lesar et al., 1990).

Only a few studies have focused on drug reactions leading to admission to psychiatric hospitals. Adverse drug reactions account for 5–7.5% of psychiatric admissions (Hermesh, Shalev, & Munitz, 1985; Stewart, Springer, & Adams,

1980). Between one half and one third of such cases are constituted by extra-pyramidal side effects; older age, polypharmacy, use of high dosage, and parenteral administration were significant risk factors (Wolf, Grohmann, Schmidt, & Ruther, 1989).

MECHANISMS

Drug-induced adverse effects may represent exaggeration of expected or intended pharmacological effects, or problems unrelated to the desired pharmacological effects. The latter may result from direct toxic effects or abnormal immune responses. Most of the adverse effects in psychopharmacology are of the first type, and although potentially expected, the effects are not always predictable for any single individual. The potential for this type of adverse side effect can be usually identified by the battery of tests carried out during the drug's development. The groups of patients who are likely to develop such adverse effects include those in whom the metabolism of the drug is altered by hepatic or renal disease or genetic alterations leading to quantitative changes in drug effects; adjustment of the dosage without necessarily discontinuing the drug often helps to treat such problems. The second group, the adverse effects mediated by toxic or immune mechanisms, are unpredictable—or "idiosyncratic"—and may require discontinuation of the drug. Idiosyncrasy usually represents qualitatively altered response by the patient to the drug; clozapine-included agranulocytosis and barbiturate-induced porphyria are examples. Skin rashes and other allergic reactions are most often unpredictable and idiosyncratic. As information accrues allowing prediction of any individual's risk to develop specific "adverse" responses, the adverse potential ceases to be idiosyncratic.

DIAGNOSIS

It is important to have a high index of suspicion to first identify adverse drug effects. Often, the adverse drug effect may be mistaken for symptoms of the illness being treated (e.g., akathisia may be mistaken for psychotic agitation). Knowledge concerning the natural history and phenomenology of specific adverse events and the illness being treated is helpful in allowing accurate differentiation of the cause. Disappearance of the adverse reaction with discontinuation of the drugs usually offers a good initial confirmation of the drug's causal role. When doubt exists and therapeutic options are absent, it may be necessary to cautiously readminister the drug. Because dealing with an allergic or idiosyncratic reaction is potentially dangerous, specific informed consent, provision of adequate conditions to assure necessary medical supervision, and a second opinion are indicated.

PREVENTION

A substantial proportion of iatrogenic injury to patients results from negligent medical management (Brennan et al., 1991). The majority of adverse iatrogenic events including drug reactions are, therefore, preventable; less than 20% of all adverse reactions are caused by hypersensitivity or idiosyncrasy, which are difficult to predict. Avoidable causes of drug-induced adverse reactions include those related to inappropriate prescriptions and those resulting from errors in prescribing (Lesar et al., 1990). The following is a discussion of the "ten commandments" of wise drug prescribing and can help to avoid many clinically significant and adverse drug reactions.

Know the Patient Well before Beginning Treatment

Cicero said, "The competent physician, before he attempts to give medicine to his patient, makes himself acquainted not only with the disease, but also with the habits and constitution of the sick man." (Quoted by Shader & Dimascio, 1970.) Good pharmacotherapy begins with a comprehensive assessment of patients. This involves developing a framework for care including a careful diagnosis, assessment of baseline historical and laboratory data, identification of target symptoms, and delineation of goals of treatment. Before initiation of therapy, the physician should establish a therapeutic relationship with the patient and/or, if unable because of severity of state, establish a therapeutic relationship with the patient's significant others.

Offer a Treatment Package, Not Just a Prescription

Most psychiatric disorders benefit from some form of psychotherapy, which may take the form of supportive counseling, crisis intervention, dynamic or behavioral psychotherapy, or family-systems therapy. Psychotherapeutic treatments frequently work synergistically with pharmacotherapy (Schooler & Hogarty, 1987). A judicious combination of these helps not only to minimize the tendency to overprescribe drug treatments, but also to promote compliance and improve the physician-patient relationship.

Another frequent error is for clinicians to withhold, on principle, medication for a patient with a medication-responsive but reactive (stress-related) syndrome. When well considered, medication therapy often can assist the patient to obtain remission from immediate distress, while efforts to adapt to changed circumstances occur in the context of psychotherapy.

Educate the Patient

According to the Hippocratic tradition, physicians were obligated not to alarm the patients by revealing knowledge about illness or its treatment (Gregory, 1817). This is no longer advisable in modern day medicine; the physician and patient increasingly share in decisionmaking. Central to the educative process is the discussion of the risks and benefits of the treatment and the informed consent (see Chapter 2 for a further discussion).

Choose the Right Medicine

Several factors govern the choice of the appropriate drug for a given patient. In general, the drug with the most favorable risk/benefit ratio should be chosen. A drug with a known prior effectiveness in the patient is likely to be a better choice, but this should not be the sole determinant of choice of therapy. Another factor in the choice of the drug is the question of which side effects are desired and which are to be avoided. For example, an antidepressant with a significant anticholinergic profile might be useful under certain circumstances in a depressed patient with parkinsonism, whereas a low-potency antipsychotic with prominent anticholinergic and adrenergic blocking effects such as chlorpromazine is not the best first line therapy in an elderly woman with osteoporosis and risk of falls and fractures. Finally, a drug of which the physician has personal knowledge and experience is to be preferred to one that is new and "just on the market," unless the new drug is established beyond doubt to be a real advance. This should not be taken to imply that physicians should avoid prescribing newer medications that offer better side effects profiles or continue routine prescribing of older, less advantaged medication.

Ensure That the Patient Takes the Medication

Noncompliance is very common in psychopharmacological practice. The first step in the management of noncompliance is to initially establish a contract of expectations between the physician and the patient; next, it is important to identify the presence of noncompliance, and the reason(s) why the patient is not following the prescribed treatment. Noncompliance may be a result of the complexity of the medication regime, inadequate supervision by the patients' significant others or the physician, inappropriate health beliefs or attitudes to illness, or adverse effects. The cause of noncompliance, if found, may be remediable by modifying the therapeutic regime, improving the doctor-patient relationship, or enhancing supervision of treatment.

It is also equally important to ensure that the prescribed medication is dispensed, and taken by the patient, *correctly.* Errors in this regard are common; review of medication orders by pharmacists, "double checking" by physicians and nurses, and periodic monitoring of errors in the hospital provide important "checks and balances" and help reduce risk (Lesar et al., 1990).

Use as Few Drugs as Possible

Polypharmacy is one of the ideal settings for adverse drug reactions and drug interactions. This practice has been satirized by Moat (1969) in an article in the *Daily Telegraph* (Supplement 255). He described the treatment taken by a guest at home:

> The other day a friend from the big world came to stay, and when I took him his breakfast I found him swallowing pills. He'd been depressed recently, which was why he took the yellow pills, antidepressants. The white pills were tranquillizers, and he took those because the yellow pills were inclined to agitate him. The mixture affected his vision, hence the blue pills. He found this particular dosage of pills constipating, and for that he took a strong aperient. 'And just look at these' he said excitedly, waving at me a bottle of large multicoloured pills. 'And what are those?' I asked. 'I don't know,' he said, 'but I like to keep them till last.'
>
> I then asked him how he was feeling. He said he felt fine, except that the pills made him lethargic, which he personally found depressing. (Quoted by D'arcy & Griffin, 1972, pp. v-vi)

The pharmacological basis of some adverse effects with polypharmacy is discussed in detail in Chapter 3.

Tailor the Treatment to the Patient's Needs

The nature of adverse effects is influenced both by factors intrinsic to the drug and by factors intrinsic to the individual (e.g., age, genetics, tendency to allergy, nature of disease, personality, and habits). It is important to consider these in choosing the appropriate treatment. The physician also needs to pay particular attention to the patient's body weight and metabolic (hepatic, renal, and respiratory, etc.) status in individualizing the treatment to each patient.

Familiarize Yourself with the Drug

It is important to learn the metabolism, routes of excretion, half-life, and major adverse effects of the drug being used. Some drugs require periodic monitoring of specific laboratory parameters (e.g., lithium, carbamazepine, clozapine). The need for improved physician training to reduce erroneous medication prescribing has been well recognized (Health and Public Policy Committee, 1988).

Have a High Index of Suspicion

We believe many adverse reactions are unrecognized; this is often a result of the prescriber not suspecting that the patient's complaint is an adverse occurrence. Laboratory data or new symptoms that do not fit the expected course of the disease should rouse suspicion of possible adverse drug effects. Keeping up to date about the current literature regarding drug effects and side effects is important.

Consider the Patient's Viewpoint

It is important to realize that the patient is often the authority on his or her illness. Similarly, the patient frequently knows very well his or her reaction to drugs (Blaska, 1990; Staff, 1990). The patient's views should therefore be taken seriously while prescribing medications. In one study of relapse with maintenance antipsychotic treatment (Manchanda & Hirsch, 1986), the authors concluded that the patients may be "as able as the psychiatrist in predicting . . . the benefit of continued maintenance treatment."

Physicians should report unusual drug reactions to the manufacturing firm and, when appropriate, to the Food and Drug Administration (FDA). Although often a burdensome process results, this helps in wider dissemination of knowledge about drug reactions, broader recognition and prevention, and advancement of our understanding and treatment of the patients we are entrusted to assist.

MANAGEMENT

If an adverse reaction does occur, the type of the reaction and any triggering factors (e.g., lithium intoxication occurring during diuretic therapy) need to be elucidated. With dose-related adverse effects, adjustment of the dose helps; it is also important to pay attention to the possible precipitating factors. With the idiosyncratic side effects, the drug should be discontinued. In case of toxicity, immediate treatment should consist of temporarily holding further exposure to the drug, supporting the vital physiological functioning such as respiration and circulation, removing the offending agent from the patient (e.g., forced diuresis, peritoneal or hemodialysis, gastric lavage), and using physiological antidotes if indicated (e.g., naloxone for opiate poisoning).

REFERENCES

Blaska B, 1990: The myriad medication mistakes in psychiatry: A consumers view. *Hospital and Community Psychiatry, 41,* 993–998.

Borda IT, Slone D, Jick H, 1968: Assessment of adverse drug reactions within a drug surveillance program. *Journal of the American Medical Association, 205,* 645.

Brennan TA, Leape, LL, Laird NM, Hebert L, Localio AR, Lawthers AG, Newhouse JP, Weiler PC, Hiatt HH, 1991: Incidence of adverse events and negligence in hospitalized patients: Results of the Harvard Medical Practice Study I. *New England Journal of Medicine, 324*(6), 353–376.

D'arcy PF, Griffin JP, 1972: *Preface. Iatrogenic diseases.* London: Oxford University Press.

Gregory J, 1817: *Lectures on the duties and qualifications of a physician.* Philadelphia: M. Carey & Son.

Health and Public Policy Committee, American College of Physicians, 1988: Improving medical education in therapeutics. *Annuals of Internal Medicine, 108,* 145–147.

Hermesh H, Shalev A, Munitz H, 1985: Contribution of adverse drug reaction to admission rates in an acute psychiatric ward. *Acta Psychiatrica Scandinavica, 72,* 104–110.

Lesar TS, Briceland LL, Delcoure K, Parmalee JC, Masta-Gornic V, Pohl H, 1990: Medication prescribing errors in a teaching hospital. *Journal of the American Medical Association, 263*(17), 2329–2334.

Manchanda R, Hirsch SR, 1986: Low dosage maintenance for schizophrenia. *British Medical Journal, 293,* 515–516.

Melman KL, 1971: Preventable drug reactions—causes and cures. *New England Journal of Medicine, 284,* 1361–1368.

Schooler NR, Hogarty GE, 1987: Medication and psychosocial strategies in the treatment of schizophrenia. In: *Psychopharmacology: The third generation of progress,* edited by HY Meltzer. New York: Raven Press.

Shader RI, Dimascio A, 1970: Preface. *Psychotropic drug side effects.* Baltimore: Williams and Wilkins.

Staff, 1990: Common prescribing errors and their effects. *International Drug Therapy Newsletter, 25,* 34–36.

Stewart RB, Springer PK, Adams JE, 1980: Drug-related admissions to an inpatient psychiatric unit. *American Journal of Psychiatry, 137,* 1093–1095.

Wolf B, Grohmann R, Schmidt LG, Ruther E, 1989: Psychiatric admissions due to adverse drug reactions. *Comprehensive Psychiatry, 30*(6), 534–545.

Woods AJJ, Oates JA, 1987: Adverse drug reactions to drugs. In: *Harrison's principles of internal medicine,* edited by E Braunwald, KJ Isselbacher, RG Petersdorf, JD Wilson, JB Martin, AS Fauci. New York: McGraw-Hill.

2

Legal Aspects of Prescribing

Robert M. Wettstein

As in most areas of psychiatric practice, the prescription of psychotropic medication involves many legal issues and presents many potential clinical-legal problems. This chapter addresses just a few of these. The initial discussion is of tort liability issues in psychopharmacology; the text then centers on a discussion of the legal and clinical issues pertinent to the area of treatment refusal. Those interested in the many other legal aspects of psychopharmacology are referred elsewhere (e.g., Brackins, 1985; Dukes & Swartz, 1988; Mathieu, 1991).

PSYCHOPHARMACOLOGY LITIGATION

Prescribing psychoactive medication exposes the psychiatrist to significant professional liability claims (Brackins, 1985; Dukes & Swartz, 1988; Wettstein, 1985). Indeed, improper medication was the most common allegation against psychiatrists insured with the American Psychiatric Association's (APA) professional liability insurance program from 1973–1984 (Slawson, 1989). The psychiatrist's prescription liability mostly pertains to two areas in law and medicine, negligence and informed consent. But psychiatrists, like other physicians, are subject to criminal sanctions and license revocations when they inappropriately prescribe or document their use of controlled medications such as opioids, and more recently benzodiazepines or psychostimulants in some jurisdictions (*Kollmorgen v. Board of Medical Examiners*, 1987). In many legal cases, improper treatment includes allegations of undertreatment, or failure to use medication, rather than simply the improper use of medication.

Since improper medication use often results in somatic injuries, allegations of improper use are more persuasive to courts and juries than damages from improper psychotherapy, which are emotional in type. The latter are difficult to verify and quantify and tend to be discounted by laypersons except in extreme cases.

According to the law of torts (i.e., civil wrongs), a negligence action against a psychiatrist is successful when the plaintiff proves by a preponderence of the evidence (the plaintiff's case is more convincing than that of the defendant) that: (1) the psychiatrist had a legal duty to care for the patient according to the standard of care; (2) the psychiatrist, in his care of the patient, deviated from that duty

---

This chapter is not a substitute for an attorney; nor does it attempt to answer specific clinical-legal questions about patient care. The reader is advised to consult an attorney for appropriate legal advice on specific legal problems, and a clinical-legal consultant for advice about specific clinical problems, as needed.

either through an omission or commission; and (3) the patient suffered physical or emotional damage as a result of the psychiatrist's violation of the standard of care to the patient (King, 1986).

Prescribing psychiatrists risk negligence liability in a variety of areas when they prescribe psychoactive medication. These areas include: (1) failure to take an adequate history; (2) failure to obtain an adequate physical examination; (3) failure to obtain an adequate laboratory examination; (4) lack of indication for a prescription; (5) contraindication for a prescription; (6) prescription of an improper dosage; (7) prescription for an improper duration; (8) failure to recognize, monitor, and treat medication side effects; (9) failure to abate drug reactions and interactions; and (10) failure to consult with other physicians (Wettstein, 1983, 1988).

Psychiatrists are also subject to litigation for failure to obtain informed consent to treatment with psychotropic medication (Rozovsky, 1990; Tietz, 1986; Wettstein, 1988). According to the legal doctrine of informed consent, in addition to obtaining the patient's consent to treatment, the prescribing psychiatrist must also inform the patient or his legal guardian about the nature of the proposed treatment, its risks, benefits, and alternatives, as well as the risks and benefits of the alternatives, including no treatment (Appelbaum, Lidz, & Meisel, 1987; Faden & Beauchamp, 1986). Such informed consent disclosures are dictated by state law (statute or case), which describes whether disclosure should be governed by what psychiatrists ordinarily disclose to patients in such circumstances, or by what reasonable patients would want to hear in such circumstances. There are limited exceptions to the informed consent requirements such as an emergency or waiver by the patient (Meisel, 1979). Liability for failure to obtain informed consent to treatment occurs when the psychiatrist failed to disclose a risk of treatment, the risk eventuates in an injury to the patient, and the patient-litigant convinces the jury that he would not have consented to the treatment had he been informed of that particular risk.

Case Examples of Negligence and Informed Consent

Litigation in psychopharmacology has involved a variety of psychotropic medications and iatrogenic results. A few cases will help to illustrate some of the aforementioned principles. The facts in each case are obtained solely from publicly available documents, so that other relevant details are not necessarily available.

In a Michigan case, a psychiatrist prescribed 50 10-mg diazepam tablets for a man who, while driving his car the next day, collided head on with a motorcycle. It was alleged that the patient was under the influence of beer and diazepam, which he had obtained for nonmedical purposes. The plaintiff, who sustained serious injuries, also alleged that the prescription to a person who was likely to abuse drugs was negligent. A $410,000 out-of-court settlement was reached with the psychiatrist and other parties (*Munsell v. Lynk,* 1983).

In *Miller v. United States* (1976), a male patient on admission to the hospital informed the staff that he was allergic to antihistamines because they caused urinary retention. On discharge, he was nevertheless provided with hydroxyzine (100 mg q.i.d.) and trifluoperazine. When urinary retention again developed, the hydroxyzine was reduced and later discontinued. Complications entailed a prostatic infection, Foley catheter for 4 years, and eventual prostatic resection. There was expert testimony that the hydroxyzine prescription was negligent given the patient's history and that the hydroxyzine caused the bladder damage. A judgment of $20,000 was awarded to the plaintiff.

In *Brown v. State* (1977), a 35-year-old male patient became violent the morning after he was admitted to a state hospital. He was treated with 200 mg of chlorpromazine in an upright position, had to be subdued by the police, and was transferred to another building. There he was not monitored for 1 1/4 hours, was found in a respiratory arrest, but could not be resuscitated. The court found negligence for the failure to monitor the patient "during the period of time that defendant knew serious side effects might have been manifested by the administration of thorazine."

An inpatient at a teaching hospital, treated in a team approach, was given four different antipsychotics, as well as diphenhydramine and anticholinergics, for what was thought to be a schizophreniform disorder. In an anticholinergic crisis, she suffered a cardiopulmonary arrest after 5 weeks' hospitalization, with a rectal temperature of 108°. The patient survived with severe brain damage. Although the plaintiff claimed over 10 million dollars in damages, she was awarded the statutory maximum of $500,000 (*Sibley v. Board of Supervisors*, 1983, 1985).

In *Hedin v. United States* (1985), after a hospitalization for treatment of alcohol abuse, the plaintiff was treated with thioridazine and then chlorpromazine as an outpatient. He continued to take 600 mg chlorpromazine daily for nearly 4 years before his physicians noted his movement disorder and discontinued the medication. Although the patient had been aware of the movements, which involved the face, mouth, trunk, and extremities, he testified that he was unaware they were a result of the medication. The defendant admitted that he had been negligent in prescribing excessive amounts of medication over a prolonged period of time without proper supervision. Damages of nearly $2.2 million were awarded to the plaintiff who had become functionally disabled because of the tardive dyskinesia.

A severely mentally retarded man, institutionalized for his entire life, had been stabilized on 4 mg per day of haloperidol for self-abusive behavior. On his transfer to a community facility, he was treated by a new psychiatrist, the defendant. The patient did well for 16 months, and the psychiatrist changed his medication to 2 mg only as needed. The psychiatrist indicated that the medication withdrawal was prompted by a state audit regarding medication use in this patient population, as well as the risk of tardive dyskinesia, which the patient did not have. Within 1 month of medication withdrawal, the patient regressed, requiring hospitalization and much larger doses of haloperidol. He was returned to the state developmental center, developed flexion contractures of his extremities, and became confined to a wheelchair. The jury found that the psychiatrist was negligent in reducing the medication so abruptly, failing to review the patient's history, and failing to obtain the patient's complete medical records from the transferring agency (*Leal v. Simon*, 1989).

A psychiatrist unsuccessfully contested the suspension of his license after he was found of guilty of grossly inappropriate practice in prescribing controlled substances and recordkeeping for such. This included postdating prescriptions, prescribing for habitual users, prescribing without conducting physical examination, and prescribing not in the course of practice. Allegations included fraudulent practice, gross negligence, and unprofessional conduct (*Nadell v. Ambach*, 1988).

In *Clites v. Iowa* (1980), the parents of a mentally retarded man at a state residential facility sued the state for negligence and lack of informed consent. The patient had been treated with antipsychotic medication since age 18 for "aggressive behavior" by several physicians. Medication continued for 5 years before tardive dyskinesia of the face and extremities was diagnosed. In addition to a ruling that medication had been inappropriately used, the court held that the patient was improperly monitored because "he was not regularly visited by a physician and physical exams had not been conducted for a 3-year period; further, the attending physician, being unfamiliar with tardive dyskinesia, failed to obtain consultation." The trial court also ruled that the patient's parents, his legal guardians, "were never informed of the potential side effects of the use, and prolonged use, of major tranquilizers, nor was consent to their use obtained," thus violating the "standard that requires some form of informed consent prior to the administration of major tranquilizers." Since the parents had not been informed of the risks attendant to the treatment program, the trial court rejected the defendant's argument that the parents had implicitly consented to the treatment. The trial court ruled for the plaintiff and awarded $385,165 for future medical expenses and $375,000 for past and future pain and suffering. The district court's ruling was later upheld in the Iowa Court of Appeals (1982).

Clinical-Legal Management Issues

These cases, and others, give reason to consider the following principles when prescribing psychotropic medication. Although there can be no assurance that a lawsuit will not be filed should an adverse clinical result occur, compliance with principles of good care may help to minimize the likelihood or success of litigation against the psychiatrist.

1. Avoid polypharmacy, unconventional dosages or medication combinations, or frequent changes in regimens that do not permit a rational assessment of the patient's response to treatment.
2. Be intimately familiar with a few medications of each class rather than less familiar with many medications. Prescribing physicians are expected to be familiar with the intended and potential adverse effects of each prescribed medication. The physician is expected to know the precautions and warnings that have been published in the professional literature and the manufacturer's mailing address, available from sources such as the *Physicians' Desk Reference.*
3. Be familiar with organizational guidelines on medication use and abuse. Organizations such as the APA have published monographs on tardive dyskinesia and benzodiazepine abuse, which provide much useful information on these topics (APA, 1990; APA, in press). Compliance with organizational guidelines is taken as evidence that the care provided was in accordance with accepted principles and practices.
4. Discontinue medications with care. Recent litigation has addressed the propriety and procedures of discontinuing psychotropic medication (*Leal v. Simon,* 1989; *Soileau v. Health Care of America Health Services,* 1989). The prescribing psychiatrist should be familiar with the ever increasing clinical literature on the effects of medication withdrawal and the procedures for doing so.
5. Clarify the ambiguity of PRN orders. It is often unclear whether an "as

needed" order refers to the nursing determination or the patient's request for treatment. This should be clarified in advance in the psychiatrist's orders.

6. Obtain consultation in complex cases. Given the increasing knowledge and complexity of clinical psychopharmacology, consultation with an expert in this area may be helpful in patient management. These consultations can be formal, in which the psychiatrist examines the patient, or informal.

7. Obtain consent from the patient or guardian (Rozovsky, 1990). The patient or his legal guardian must agree to undergo the course of treatment recommended by the psychiatrist, including any changes thereafter.

8. Provide information about the treatment and its alternatives to the patient or legal guardian as soon as clinically feasible (Appelbaum et al., 1987; Benson, 1984; Kleinmann et al., 1989; Munetz, 1985; Munetz & Roth, 1985; Wettstein, 1988). Informed consent liability occurs most often when the psychiatrist fails to describe treatment alternatives or treatment risks. With regard to disclosure of treatment risks, those that are more serious or more common should be reviewed with the patient. For example, when prescribing antipsychotic medication, the psychiatrist should specifically inform the patient of the risk of developing tardive dyskinesia. When prescribing psychotropic medication to a woman of childbearing years, the patient should be informed of the risk of teratogenesis with treatment. Since prescription in both of these cases requires that the patient carefully weigh the benefits and risks of treatment, this can be accomplished over time in long-term care settings by repeatedly reviewing this information. It is often necessary to do so because of cognitive incapacity resulting from the patient's psychiatric disorder (Ganguli & Raghu, 1985; Geller, 1982; Grossman & Summers, 1980; Gurian, Baker, Jacobson, Lagerbom, & Watts, 1990; Irwin et al., 1985; Kleinman, Schacter, & Koritar, 1989). Especially in psychiatric treatment, informed consent is a process that occurs over time, rather than a single event. Psychiatrists need not fear that information disclosure will be harmful to the patient or even that the patient will subsequently refuse the treatment (Munetz & Roth, 1985; Quaid, Faden, Vining, & Freeman, 1990).

9. Monitor the patient for the development of, or change in, adverse medication effects. The psychiatrist's obligation to the patient does not end with the decision to prescribe medication. In many cases, the psychiatrist delegates this responsibility to nonphysicians such as nurses, pharmacists, or social workers (Munetz & Benjamin, 1990) (e.g., administering the Abnormal Involuntary Movement Scale (AIMS) for patients on long-term antipsychotics), but the psychiatrist is still ultimately responsible for the patient's treatment.

10. Be aware of the risks of prescribing medications unapproved for a particular use (Shapiro, 1979). In the United States, prescription medications are approved by the Food and Drug Administration for a particular use. Once a drug is on the market, licensed physicians may prescribe it for other purposes, even though the medication is not formally approved for such use. This is a common practice in psychopharmacology and it carries some additional risk, especially when unsupported by research or clinical literature. Patients should also be informed of this practice as it occurs. Individual facilities may also have specific policies and procedures in such cases that regulate the psychopharmacological practice.

11. Attend to medication recordkeeping. Medical records are legal and administrative documents in addition to clinical ones. They provide the only objective

account of the patient's psychiatric care. Medical records do not later develop amnesia as may the patient, family, or service providers. Records may be reviewed by peer review committees, utilization review agencies, third party payors, attorneys, and ultimately judges and juries. Medication errors occur with surprising frequency, often for simple and avoidable reasons. Consider using medication sheets to summarize prescriptions in the hospital or clinic. Place carbon copies of prescriptions in the outpatient record and routinely record refills (dosage, amount, method of administration). Document relevant telephone contacts with patients and third parties (family, pharmacy, hospital, laboratory). Write legibly, and, most importantly, document decisionmaking regarding treatment approaches, especially polypharmacy or unconventional treatments.

12. Know the pitfalls of written consent forms for medication, and resist the temptation to use written forms, if possible (Grundner, 1980; Morrow, 1980; Rozovsky, 1990). Written consent forms are not typically recommended in medical practice in any medical speciality in which standard or routine medication is prescribed. They have limited defensive value from a legal perspective and may inadvertently substitute for or interfere with the psychiatrist-patient dialogue known as informed consent. However, they may be necessary to comply with hospital administrative procedures or applicable law. When written consent forms are used, the psychiatrist must still discuss with the patient the relevant informed consent issues (e.g., tardive dyskinesia from antipsychotics), both initially and also periodically thereafter. Written medication information sheets or brochures are useful supplements to the oral discussion with the patient.

13. Dispense only that quantity of medication reasonably necessary under the circumstances. This may be difficult to ascertain, and a certain amount of risk taking is inherent in outpatient prescription (e.g., intentional antidepressant overdose). Also, third party payment programs increasingly encourage the patient to obtain larger prescriptions (e.g., a 3-month supply) to reduce cost. The psychiatrist should be mindful of these issues.

THE RIGHT TO REFUSE PSYCHOTROPIC MEDICATION

Perhaps the most significant development in mental health law in the last 15 years relates to the patient's right to refuse treatment with psychotropic medication.

Legal Aspects of Medication Refusal

Until individual and class action lawsuits were filed in the 1970s, patients in state psychiatric hospitals in the United States were medicated at the discretion of the treating physician. Patients generally did not have a legal right to refuse medication once hospitalized. In right-to-refuse-treatment cases, federal and state courts have considered not only the benefits of treatment to the patient and others but also the seriousness of the possible side effects to antipsychotic medication, including tardive dyskinesia. Some courts tended to overvalue the risks of treatment in contrast to its benefits (Gutheil & Appelbaum, 1983) and raised fears of such results as "mind control" by psychotropic medication. To support the patient's right to refuse treatment, legal arguments have been based on state statutory rights, federal constitutional grounds of the First Amendment (freedom of speech, freedom of expression, freedom of religion), the Eighth Amendment (prohibiting cruel and unusual punishment), the Fourteenth Amendment's procedural due process (right to a hearing, to present and crossexamine witnesses, to an independent decisionmaker), and the right of privacy (freedom from bodily intrusion) (Perlin, 1989). The right to refuse treatment is variously implemented by federal and state statute, case law, regulation, or administrative policies and procedures.

The right of a patient to refuse psychotropic medication depends on the patient's legal and clinical status. Both statutes and courts have provided that voluntarily hospitalized patients have a right to refuse psychotropic medication in nonemergency situations. On the other hand, both voluntarily hospitalized and civilly committed patients can be involuntarily medicated in psychiatric emergencies, for the duration of the emergency. Applicable law may or may not provide a useful definition of emergency, or the duration of emergency, for medication purposes.

The greatest controversy about medication refusal occurs in those patients who have been involuntarily hospitalized (Appelbaum, 1988). Following the series of decisions in Massachusetts (*Rogers v. Okin*), an increasing number of state supreme courts have ruled that a legally competent patient, even though civilly committed, has the right to refuse psychotropic medication (usually antipsychotics) in nonemergencies. In such jurisdictions, patients may only be involuntarily medicated following a judicial hearing in which the patient is adjudicated incompetent to consent to or refuse medication. A guardian is then appointed to make the substituted treatment decision on behalf of the patient, and then, in some cases, monitor the patient's treatment. In Massachusetts, this procedure has resulted in increased direct and indirect costs of litigation and lengthy delays before treatment can begin; nevertheless, in almost all cases, the court has adjudicated the patient incompetent and ordered treatment (Hoge et al., 1990; Schouten & Gutheil, 1990; Veliz & James, 1987). An alternate approach to reviewing treatment refusals, described in the New Jersey *Rennie v. Klein* series of decisions, approved a nonjudicial determination made by the medical director of the facility or his delegate. Still other approaches to managing refusals involve a treatment review panel of hospital staff and/or clinical administrators (Appelbaum, 1988).

In contrast to the approach taken by many state supreme courts to recognize the right of competent though committed patients to refuse treatment, the federal courts in several cases have recently shown a greater willingness to authorize involuntary medication. The Fourth Circuit Court of Appeals, ruling on a case involving a hospitalized criminal defendant adjudicated incompetent to stand trial, permitted the physician to make the involuntary medication decision using professional judgment (*United States v. Charters,* 1988). Subsequent judicial review is only available to determine if the decision to treat was made arbitrarily.

In addition, the United States Supreme Court, ruling on a Washington state prison inmate's right to refuse medication in the absence of a judicial determination of incompetency, permitted compulsory treatment by the prison authorities when the mentally ill inmate was considered dangerous to himself or others (*Washington v. Harper,* 1990). The court held that adequate due process was provided by an administrative hearing at the prison, conducted by an in-house committee of a staff psychiatrist, staff psychologist, and an administrator from the institution, none of whom were currently involved in the inmate's care. Of great significance was the holding that a judicial review of the inmate's medication refusal, particularly an inquiry into the inmate's competency to refuse treatment, was not required by federal law. Whether this decision will be applied to the civil commitment context remains to be determined.

Clozapine, a new antipsychotic medication with a different risk/benefit profile than standard antipsychotic medications, presents somewhat different legal issues in the context of treatment refusals. These have not yet been addressed by the legislatures or the courts. With an annual 2% incidence of agranulocytosis, patients on clozapine must be carefully monitored during treatment for leukopenia and agranulocytosis, so that treatment can be interrupted to obviate any fatality. When a guardian or court determines whether a patient can be involuntarily medicated with clozapine, the substitute decisionmaker should be informed of the specific risks and treatment plan required. On the other hand, when the law permits physicians and consultants to make the substitute decision for overriding medication refusal, prescribing psychiatrists are entering into a legal vacuum with regard to clozapine. An alternate approach under such circumstances is to petition the court to make the treatment decision or at least appoint a substitute decisionmaker outside of the facility.

Clinical Aspects of Medication Refusal

The management of patients who refuse psychotropic medication often requires much clinical skill and patience. The following are some relevant issues:

1. Consider the effect of refusal on ward atmosphere (Hoge et al., 1990). Treatment refusal by one patient can often surprisingly affect the attitudes and compliance with treatment for the entire hospital ward. Refusals often appear contagious.

2. Assess reasons for refusal. Patients refuse medication for a variety of reasons, and it is important to identify the particular reason for a given patient (Appelbaum & Gutheil, 1982; Van Putten, 1974). These include problems in the doctor-patient relationship, transference problems, side effects of treatment, and psychopathology ("symptomatic refusals") in the patient or the family. Further complicating the issue is that, although a patient may assert that he is refusing because of side effects, a closer examination reveals that he is in fact refusing for symptomatic reasons.

3. Assess competence to refuse treatment (Beck, 1988; McKinnon, Cournos, & Stanley, 1989). Since the law in some jurisdictions requires that involuntary treatment can proceed only if the patient is incompetent to refuse, the patient's decisionmaking ability regarding treatment must be assessed in those states. This requires investigation into the patient's basis for refusal, knowledge of risks and benefits of treatment, ability to comprehend risks and benefits of treatment, ability to weigh risks and benefits of treatment, and ability to communicate his decisionmaking. Family members may be helpful in this assessment.

4. Assess dangerousness. The law may also require that dangerousness to self or others be assessed to implement involuntary treatment. This requires taking an extensive history, reviewing records, and assessing the patient's ideation, inten-

tion, and impulsivity. In addition, delays in treatment required by administrative or judicial review proceedings result in increased risk of violence.

5. Consider obtaining consultation. A consultant experienced in the patient population at issue, as well as law and psychiatry, may be helpful in assessing the patient's symptoms, diagnosis, need for medications, decisionmaking ability, and dangerousness.

6. Provide therapy for the refusal. Depending on the patient's reason for refusal, this may entail understanding the psychodynamics of the refusal, reassurance and education about treatment, and perhaps coaxing from the staff. Family members who have an alliance with the staff can also be helpful in convincing the patient to proceed with treatment. It is usually necessary to be firm rather than tentative or fearful when dealing with ambivalent patients.

7. Know the law. Because of the complex and changing nature of mental health law in this area, it is necessary to know the procedures and standards of medication refusal to avoid undertreatment or overtreatment. This means knowing the definition of such terms as "competent," "emergency," and "treatment," which the law may define differently than the clinician. It may be helpful to have a copy of the statute, case law, or applicable regulations for reference.

8. Know when to respect the refusal. It may not be advisable to involuntarily treat a patient even if the law permits it. It is important to weigh the potential consequences of overriding treatment refusals such as antagonizing the patient and alienating the patient or other patients from future medication approaches.

9. Know the facility policy and procedures about treatment refusal. Particular facilities may adopt more strict policies or procedures in the treatment refusal area than is required by law. The staff should be familiar with these and comply with them. This may include documentation requirements of the physician's assessment and any necessary committee meetings or consultations. Violation of hospital policies may be viewed by the courts as evidence of negligence.

10. Tell patients their rights. Some refusals result from patients' testing their staff just to prove that they do in fact have a right to refuse. Once the staff simply agree that the patient has a legal right to refuse treatment, such patients often agree to take the medication.

11. Deal with the staff's countertransference. The staff may be divided about the patient's decisionmaking ability, dangerousness, or need for treatment, especially if involuntary. The staff may not agree about the ethics or law of involuntary medication. Character disordered patients will also split the staff against one another. Other patients will invite punitive or protective measures from the staff. These issues should be identified and dealt with as soon and directly as possible.

12. Involve family and legal guardians in the treatment refusal and its management. Family members are often more successful than the staff in facilitating the patient's compliance with treatment, either by reassuring the patient or by more forceful means. Later, if the court appoints a guardian ad litem or personal guardian to make treatment decisions or monitor treatment, then the staff will need to contend with a third party in the treatment negotiations. This can be difficult when the guardian is ambivalent about treatment or uninvolved with the patient's care.

13. Use a show of force before forcing medication. When the staff implements the decision to involuntarily medicate a patient, many patients will not physically resist the staff's plan once they see the assemblage of large, male staff members

ready to enforce the physician's order. This is likely to reduce the risk of physical injuries to the staff or the patient.

REFERENCES

American Psychiatric Association Task Force, 1990: *Benzodiazepine dependence, toxicity, and abuse.* Washington, DC: American Psychiatric Press.

American Psychiatric Association Task Force, in press: *Tardive dyskinesia, 2nd edition.* Washington, DC: American Psychiatric Press.

Appelbaum PS, 1988: The right to refuse treatment with antipsychotic medications: Retrospect and prospect. *American Journal of Psychiatry, 145,* 413–419.

Appelbaum PS, Gutheil TG, 1982: Clinical aspects of treatment refusal. *Comprehensive Psychiatry, 23,* 560–566.

Appelbaum PS, Lidz CW, Meisel A, 1987: Informed consent: Legal theory and clinical practice. New York: Oxford University Press.

Beck JC, 1988: Determining competency to assent to neuroleptic drug treatment. *Hospital and Community Psychiatry, 39,* 1106–1108.

Benson PR, 1984: Informed consent: Drug information disclosed to patients prescribed antipsychotic medication. *Journal of Nervous and Mental Disease, 172,* 642–653.

Brackins LW, 1985: The liability of physicians, pharmacists, and hospitals for adverse drug reactions. *Defense Law Journal, 34,* 273–344.

Brown v. State, 44 N.Y.2d 1006 (1977).

Clites v. Iowa, Law #46274, Iowa District Court, Pottawattamie County, August 7, 1980.

Clites v. Iowa, 322 N.W.2d 917 (Iowa, 1982).

Dukes MNG, Swartz B, 1988: *Responsibility for drug-induced injury.* Amsterdam: Elsevier.

Faden RF, Beauchamp TL, 1986: A history and theory of informed consent. New York: Oxford University Press.

Ganguli R, Raghu U, 1985: Tardive dyskinesia, impaired recall, and informed consent. *Journal of Clinical Psychiatry, 46,* 434–435.

Geller JL, 1982: State hospital patients and their medication-do they know what they take. *American Journal of Psychiatry, 139,* 611–615.

Grossman L, Summers F, 1980: A study of the capacity of schizophrenic patients to give informed consent. *Hospital and Community Psychiatry, 31,* 205–206.

Grundner TM, 1980: On the readability of surgical consent forms. *New England Journal of Medicine, 302,* 900–902.

Gurian BS, Baker EH, Jacobson S, Lagerbom B, Watts P, 1990: Informed consent for neuroleptics with elderly patients in two settings. *Journal of the American Geriatrics Society, 38,* 37–44.

Gutheil TG, Appelbaum PS, 1983: "Mind control," "synthetic sanity," "artificial competence," and genuine confusion: Legally relevant effects of antipsychotic medication. *Hofstra Law Review, 12,* 77–120.

Hedin v. United States of America, No. 5–83 CIV 3 (D. Minn. 1985).

Hoge SK, Appelbaum PS, Lawlor T, Beck JC, Litman R, Greer A, Gutheil TG, Kaplan E, 1990: A prospective, multicenter study of patients' refusal of antipsychotic medication. *Archives of General Psychiatry, 47,* 949–956.

Irwin M, Lovitz A, Marder Sr, Minz J, Winslade W, van Patten T, Mills M, 1985: Psychotic patients' understanding of informed consent. *American Journal of Psychiatry, 142,* 1351–1354.

King JH, 1986: *The law of medical malpractice, 2nd edition.* St. Paul, MN: West Publishing.

Kleinman I, Schacter D, Koritar E, 1989: Informed consent and tardive dyskinesia. *American Journal of Psychiatry, 146,* 902–904.

Kollmorgen v. Board of Medical Examiners, 416 N.W.2d 485 (Minn. App. 1987).

Leal v. Simon, 542 N.Y.S.2d 328 (A.D. 1989).

Mathieu M, 1991: *New drug development: A regulatory overview.* Cambridge, MA: Parexel.

McKinnon K, Cournos F, Stanley B, 1989: *Rivers* in practice: Clinicians' assessments of patients' decision-making capacity. *Hospital and Community Psychiatry, 40,* 1159–1162.

Meisel A, 1979: The exceptions to the informed consent doctrine: Striking a balance between competing values in medical decisionmaking. *Wisconsin Law Review, 1979,* 413–488.

Miller v. United States, 431 F. Supp. 988 (S.D. Miss. 1976).

Morrow GR, 1980: How readable are subject consent forms? *Journal of the American Medical Association, 244,* 56–58.

Munetz MR, 1985: Overcoming resistance to talking to patients about tardive dyskinesia. *Hospital and Community Psychiatry, 36,* 283–287.

Munetz MR, Benjamin S, 1990: Who should perform the AIMS examination? *Hospital and Community Psychiatry, 41,* 912–915.

Munetz MR, Roth LH, 1985: Informing patients about tardive dyskinesia. *Archives of General Psychiatry, 42,* 866–871.

Munsell v. Lynk, Genesee County (Mich.) Circuit Court, No. 80-58801-NI, June 1, 1983.

Nadell v. Ambach, 523 N.Y.S.2d 637 (A.D. 1988).

Quaid KA, Faden RR, Vining EP, Freeman JM, 1990. Informed consent for a prescription drug: Impact of disclosed information on patient understanding and medical outcomes. *Patient Education and Counseling, 15,* 249–259.

Perlin ML, 1989: *Mental disability law: Civil and criminal.* Charlottesville, VA: Michie.

Rennie v. Klein, 462 F. Supp. 1131 (D.N.J. 1978), suppl., 476 F. Supp. 1294 (D.N.J. 1979), modified 653 F.2d 836 (3rd. Cir. 1981), vacated and remanded, 458 U.S. 1119 (1982), on remand, 720 F.2d 266 (3rd. Cir. 1983).

Rogers v. Okin, 478 F. Supp. 1342 (D. Mass. 1979), modified 634 F.2d 650 (1st Cir. 1980), sub nom Mills v. Rogers 457 U.S. 291 (1982), 102 S.Ct. 2442 (1982), sub nom Rogers v. Commissioner, 458 N.E.2d 308 (Mass. Sup. Jud. Ct. 1983), on remand 738 F.2d 1 (1st Cir. 1984).

Rozovsky F, 1990: *Consent to treatment: A practical guide,* 2nd edition. Boston: Little, Brown.

Schouten R, Gutheil TG, 1990: Aftermath of the *Rogers* decision: Assessing the costs. *American Journal of Psychiatry, 147,* 1348–1352.

Shapiro SA, 1979: Limiting physician freedom to prescribe a drug for any purpose: The need for FDA regulation. *Northwestern University Law Review, 73,* 801–872.

Sibley v. Board of Supervisors, 446 So.2d 760 (La. App. 1983); affirmed 462 So.2d 149 (Sup.Ct.La. 1985).

Slawson P, 1989: Psychiatric malpractice: Ten years' loss experience. *Medicine and Law, 8,* 415–427.

Soileau v. HCA Health Services, 539 So.2d 662 (La. App. 1989).

Tietz GF, 1986: Informed consent in the prescription drug context: The special case. *Washington Law Review, 61,* 367–417.

United States v. Charters, 863 F.2d 302 (4th Cir. 1988).

Van Putten T, 1974: Why do schizophrenic patients refuse to take their drugs? *Archives of General Psychiatry, 31,* 67–72.

Veliz J, James WS, 1987: Medicine court: *Rogers* in practice. *American Journal of Psychiatry, 144,* 62–67.

Washington v. Harper, 110 S.Ct. 1028 (1990).

Wettstein RM, 1983: Tardive dyskinesia and malpractice. *Behavioral Sciences and the Law, 1,* 85–107.

Wettstein RM, 1985: Legal aspects of neuroleptic-induced movement disorders. In: *Legal medicine,* edited by CH Wecht. New York: Praeger.

Wettstein RM, 1988: Informed consent and tardive dyskinesia. *Journal of Clinical Psychopharmacology, 8*(suppl), 65S–70S.

3

Drug Interactions
in Psychopharmacology

Shitij Kapur and R. Krishna Kambhampati

The use of multiple medications simultaneously, usually managed by more than one physician, is becoming increasingly common. This reality places the patient at a higher risk of adverse consequences resulting from drug-drug interactions. Iatrogenic complications are potentially avoidable; it is important for the clinician to be aware that polypharmacy results in ever-increasing permutations of potential adverse drug-drug interactions.

The magnitude of this problem may be estimated from one survey of intermediate care facilities where the patients received an average of 8.1 medicines. Of these patients, 50% received psychotropic medications (Beers, 1988). Surveys among psychiatric facilities have yielded similar results. In a study of long-term hospitalizations, 28% of psychiatric patients in the United States, 69% in Finland, and 68% in Britain received multiple psychotropic medications (Muijen & Silverstone, 1987). Fortunately, most interactions are benign and easily avoided or managed; yet, some interactions are potentially fatal.

MECHANISMS OF INTERACTIONS

Given the seemingly endless plethora of interactions and the continuous report of new ones, it is unlikely that a clinician can be familiar with all described interactions. However, the knowledge of the pharmacological basis of interactions serves to alert the clinician to possible interactions and consideration of optimal management strategies. As outlined in Chapter 1, there are three types of drug interactions: (1) pharmacokinetic interactions, (2) pharmacodynamic interactions, and (3) idiosyncratic interactions, which by definition is a less well-understood category.

Pharmacokinetic Interactions

Pharmacokinetics deal with the absorption, distribution, biotransformation, and excretion of drugs. Drug interactions involving any of these processes are called pharmacokinetic interactions.

Absorption

Most psychotropic drugs are administered orally and are absorbed through the gastrointestinal epithelium. Any alteration in the formulation of the medications and the chemical or ionic nature of the drug may influence absorption. A well known example of this phenomenon is the decrease in the levels of chlorpromazine when coadministered with antacids; this is attributed to the chelation of the antipsychotic by the antacid, leading to a decrease in the amount absorbed. Liquid elixirs of fluphenazine, haloperidol, and chlorpromazine form insoluble precipitates when given with citrus fruit juice, tea, or coffee. However, clinical studies of neuroleptic levels and clinical effects of a given dose do not suggest that this phenomenon is clinically relevant (Wallace, Suveges, Blackburn, Korchinski, & Midha, 1981). Drugs that alter the motility characteristics of the gut or compromise the integrity of the active transport mechanism may influence absorption. Anticholinergic drugs, by reducing motility, may delay absorption. Most tablets or capsules contain not only the active principles but also binders, filling agents, and protective coats. These ingredients may influence the bioavailability of the active principle such that less drug is absorbed or the time course of absorption is altered. This issue becomes potentially important when a patient is using different proprietary and generic preparations of a given drug.

Distribution

Once absorbed, a drug is distributed throughout the various body compartments. The physicochemical properties of the drug, composition of the body, and the affinity of the drug for the various compartments determine its final distribution. Interactions primarily resulting from the changes in drug distribution are known for some drugs; the interaction between guanethidine and tricyclic antidepressants as well as that between warfarin and chloral hydrate are prime examples. Guanethidine is actively transported into the axon-terminals where it exerts its actions. Tricyclic antidepressants block the uptake of guanethidine into the axon-terminals and hence antagonize its ability to lower blood pressure. Warfarin is a drug that is highly protein-bound. Trichloroacetic acid, a metabolite of chloral hydrate, displaces warfarin from its binding site on the plasma proteins. It is the unbound (or the free fraction) drug that is pharmacologically active. A higher free fraction of the drug produced by the addition of chloral hydrate causes an enhancement of the anticoagulant effect of a given dose of warfarin.

Metabolism

Most drugs are altered by an enzymatic process before excretion. The liver is the most common site of metabolism. The process of metabolism usually proceeds in two phases. In phase 1 the drug is detoxified through oxidation, hydroxylation, sulfoxidation, and demethylation, processes that involve the enzyme system called the microsomal enzyme oxidase system (MEOS)—also known as mixed function oxidase or cytochrome P450. In phase 2 the metabolite is then conjugated so that it can be eliminated. Since these processes are enzyme-mediated, drugs that alter the kinetics of these enzymes may alter the metabolism of other drugs that use the same enzymatic pathways. In humans, barbiturates, chronic ethanol intake, phenytoin, theophylline, and smoking induce some of the liver enzymes, usually leading to a enhanced metabolism and decreased levels of drugs, which are metabolized by these pathways. Carbamazepine is another enzyme-inducing agent. When carbamazepine is added to haloperidol at a steady state, it may decrease the levels of haloperidol by as much as 60%. This has been associated with reemergence of psychosis (Davis & Dysken, 1989). Some medicines may inhibit the metabolism of other drugs. Cimetidine, disulfiram, acute alcohol intake, and chloramphenicol inhibit the MEOS enzyme system, causing an increase in levels of some drugs and increased potential for toxicity. The addition of cimetidine to a steady-state regimen of imipramine increased imipramine levels by greater than 40% (Davis & Dysken, 1989). Enzymatically mediated effects may take up to 2 weeks to be completely exhibited (Stockley, 1981; Oates & Wilkinson, 1987).

Excretion

Most drugs are excreted by the body either in a lipid soluble form via the bile or in a water soluble form via the kidneys. Thiazide diuretics decrease the excretion of lithium by the kidney and can increase levels, precipitating toxicity. Many drugs are excreted as weak bases or weak acids. Such medicines are susceptible to the effects of small changes in their state of ionization. Small pH changes in the urine can significantly alter rate of excretion. Phenobarbital, which is a weak acid, is more rapidly excreted in alkaline urine than it is in acid urine. Awareness of this effect has led to alkalinization of urine being used in the management of barbiturate overdose. This example demonstrates that some medicines, which alter the pH of urine, can affect excretion of other drugs.

Pharmacodynamic Interactions

Pharmacodynamics describe the action of a drug on the target organ. Drugs that interact to alter the effects produced at end organs, without significantly altering the available drug levels at the receptor, are said to interact pharmacodynamically.

Most psychotropic drugs have overlapping effects on multiple neurotransmitters and neural substrates. For example, tricyclic antidepressants, antipsychotics, and antiparkinsonian drugs have anticholinergic actions. Patients requiring treatment with all three medications may have additive anticholinergic effects and are at increased risk for anticholinergic toxicity. On the other hand, drugs with dissimilar and opposing mechanisms can antagonize each others' actions. A classic example is the enhancement of dopaminergic transmission with levodopa and the decrease in dopaminergic transmission with the antipsychotics. Patients receiving levodopa for parkinsonism may experience psychotic symptoms as a side effect of dopamine replacement therapy, and the prescription of typical antipsychotics often worsens or causes a recurrence of extrapyramidal symptoms. Conversely patients with psychotic disorders can have worsening of their psychosis with the administration of levodopa (Bernstein 1981; Stockley 1988).

From the perspective of adverse drug interactions, the elderly are a particularly high risk group. First, the aging brain has an enhanced inherent susceptibility to the effects of psychoactive medications (Thompson, Moran, & Nies, 1983). Second, the elderly commonly suffer from more than one disease, have more than one physician, and are on more than one prescribed or over-the-counter medication at any given time. A combination of these factors explains in part the high incidence of iatrogenic delirium seen in this developmentally distinct population.

SPECIFIC INTERACTIONS

There are many reasons underlying the limitations to our understanding of drug interactions. The sources of information for much of the interactions involving older drugs are case reports; it is only recently that rigorous investigation of drug interactions has become an integral component of drug approval for marketing. The information is not infrequently obtained or extrapolated from in vitro or laboratory animal experiments of uncertain clinical relevance. Additionally, generalizations about a class of drugs have often been made from observing interactions with only one member of that class. Although the approach of generalizing from a single member of a class to all members of a class may be useful when the mechanism of the underlying interaction is understood, the value of this approach in other instances is less certain. In this regard, rare interactions may reflect observer bias or represent idiosyncratic responses of the reported patients to a given drug or combination (Davis & Dysken, 1989) and may not be relevant to the entire class of drugs.

Sedative Hypnotics and Anxiolytics

Barbiturates are being used less frequently as sedative hypnotics because of the high addictive potential, adverse drug interactions, and the availability of benzodiazepines. Barbiturates, especially the long acting ones like phenobarbital, are potent inducers of the MEOS. Patients at steady state on medications metabolized by the liver MEOS, such as phenytoin, phenothiazines, butyrophenones, and heterocyclic antidepressants, experience a decrease in levels on addition of a barbiturate (Csernansky & Whiteford, 1987). As a corollary, patients receiving higher than usual dosage of such medicines to compensate for concomitant administration of a barbiturate are at a risk of toxicity when the barbiturate is discontinued and the MEOS returns to baseline. At a pharmacodynamic level the barbiturates are potent depressants of the central nervous system (CNS) with effects on arousal, attention, and respiratory drive. When combined with other drugs with sedative-hypnotic effects, such as anticonvulsants, alcohol, benzodiazepines, tricyclics, and antipsychotics, there is a risk of severe sedation and respiratory depression or arrest.

Benzodiazepines have largely replaced barbiturates for use as sedative hypnotics. Most benzodiazepines are metabolized by the liver MEOS using phase 1 and phase 2 (conjugation) mechanisms discussed earlier. The phase 1 of this process is susceptible to enzyme induction (barbiturate, smoking, alcohol) and enzyme inhibition (disulfiram, cimetidine), whereas phase 2 is unaffected. Benzodiazepines like oxazepam, temazepam and lorazepam, which do not require phase 1 metabolism, may be alternatives if pharmacokinetic interactions are clinically significant. The effect of cimetidine causing prolonged elimination half-life of benzodiazepines is of significance, especially in the elderly and patients with liver dysfunction. Additive sedative interactions are also a practical concern, especially in the elderly.

Buspirone, an anxiolytic unrelated to benzodiazepines or barbiturates, has been used extensively. Few adverse drug interactions have been reported. A beneficial interaction is that, in controlled experimental situations, the drug antagonizes alcohol-related psychomotor impairment (Mattila, Aranko & Seppala, 1982). Concomitant administration of buspirone and haloperidol can result in increased serum haloperidol concentrations. The clinical significance of this finding is unclear (*Physician's Desk Reference*; Medical Economics Company, 1989).

Lithium (Table 1)

Antidepressants

Lithium and tricyclics have been used extensively in combination with good therapeutic effect and a safe record. However, at least one case of seizures has been reported on the combination. The seizure remitted on discontinuing lithium and recurred on reinstitution (Hansten & Horn, 1989; Solomon, 1979). Seizures are a potential concern in combination therapy of other antidepressant classes also. Use of lithium with agents such as maprotiline and bupropion, which are known to lower the seizure threshold, should be undertaken with appropriate awareness of the possible risk, even though seizure episodes to our knowledge have not yet been reported.

Antipsychotics

Patients with mania often receive both antipsychotics and lithium during the acute stages of management. Patients with schizophrenia or schizoaffective disorders may also receive lithium together with an antipsychotic. This has raised concern regarding possible neurotoxicity to patients taking both lithium and an antipsychotic. Patients on high doses of both have been reported to be at risk to developing an encephalopathic syndrome of fever, lethargy, confusion, extrapyramidal, and cerebellar signs (Cohen & Cohen, 1974). The exact mechanism of this interaction is unknown but may be related to lithium-induced dopamine blockade (Addonizio, Roth, Stokes, & Stoll, 1988), increases in phenothiazine levels (Stockley, 1981), and/or increases in tissue lithium uptake (Hansten & Horn, 1989). Although little studied, it has been suggested that when the two drugs are given together, neurotoxicity (encephalopathic syndrome, extrapyramidal effects,

Table 1 Interactions with lithium

Drug	Mechanism	Clinical outcome
Tricyclic antidepressants	Lower seizure threshold	Grand mal seizures
Antipsychotics	Increased tissue lithium uptake Increased levels of antipsychotics	Increased neurotoxicity
Carbamazepine	Unknown	Increased neurotoxicity
Phenytoin	Unknown	Increased neurotoxicity
ECT	Unknown	Increased post-ECT confusion Increased memory loss
Diuretics	Increased reabsorption	Increased levels of lithium Increased adverse effects
ACE inhibitors	Increased lithium levels	Increased adverse effects
NSAID	Decreased renal clearance	Increased levels of lithium Increased adverse effects

cerebellar effects, and EEG abnormalities) is observed more often than either drug alone (Miller & Menninger, 1987), and that antipsychotic-induced extrapyramidal side effects may worsen on addition of lithium to the regimen (Addonizio et al., 1988). A recent review of this issue concluded that the safe coadministration of lithium and antipsychotics is feasible. Interactions are infrequent and not necessarily associated with residual neurological impairment; it was suggested that the doses of the two drugs should be kept at the lowest effective level (Miller & Menninger, 1987).

Anticonvulsants

Carbamazepine is being increasingly used as an antimanic agent in bipolar patients, often with lithium for synergistic effect. A possible positive interaction with the lithium-induced leukocytosis overriding the carbamazepine-induced bone marrow suppression has been noted (Brewerton, 1986). A negative interaction, with carbamazepine enhancing the lithium-related tremors, ataxia, and other features of neurotoxicity has been consistently observed, at times even with therapeutic levels of both drugs (Shukla, Godwin, Long, & Miller, 1984; Price & Giannini, 1985). Phenytoin, another anticonvulsant, is known to enhance lithium-related ataxia and neurotoxicity. The mechanism is not known, and this effect may be seen without an increase in the levels of lithium and in the absence of toxic levels of phenytoin (Raskin, 1984).

Electroconvulsive Therapy

Many patients being treated with lithium may need electroconvulsive therapy (ECT) for their psychiatric condition. Studies have demonstrated increased post-ECT confusion, memory loss, increased atypical neurological findings, and impairment on neuropsychological testing in patients who continue to receive lithium during the course of ECT (Blackwell & Schmidt, 1984; Small, Kellams, Milstein, & Small, 1980). Lithium also causes a prolongation of the succinylcholine-induced muscle relaxation, possibly by its action on the neuromuscular junction, a concern during modified ECT and surgical procedures (Reimherr, Hodges, Hill, & Wong, 1977). Given these concerns, withholding lithium before starting ECT is recommended. If lithium is needed during ECT therapy, the patient's electrolyte and mental status should be frequently reviewed for unwanted changes.

Diuretics

Lithium is orally administered, readily absorbed, and excreted unchanged by the kidney. Since lithium has a narrow therapeutic window and its levels are readily affected by alterations in renal function, drugs altering renal function need to be used with caution. Some diuretics, particularly thiazides, impede lithium excretion. With chronic diuretic administration, a state of relative hypovolemia may occur, and resultant compensatory drives tend to conserve sodium via the proximal tubule; this leads to an enhanced concomitant reabsorption of lithium and frequently significantly increased levels (Stockley, 1981). This is a clinically relevant interaction and is commonly responsible for the precipitation of lithium toxicity in patients. In contrast, osmotic diuretics such as mannitol and urea, as well as certain compounds with diuretic activity such as theophylline, aminophylline, and acetazolamide, may enhance the clearance of lithium. The mechanism and the clinical significance of this are unclear.

Antihypertensive Agents

Interactions have been noted when the angiotensin converting enzyme (ACE) inhibitors, enalapril and captopril, were added to the medication regimes of patients on steady-state lithium. The effect is acute, may at times double the lithium plasma levels, and precipitate toxicity (Gelenberg, 1988). Verapamil, a calcium-channel blocker, has been reported to cause severe bradycardia and an encephalopathic syndrome when added to therapeutic steady-state doses of lithium (Dubovsky, 1986; Price & Giannini, 1986).

Nonsteroidal Antiinflammatory Drugs

Nonsteroidal antiinflammatory drugs (NSAID) have been noted to decrease renal clearance of lithium and increase levels. A possible mechanism is the NSAID-induced renal prostaglandin inhibition with decreased glomerular filtration rate. Indomethacin, ibuprofen, naproxen, mefenamic acid, and piroxicam have all been implicated. However, sulindac does not appear to produce this effect (Raghels & Powell, 1986).

Antipsychotics (Table 2)

Since the introduction of chlorpromazine, antipsychotics have grown in clinical applications. Antipsychotics have clearest indication in the treatment of schizophrenia, brief reactive psychosis, mania, and agitation states. Commonly encountered side effects of the typical antipsychotics are sedation, anticholinergic side effects (acute glaucoma, dry mouth, urinary retention, constipation), orthostatic hypotension, and extrapyramidal symptoms. The antipsychotics can be divided into two groups on the basis of potency: low potency (clozapine, chlorpromazine, and thioridazine) and high potency (perphenazine, trifluperazine, fluphenazine, thiothixene, and haloperidol). The low potency antipsychotics frequently cause prominent sedation, orthostatic hypotension, and severe anticholinergic side effects but produce relatively less extrapyramidal symptoms with equipotent doses. Thioridazine and clozapine are particularly remarkable for exhibiting the lowest extrapyramidal symptoms. The high potency neuroleptics cause less sedation and

Table 2 Interactions with antipsychotics

Drug	Mechanism	Clinical outcome
Anticholinergic agents	Additive actions	Increased anticholinergic side effects
Antidepressants	Mutual inhibition of metabolism Additive anticholinergic and antiadrenergic effects	Increased side effects—especially anticholinergic and orthostatic side effects
Lithium	Increased tissue lithium uptake Increased levels of antipsychotics	Increased neurotoxicity
Anticonvulsant (carbamazepine)	Increased enzymatic metabolism	Decreased antipsychotic levels Possible loss of efficacy

orthostatic and anticholinergic symptoms but more frequently cause disabling extrapyramidal symptoms.

Anticholinergic Agents

Anticholinergic agents such as benztropine, trihexyphenidyl, and biperiden are often combined with antipsychotics to control extrapyramidal side effects. These medicines may decrease gastrointestinal motility delaying absorption and decreasing blood levels of the antipsychotic (Gautier et al., 1977). The addition of anticholinergic agents, especially in the elderly, predispose them to the development of serious anticholinergic side effects: paralytic ileus, heat stroke, and the precipitation of an anticholinergic delirium have been noted (Hansten & Horn, 1989). This situation may often be avoided by using low doses of higher potency antipsychotic agents with fewer anticholinergic effects. Antiparkinsonian anticholinergic drugs should not be added routinely, but only after signs of extrapyramidal syndrome are manifested (Bohacek et al., 1990; Hansten & Horn, 1989).

Antidepressants

Antipsychotics are frequently combined with antidepressants, especially in the treatment of delusional depression. Fixed-dose combinations like Triavil (amitriptyline and perphenazine) are often used. Coadministration of antipsychotics and antidepressants has been observed to yield higher individual levels; the mechanism, although not clearly understood, may be related to mutual inhibition of enzymatic metabolism. Antipsychotic and antidepressant combinations may result in additive anticholinergic and sedative effects. An increased incidence of arrhythmias and myocardial depression is seen when the calcium-channel blocking antipsychotic thioridazine is combined with antidepressants like imipramine, which have quinidine-like properties (Bernstein, 1988). The elderly may develop (with greater frequency than younger individuals) a pronounced orthostatic hypotension with combination therapy, leading sometimes to the development of a hypotensive "shock" syndrome. This problem is noted especially with low potency neuroleptics combined with monoamine oxidase inhibitors. This is a particularly tricky situation as pressors, usually administered to reverse severe hypotension, are contraindicated in the presence of established monoamine oxidase inhibition (Bernstein, 1988; Blackwell, 1984).

Lithium

Please see pages 25-26.

Antihypertensives

By a mechanism similar to that described previously for tricyclic antidepressants, antipsychotics may reduce the antihypertensive effects of guanethidine (Blackwell & Schmidt, 1984; Janowsky, El-Yousef, & Davis, 1973). Patients on antipsychotics may receive beta blockers to treat hypertension, akathisia, or as an adjunct in the management of schizophrenia. Administration of propanolol to patients on thioridazine caused a three-fold increase in levels of the latter, even though no clinical toxicity was observed (Stockley, 1981).

Heterocyclic Antidepressants (Table 3)

Monoamine Oxidase Inhibitors (MAOIs)

Combined monoamine oxidase inhibitor (MAOI) and tricyclic antidepressant therapy is efficacious in certain patients who are resistant to other forms of antidepressant therapy. Although this combination is potentially hazardous, several recent studies have reported the safe use of this combination.

Since both MAOIs and tricyclics increase CNS noradrenergic and serotonergic transmission via different mechanisms, the coadministration can cause a synergistic neurotransmitter "overflow" leading to excitatory side effects (Stockley, 1981). Despite these potentially serious effects, the coadministration is *not* contraindicated and judicious administration is possible if there are obvious benefits of the combination. The following guidelines are suggested (Hansten & Horn, 1989; Stockley, 1981; White & Simpson, 1981; Blackwell & Schmidt, 1984; Pare, 1985; Feighner, Herbstein, & Damlouji, 1985) for coadministration of heterocyclic antidepressants and MAOIs: (1) use only in patients who are refractory to other treatments; (2) use only oral drugs; (3) avoid large doses and titrate slowly upward; (4) avoid clomipramine, desipramine, and imipramine, but use amitriptyline, nortriptyline, or trimipramine. (Avoid tranylcypromine in favor of phenelzine or isocarboxazid. No combination has been convincingly shown to be the safest or the most efficacious. See also chapter 3.); (5) continually reassess the need for both medications; (6) the patient may be asked to carry 100 mg of chlorpromazine, which the patient may self-administer if medical help is not readily accessible in the event of a hypertensive crisis. This practice is potentially risky and should be avoided if possible; (7) establish the heterocyclics therapy first and add the MAOIs thereafter. Combined therapies as outlined above should only be carried out by physicians experienced in this approach.

Pressor Agents

Tricyclics decrease reuptake and thus enhance the action of neurotransmitters at the synapse. In patients receiving antidepressants, unexpected increases in blood pressure can be observed with the use of direct and indirect pressor agents. This interaction has been known to result in fatalities after the administration of local anesthesia containing epinephrine in patients on tricyclics (Blackwell & Schmitt, 1984).

Cimetidine

This drug has been shown to prolong the half-life of tricyclic antidepressants by impairing their metabolism. The impairment of metabolism results in an increase in the tricyclic levels and may produce increased adverse effects (Miller & Macklin, 1983). This interaction can be avoided by using ranitidine, which has a significantly less effect on the MEOS (Webster et al., 1984).

Neuroleptics

Please see pages 28–29.

Stimulants

Many patients receive methylphenidate to augment the effect of tricyclic antidepressants especially in anergic depression. Methylphenidate is known to increase tricyclic levels by inhibiting its metabolism. This increase in levels may enhance the effect of the tricyclics but may precipitate toxicity in some patients (Hansten & Horn, 1989; Stockley, 1981, Zeidenberg, Perel, Kanzler, Wharton, & Malitz, 1971).

Newer, Atypical Antidepressants

Fluoxetine

This is a new bicyclic antidepressant, which selectively inhibits serotonin reuptake and is effective in major depression and obsessive compulsive disorder. Fluoxetine is free of anticholinergic, orthostatic, or significant cardiac effects. The most common adverse reactions include anxiety, nervousness, insomnia, and gastrointestinal complaints like nausea, anorexia, and diarrhea. Fluoxetine has a prolonged half-life, which ranges from 2 to 9 days; it takes over a month after discontinuation of the drug for it to clear from the system.

Adverse interactions have been noted between fluoxetine and other antidepressants. Addition of fluoxetine to steady level tricyclics (specifically nortriptyline and desipramine) has led to an increase in levels, often leading to increased side effects and toxicity (Downs et al., 1989; Vaughan, 1988; Aranow et al., 1989). Several cases of the hypertensive-hypermetabolic reaction has been reported in patients receiving both fluoxetine and MAOIs. Therefore, based its pharmacokinetics, fluoxetine should be started at least 15 days after MAOI therapy is stopped and MAOIs started at least 35 days after fluoxetine has been stopped (Sternbach, 1988).

Pharmacokinetic interactions have been reported between fluoxetine and diazepam. Fluoxetine decreases the metabolism of diazepam to desmethyldiazepam,

Table 3 Interactions with heterocyclic antidepressants

Drug	Mechanism	Clinical outcome
MAOIs	Synergistic neurotransmitter enhancement	Hypertensive reactions
Cimetidine	Decreased metabolism	Increased heterocyclic levels Increased adverse effects
Antipsychotics	Mutual inhibition of metabolism Additive anticholinergic and antiadrenergic effects	Increased side effects Especially anticholinergic and orthostatic side effects
Stimulants	Inhibition of antidepressant metabolism	Increased heterocyclic levels Increased side effects
Fluoxetine	Inhibition of metabolism of antidepressants	Increased heterocyclic levels Increased side effects
Lithium	Lower seizure threshold	Grand mal seizures
Pressor agents	Increased central adrenergic transmission	Unexpected hypertension

causing an increase in the level of diazepam and decrease in the level of its active metabolite. However, no psychomotor adverse effects have been noted, possibly related to the fact that the level of total benzodiazepines (i.e., diazepam and desmethyldiazepam) remains unchanged (Lemberger, Rowe, Bosomworth, Tenbarge, & Bergstrom, 1988).

Tryptophan, which can increase brain serotonin, has sometimes been given with fluoxetine to further augment serotonergic transmission. However, in certain cases, tryptophan has caused a reversible increase in agitation, restlessness, anxiety, depression, and obsessive compulsive symptoms along with gastrointestinal adverse effects (Steiner & Fontaine, 1986). Fluoxetine has been reported to be associated with a worsening of neuroleptic-related extrapyramidal symptoms and an increase in lithium levels with an associated increase in side effects (Tate, 1989). The drug-drug interactions of fluoxetine are currently being systematically evaluated.

Bupropion

This new antidepressant is biochemically distinct from tricyclics and MAOIs. Its efficacy may be related to its presynaptic dopaminergic activity (Ayd, 1984). It does not potentiate the sedative effects of alcohol and has also been shown to decrease benzodiazepine-induced cognitive impairment (Peck & Hamilton, 1984). Coadministration of bupropion with levodopa is associated with increased nausea and agitation (Watsky & Salzman, 1991). Bupropion has a tendency to lower the seizure threshold and should therefore be used with caution with other drugs that lower the threshold and in populations at higher risk for seizures.

Monoamine Oxidase Inhibitors (Table 4)

MAOI antidepressants have a well-known potential for serious adverse interactions. Dopamine, norepinephrine, and serotonin have their action terminated by reuptake and subsequent metabolism by monoamine oxidase. MAOIs inhibit this enzyme irreversibly and thus enhance dopaminergic, noradrenergic, and serotonergic transmission. The currently available MAOIs can be classified as hydrazine (phenelzine and isocarboxazid) and nonhydrazine derivatives (tranylcypromine). Tranylcypromine is structurally similar to amphetamine and has a

Table 4 Interactions with MAOIs

Drug	Interactions	Clinical outcome
Heterocyclic antidepressants	Synergistic "neurotransmitter" enhancement	Hypertensive reaction
Fluoxetine	Synergistic serotonergic enhancement	Hypertensive–hyperthermic reaction
Tyramine rich foods	Increased synaptic availability of tyramine	Hypertensive reaction
Pressor agents	Increased synaptic availability of pressor agents	Hypertensive reaction
Recreational drugs	Enhanced sympathomimetic effect	Hypertensive reaction
Narcotics	Possibly enhanced serotonergic transmission	Hypertensive–hyperthermic reaction

direct stimulant effect in addition to its MAOI effect. The interactions seen with MAOIs include hypertensive crises associated with foods rich in tyramine and some drugs (see chapter 23) and effects resulting from potentiation of the common side effects of other agents, such as sedation and orthostatic hypotension.

Foods

MAOIs can have serious potential for adverse interactions with foods rich in tyramine. The effect is usually a hypertensive crisis, which can lead to severe headache at best and, at worst, confusion, agitation, excitement, congestive heart failure, retinal hemorrhages, cerebrovascular accidents, seizures, coma, and even death. Fermented foods may contain high levels of tyramine (a product of decarboxylation of tyrosine), which is an indirectly acting sympathomimetic. Under usual circumstances, the tyramine in such foods is rapidly degraded by MAO in the intestinal wall and liver. In the presence of MAO inhibition, large quantities of tyramine gain access to systemic circulation and synaptic terminals where they cause exaggerated release of excitatory transmitters (Hansten & Horn, 1989; Stockley, 1981; Czernansky & Whiteford, 1987). Cheese, red wine, chicken liver, aged meats like pepperoni and salami, pickled herring, broad fava beans, and yeast extracts are all potentially dangerous. Prediction of a potential interaction is difficult as the degree of enzyme inhibition varies among individuals even on a similar dose of MAOI, and the length of treatment and the amino acid composition of different batches of the same food item vary greatly. Enzyme inhibition is prolonged and may persist and cause side effects for up to 3 weeks after discontinuing an MAO inhibitor. A list of foods and medicines of concern are outlined in Chapter 23, Table 1.

Pressor Agents

Direct and indirect pressors cause exaggerated responses in the presence of MAO inhibitors. Phenylephrine (a direct sympathomimetic), pseudoephedrine and metaraminol (which are indirect sympathomimetic agents), ephedrine and phenylpropanolamine (which have both direct and indirect effects) can all cause hypertensive crises. Levodopa is metabolized in the body to dopamine and norepinephrine; in the presence of an MAOI it can cause an increased release of dopamine, norepinephrine, or both (Bernstein, 1988). Some authors have suggested that the directly acting pressor agents like norepinephrine and epinephrine may be safer since the MAOIs exert their action intraneuronally and not at the synaptic junction (Janowsky & Janowsky, 1985).

Over-the-Counter (OTC) Drugs

Nasal or oral decongestants, diet pills, or "pep" pills may contain pressors. A patient may obtain these without prior discussion with the physician, and serious interactions and fatalities have been reported. The majority of fatalities reported lately have resulted from the interaction of MAOIs and sympathomimetic OTC drugs (Harrison, McGrath, Stewart, & Quitkin, 1989). This suggests that physicians should emphasize this as a potential problem during informed consent discussions.

Recreational Drugs

With the increasing use of so-called recreational drugs, especially amphetamine and cocaine, drug abusers run a risk of having hypertensive crises. Such risk may persist for several weeks after the patient has discontinued MAOI therapy. (Devabhaktuni & Jampala, 1987)

Tricyclic Antidepressants

Refer to page 29.

Narcotics

Narcotics, meperidine in particular, have produced serious interactions with MAOIs. The reaction may be CNS excitation causing agitation, sweating, rigidity, and hypertension or CNS depression with coma and shock. Dextromethorphan can also give rise to a similar interaction. The mechanism has been hypothesized to be related to excessive serotonergic drive (Stockley, 1981).

Anesthetics

Patients on MAO inhibitors may require anesthesia for planned surgical procedures, ECT, or emergency procedures. Even though the safe administration of anesthesia has been documented (Janowski & Janowski, 1985; Remik, Jewesson, & Ford, 1987), this situation is best avoided if possible. MAOIs (especially phenelzine) are known to decrease plasma pseudocholinesterase activity; thus, prolonged neuromuscular blockade has the potential to occur with direct depolarizing relaxants like succinylcholine (Janowski & Janowski, 1985; Stockley, 1981). Patients on MAOIs developing a hypotensive episode during surgery may require a pressor agent and consequently encounter the risk of a hypertensive crises. Caution should also be used regarding the use of narcotic analgesics for pre- and postoperative pain in patients on MAO inhibitors.

Anticonvulsants

Anticonvulsants are being increasingly used in psychiatry. Carbamazepine is now an established treatment for mania and prophylaxis of bipolar disorder. Carbamazepine stimulates the MEOS and consequently stimulates its own metabolism, a process called autoinduction. This causes a decrease in the levels of carbamazepine after an initial achievement of steady state. This phenomenon has been observed to cause breakthrough seizures in patients who are receiving the drug for control of seizures (MacPhee & Brodie, 1985). The impact of this effect in prophylactic management of bipolar disorder has not been empirically established, but clinicians need to be aware that a decrease in carbamazepine levels during the initial weeks of therapy may represent autoinduction rather than noncompliance.

Increased adverse effects in patients taking lithium have already been discussed in the section on lithium. As discussed earlier, carbamazepine enhances the metabolism of haloperidol. Monitoring of haloperidol levels during combined therapy has been suggested to be useful, but the clinical relevance of this awaits further clarification of the clinical value of haloperidol blood levels (Arana et al., 1986). Sodium valproate is being investigated as a treatment for manic episodes and prophylaxis of bipolar disorder (Small, 1990). When administered in combination with sodium valproate, the metabolism of carbamazepine is altered with increased accumulation of the active metabolite carbamazepine 10,11 epoxide. This results in displacement of carbamazepine from its protein binding. This may increase the potential for toxicity to arise (Levy et al., 1984).

Cimetidine inhibits the metabolism of carbamazepine and sodium valproate. If dosages remain unchanged, blood levels increase and thereby the risk of toxicity is also increased. Ranitidine, another H_2 blocker, does not inhibit the MEOS and hence does not alter levels of the hepatically metabolized anticonvulsants (Webster et al., 1984). Erythromycin decreases the clearance of carbamazepine; this results in increased carbamazepine levels and may precipitate signs of intoxication (Wong, Ludden, & Bell, 1983). The calcium-channel blockers, verapamil and diltiazem, have been known to cause a precipitous increase in levels of carbamazepine with consequent toxicity. Nifedipine, which is structurally dissimilar, does not cause a similar increase in levels (Brodie & MacPhee, 1986).

GUIDELINES TO PREVENT DRUG INTERACTIONS

1. *Obtain a thorough medication history.* This should include history of any allergies, past medication history, and all present medications. An effort should be made to chcck the validity of the patient's report by way of written records, prescriptions, pharmacy, or primary physician. Special note should be made of OTC use. Recreational drugs, smoking, alcohol, and use of peculiar diets or diet pills must be explored.

2. *Avoid polypharmacy as a principle.* Since this may not always be practically feasible, avoid use of multiple drugs with same action (more than one antipsychotic or more than one benzodiazepine for same purpose). If the patient is on multiple medications, constantly reassess need for all medications. Evaluate any unexpected clinical deterioration as a possible adverse interaction. Confirmed adverse interactions should be reported to relevant agencies such as the Food and Drug Administration.

3. *Educate the patient about the potential side effects and interactions.* Personally explain and supply the patient with easy to understand educational material. Ensure that the patient has understood.

4. *Document carefully.* Since drug interactions are potentially serious and may lead to malpractice litigation, clearly document on the patient's chart all medications, their indications, and steps taken to prevent adverse consequences, especially patient information.

5. *Have a high index of suspicion for any new complaints or symptoms.* A serious interaction may be masquerading as a "somatization" in a psychiatric patient.

6. *Simplify the drug regimen.* This reduces the chances of medication errors and hence unwanted effects. Most psychiatric medications have long half-lives and can be given once a day to simplify the regimen.

7. *Identify high-risk populations.* Because of their reduced metabolic capacities and increased sensitivity to adverse effects of medications, the elderly are particularly susceptible. Patients with multiple system disease, especially hypertension, heart failure, chronic renal failure, hepatic insufficiency, and diabetes, and also patients with peptic ulcer disease and glaucoma represent a high-risk group.

8. *Keep up with the literature.* No single treatise on this subject is complete. For details, the interested reader is referred to more elaborate works (Hansten, 1989; Ciraulo, 1989; Watsky & Salzman, 1991; Ciraulo, Shader, Greenblatt, & Greelman, 1989; the AMA Drug Evaluations, *Meyler's Side Effects of Drugs Annuals, The Medical Letter, the Journal of Clinical Psychopharmacology* and *the Journal of Clinical Psychiatry).*

REFERENCES

Addonizio G, Roth SD, Stokes PE, Stoll PM, 1988: Increased extrapyramidal symptoms with addition of lithium to neuroleptics. *Journal of Nervous and Mental Disease, 176,* 682–685.

Arana GW, Goff, DC, Friedman H, Ornsteen M, Greenblatt DJ, Black B, Shader RI, 1986: Does carbamazepine-induced reduction of plasma haloperidol levels worsen psychotic symptoms? *American Journal of Psychiatry,143*(5), 650–651.

Aranow R, Hudson JI, Pope HG, Grady TA, Lange TA, Bell IR, Cole JO, 1989: Elevated antidepressant plasma levels after addition of fluoxetine. *American Journal of Psychiatry, 146,* 911–913.

Ayd FJ, 1984: Bupropion: A novel antidepressant. *International Drug Therapy Newsletter, 19,* 1–20.

Beers M, Avorn J, Sounerai SB, Event DE, Sherman DS, Salem S, 1988: Psychoactive medication use in intermediate care facility residents. *Journal of the American Medical Association, 260,* 3016–3020.

Bernstein JG, 1988: *Handbook of drug therapy in psychiatry.* Littleton, MA: PSG Publishing.

Blackwell B, Schmidt GI, 1984: Drug interactions in psychopharmacology. *Psychiatric Clinics of North America, 7*(3), 625–637.

Bohacek N, Bolwig T, Bunney WE, Coppen AJ, Gastpar M, Kielholz P, Kojima T, Hippius H, Mendlewicz J, Kemali D, Maj M, Moussaoui D, Nair NPV, Poldinger W, Potkin S, Racagni G, Ramon de la Fuente J, Sartorius N, Sethi BB, Yu-Cun S, Stefanis C, Takahashi R, Vartaniar ME, Verhoeven WMA, Yamashita I, 1990: Prophylactic use of anticholinergics in patients on long-term neuroleptic treatment: WHO consensus statement. *British Journal of Psychiatry, 165,* 412–414.

Brewerton TD, 1986: Lithium counteracts carbamazepine induced leukopenia while increasing its therapeutic effect: A case report. *Biological Psychiatry, 21,* 677–686.

Brodie MJ, Macphee GJA, 1986: Carbamazepine neurotoxicity precipitated by diltiazem. *British Medical Journal, 292,* 1170–1171.

Ciraulo DA, Shader RI, Greenblatt DJ, Greelman W, 1989: *Drug interactions in psychiatry.* Baltimore: Williams and Wilkins.

Cohen W, Cohen N, 1974: Lithium carbonate, haloperidol and irreversible brain damage. *Journal of the American Medical Association, 230,* 1283–1287.

Cscrnansky JG, Whiteford HA, 1987: Clinical significant psychoactive drug interactions. *Annual Review of Psychiatry, 6,* 802–815.

Davis JM, Dysken MW, 1989: The pharmacology of psychotropic drugs and drug-drug interactions. In: *Comprehensive textbook of psychiatry,* edited by HI Kaplan and BJ Sadock. Baltimore: Williams and Wilkins.

Devabhaktuni RV, Jampala VC, 1987: Using street drugs while on MAOI therapy. *Journal of Clinical Psychopharmacology, 7*(1), 60–61.

Downs J, Downs AD, Rosenthal TL, Deal N, Akiskal HS, 1989: Increased plasma tricyclic antidepressant concentrations in two patients concurrently treated with fluoxetine. *Journal of Clinical Psychiatry, 50,* 226–227.

Dubovsky SL, 1986: Calcium antagonists: A new class of psychiatric drugs? *Psychiatric Annals, 16,* 724–728.

Feighner JP, Herbstein J, Damlouji N, 1985: Combined MAOI, TCA and direct stimulant therapy of treatment resistant depression. *Journal of Clinical Psychiatry, 46,* 206–209.

Gautier J, Jas A, Villeneuve A, Jus K, Pires P, Velleneuve R, 1977: Influence of the antiparkinsonian drugs on the plasma level of neuroleptics. *Biological Psychiatry, 12,* 389–399.

Gelenberg AK, 1988: ACE inhibitors and lithium toxicity. *Biological Therapies in Psychiatry, 11,* 43.

Hansten PD, Horn JR, 1989: *Drug interactions: Clinical significance of drug-drug interactions,* 6th edition. Philadelphia: Lea and Febiger.

Harrison WM, McGrath PJ, Stewart JW, Quitkin F, 1989: MAOI's and hypertensive crises: The role of OTC drugs. *Journal of Clinical Psychiatry, 50,* 65–65.

Janowski EC, Janowski DS, 1985: What precautions should be taken if a patient on an MAOI is scheduled to undergo anesthesia? *Journal of Clinical Psychopharmacology, 5,* 128–129.

Janowsky DS, El-Yousef K, Davis JM, 1973: Antagonism of guanethidine by chlorpromazine. *American Journal of Psychiatry, 130*(7), 808–809.

Lemberg L, Rowe H, Bosomworth JC, Tenbarge JB, Bergstrom RF, 1988: The effect of fluoxetine on the pharmacokinetics and psychomotor responses of diazepam. *Clinical Pharmacology and Therapeutics, 43,* 412–419.

Levy RH, Moreland TA, Morselli PL, Guyot M, Brachet-Liermain A, Loiseau P, 1984: Carbamazepine/valproid acid interaction in man and rhesus monkey. *Epilepsia, 25*(3), 338–345.

MacPhee GJA, Brode MJ, 1985: Carbamazepine substitution in severe partial epilepsy: Implication of autoinduction of metabolism. *Postgraduate Medical Journal, 61,* 779–783.

Mattila MJ, Aranko K, Seppala T, 1982: Acute effects of buspirone and alcohol on psychomotor skills. *Journal of Clinical Psychiatry, 12*(2) 56–60.

Medical Economics Company, 1989: *Physician's desk reference,* 43rd edition. Oradell, New Jersey.

Miller DD, Macklin M, 1983: Cimetidine-imipramine interaction: A case report. *American Journal of Psychiatry, 140*(3), 351–352.

Miller F, Menninger J, 1987: Lithium—neuroleptic neurotoxicity is dose dependent. *Journal of Clinical Psychopharmacology, 7,* 89–91.

Muijen M, Silverstone T, 1987: A comparative hospital survey of psychotropic drug prescribing. *British Journal of Psychiatry, 150,* 501–504.

Oates JA, Wilkinson GR, 1987: Principles of drug therapy. In: *Harrison principles of internal medicine,* 11th edition, edited by E Braunwald, KJ Isselbacher, RG Petersdorf, JD Wilson, JB Martin, and AS Fauci AS. New York: McGraw-Hill.

Pare CMB, 1985: The present status of monoamine oxidase inhibitors. *British Journal of Psychiatry, 146,* 576–584.

Peck AW, Hamilton M, 1984: Psychopharmacology of bupropion in normal volunteers. *Journal of Clinical Psychiatry, 44,* 202–205.

Price WA, Giannini AJ, 1986: Neurotoxicity caused by lithium-verapamil synergism. *Journal of Clinical Pharmacology, 26,* 717–719.

Price WA, Zimmer B, 1985: Lithium carbamazepine neurotoxicity in the elderly. *Journal of American Geriatrics Society, 33,* 876–877.

Raghels M, Powell A, 1986: Lithium interaction with sulindac and naproxen. *Journal of Clinical Psychopharmacology, 6,* 150–154.

Raskin DE, 1984: Lithium and phenytoin interaction. *Journal of Clinical Pharmacology, 4*(20), 120.

Reimherr FW, Hodges MR, Hill GE, Wong KC, 1977: Prolongation of muscle relaxant effects by lithium carbonate. *American Journal of Psychiatry, 134*(2), 205–206.

Remick RA, Jewesson P, Ford RWJ, 1987: Monoamine oxidase inhibitors in general anesthesia: A re-evaluation. *Convulsive Therapy, 3,* 196–203.

Shukla S, Godwin CD, Long LEB, Miller MG, 1984: Lithium-carbamazepine neurotoxicity and risk factors, *141*(12), 1604–1606.

Small JG, Kellams JJ, Milstein V, Small IF, 1980: Complications with electroconvulsive treatment combined with lithium. *Biological Psychiatry, 15*(2), 103–112.

Small JG, 1990: Anticonvulsants in affective disorders. *Psychopharmacology Bulletin, 26,* 25–36.

Solomon JG, 1979: Seizures during lithium-amitriptyline therapy. *Postgraduate Medicine, 66*(3), 145–148.

Steiner W, Fontaine R, 1986: Toxic reactions following the combined administration of fluoxetine and L-tryptophan: Five case reports. *Biological Psychiatry, 21,* 1067–1071.

Sternbach H, 1988: Danger of MAOI therapy after fluoxetine withdrawal. *Lancet, ii,* 850–851.

Stockley, IH, 1981: *Drug interactions.* Oxford: Blackwell Scientific Publications.

Tate JL, 1989: Extrapyramidal symptoms in a patient taking haloperidol and fluoxetine. *American Journal of Psychiatry, 146,* 399–400.

Thompson TL, Moran MG, Nies AS, 1983: Psychotropic drug use in the elderly. *New England Journal of Medicine, 308,* 134–138.

Vaughan DA, 1988: Interaction of fluoxetine with tricyclic antidepressants. *American Journal of Psychiatry, 145,* 1478.

Wallace SM, Suveges LG, Blackburn JL, Korchinski ED, Midha KK, 1981: Oral fluphenazine and tea and coffee drinking. *Lancet, ii,* 691.

Watsky EJ, Salzman C, 1991: Psychotropic drug interactions. *Hospital and Community Psychiatry, 42*(3), 247–256.

Webster LK, Mihaly GW, Jones DB, Smallwood RA, Phillipa JA, Vajda FJ, 1984: Effect of cimetidine and ranitidine on carbamazepine and sodium valproate pharmacokinetics. *European Journal of Clinical Pharmacology, 27,* 341–343.

White K, Simpson G, 1983: Combined MAOI tricyclic antidepressant treatment—a re-evaluation. *Journal of Clinical Psychopharmacology, 5,* 264–282.

Wong YY, Ludden TM, Bell RD, 1983: Effect of erythromycin on carbamazepine kinetics. *Clinical Pharmacology and Therapeutics, 33,* 460-464.

Zeidenberg P, Perel JM, Kanzler M, Wharton RN, Malitz S, 1971: Clinical and metabolic studies with imipramine in man. *American Journal of Psychiatry, 127*(10), 57–62.

4

Psychotropic Drug Overdose

A. James Giannini

Psychotropic drugs are among the most common class of drugs used in over-dose attempts. In spite of the frequency of psychotropic overdoses appearing in hospital emergency rooms, the house and attending staff manning these areas are, in many cases, unfamiliar with appropriate treatment protocols. This is especially true in rural and small city hospitals. It is a problem complicated by a lack of full working knowledge by the psychiatrists and other physicians who prescribe these medications and who are consulted by the emergency room staffs (Giannini, 1986).

The propensity of each drug to produce serious toxicity in overdose varies in relation to the therapeutic index (i.e., the margin between toxic and minimum effective doses). In treating psychotropic overdoses, antidepressants, both hetero-cyclic and monoamine oxidase inhibitors, and lithium should be considered poten-tially lethal. Among the antipsychotics, those compounds with significant anticho-linergic effects (e.g., thioridazine, chlorpromazine) tend to be associated with more serious problems in overdose. Benzodiazepines are relatively safe in over-dose. Anticholinergic agents, which could pose substantial problems in overdose, are discussed in Chapter 14.

LITHIUM

Pharmacology

Lithium is the lightest of all metals on the periodic table. With an atomic number of three, it is also lighter than all elements, except hydrogen and helium. Chemically, it shares characteristics of sodium and, to a lesser degree, potassium. Pharmacologically it was first used as a treatment for gout in the early 20th cen-tury. This use was soon abandoned because of toxicity. However, in 1949, the Australian psychiatrist John F. Cade first published a paper demonstrating the efficacy of lithium carbonate in the treatment of mania. In 1954 a major follow-up study by Mogens Schou in Denmark confirmed Cade's initial findings and led to the adoption of lithium carbonate as the primary treatment for mania throughout the world with the exception of the United States. It was not until 1970 that lithium carbonate was approved in the United States.

Absorption occurs throughout the gastrointestinal (GI) tract. Maximum serum levels are achieved approximately 60–90 minutes after a dose. With the slow release preparations, peak levels are achieved in 4–4 1/2 hours. The lithium ion is small in size; distribution is body wide. Lithium has a serum half-life of about 24 hours, although this is age-dependent; the half-life tends to be longer in the elderly.

Lithium is mainly excreted by the kidneys (95%), with 80% reabsorption in the proximal tubles. One percent is excreted in the sweat and 4–5% in the feces.

Clinical Features of Toxicity

Lithium toxicity is usually not related to suicide. In fact, less than 15% of acute overdoses have been reported to be intentional. Rather, the overdoses tend to be a function of lithium's narrow therapeutic index and are second only to tricyclics in lethality among the psychotropics. It has a mortality rate of nearly 15% and a permanent neurological/renal morbidity rate of 12% (Steinhart & Peason-Shaver, 1988).

The initial signs of lithium toxicity are anxiety, fine resting tremor, diarrhea, and slurring. If untreated, this progresses to ataxia, dysarthria, fatigue, nausea, and polyuria with a noticeable decrease in sensorium. After this point, the emergence of symptoms accelerates to include akathisia, confusion, coarse tremor, emesis, hypothermia or hyperthermia, severe headache, choreiform movements, cogwheel rigidity, tinnitus, hypertonicity, vertigo, and severe abdominal pain. Failure to begin treatment at this point may result in a high mortality rate. End-stage of toxicity leads to arrhythmias, cardiovascular collapse, convulsions, flaccidity, and obtundation (DiPalma, 1987).

Some effects of lithium toxicity are not seen until after the patient has been detoxified. Some patients have been reported to have light-induced retinal damage after a toxic state (Reme, Federspiel, & Pfeilschafter, 1987). Others have reported precipitation of a neuroleptic malignant syndrome secondary to lithium overdose (Susman & Addonizzio, 1987). Lithium-related interstitial fibrosis, which usually occurs in the chronic state, can also occur because of prolonged lithium toxicity. Hypothermia and hyperthermia can occur after the acute toxic phase (Giannini & Price, 1986). Seizures can occur also in the posttoxic state (El-Mallakh & Lee, 1987). Polyuria, thirst, and a diabetes insipidus-like syndrome may also develop and are discussed further in Chapter 27.

Treatment

Treatment of lithium toxicity focuses on discontinuing lithium and hastening elimination. Further absorption of the drug should be limited by providing an emetic in the alert patient and nasogastric suction in an obtunded patient. Cardiac function should be monitored and vital signs supported. Since the sodium and water balance is disrupted by lithium toxicity, it should also be corrected. The patient should be vigorously hydrated, (i.e., 5–6 liters per day). Disrupted fluid and electrolyte imbalance, if untreated, can remain 10 to 20 days after detoxification (DiPalma, 1987).

Elimination can occur by forced diuresis or hemodialysis. Generally, hemodialysis is the treatment of choice when serum lithium levels exceed 3.0 mEq/L. Peritoneal dialysis is less effective than hemodialysis and should be considered only when the latter is unavailable. Often serum lithium levels may show a rebound. Under serum levels of 2.5 mEq/L, forced diuresis is the treatment of choice. Diuresis can be produced with an intravenous infusion of 0.9 N NaCl to run at 100–200 ml/hr. This infusion will increase the amount of sodium excretion and therefore lithium excretion since the lithium ion tends to passively follow the sodium ion. Adding potassium to the infusion will assist in maintaining balance (Klenfuss & Kripke, 1987). Osmotic diuresis with urea, 20 g I.V. 2–5 times per day, or mannitol, 50–100 g I.V. per day, may also be used. Lithium excretion may also be enhanced by aminophylline, 0.5 g q.i.d. If dialysis is indicated, repeated hemodialysis may be necessary because of the large volume of distribution of lithium.

Seizures may occur during the toxic phase or even after repeated dialysis (El-Mallakh & Lee, 1987). They tend to be associated with unilateral and bilateral spiking in the temporal lobes. Diazepam, phenytoin, and phenobarbitol are all effective and may be used in combination. A permanent seizure disorder is very rare after lithium toxicity; however, other residual neurological signs occur with greater frequency. It has been estimated that approximately one fourth of all patients with acute lithium intoxication have some prolonged evidence of organic brain syndrome and one third exhibit dysarthria. Mild to moderate ataxia and tremor occur in nearly one half of all lithium-intoxicated patients after detoxification (DiPalma, 1987).

The relation between severity of intoxication and serum lithium levels is not always reliable. Intoxication symptoms have been described with therapeutic lithium levels during chronic therapy (Hansen & Amdison, 1978).

MONOAMINE OXIDASE INHIBITORS

Pharmacology

The monoamine oxidase inhibitors (MAOIs) have been part of the antidepressant armamentarium for nearly 40 years. In 1952 Delay and Zeller independently investigated the effects of these groups in the treatment of depression. Then, based on the clinical studies of Nathan Kline, iproniazid and other related compounds became part of the general psychiatrist's formulary. Kline labeled this class of drugs as "psychic energizers" but the term "monoamine oxidase inhibitors" or "MAOIs" has been more widely accepted.

All MAOIs inhibit the oxidative deamination of the intracellular biogenic amines. The indoleamines are exclusively metabolized by MAO. All catecholamines are metabolized by both MAO and catechol-O-methyl transferase (COMT). MAOIs elevate the level of the biogenic amines, presumably depleted in depression, by slowing the rate of their breakdown. Thus, a new balance between production and destruction is created and maintained. Toxicity arises if the body is overwhelmed when the balance is upset in favor of an unmanageable amount of amines (Giannini, 1986).

Tyramine—compared to dopamine, norepinephrine, and epinephrine—is a relatively weak catecholamine. Yet in large amounts, it can overwhelm the body's homeostasis resulting in morbidity or fatality. Tyramine is a by-product of fermentation. Thus, it is found in aged meats and milk products (i.e., cheese, yogurt), dried fruits, fermented sauces, liquors, oil-packed products, and overripened fruits. Even though a MAOI may be taken in prescribed amounts, when tyramine-rich foods are eaten the effect is that of an overdose. Coadministering this class of antidepressants with medications that raise biogenic amine levels will also result in toxicity. Further details of these interactions are provided in Chapters 3 and 23 and in Table 23.1.

All MAOIs are quickly absorbed after ingestion. Peak levels are noted by the third day of ingestion, although objective clinical effects are usually not seen for several weeks. Excretion is renal; MAO activity returns to baseline 72 hours after discontinuance of the particular MAOI prescribed (Ravaris, Nies, Robinson, & Gropetti, 1978).

Toxicity

In the cases of direct overdose or the ingestion of any of the aforementioned substances with a MAOI, a number of symptoms are noted. These are all related to a sympathomimetic overload and include anxiety, chills, confusion, convulsions, edema, extreme headache, hyperthermia, myoclonus, nose bleed, palpitation, restlessness, tachycardia, and severe hypertension. Immediate treatment after overdose includes gastric lavage. The excretion of tranylcypromine can be hastened by acidification of urine (Turner, Young, & Paterson, 1967). Barbiturates may be employed for myoclonus and convulsions but dosage needs to be carefully adjusted downward since MAOIs prolong barbiturate activity. Excitation can be treated with diazepam 2–10 mg I.V. Hyperpyrexia can be controlled with cooling blankets. Phenothiazines should be avoided for this purpose since they could precipitate irreversible shock. Hypertensive crises are treated with phentolamine (2.5–5 mg) by slow I.V. push followed by 0.25—0.5 mg I.M. every 4–6 hours until hypertension is under control. A vasodilator, such as nitroprusside 1 mg/kg/min as needed, is a useful alternative. Labetolol has also been used with some success. For further details of the treatment, see Chapter 23.

ANTIPSYCHOTICS

Pharmacology

The prototypical antipsychotic drug, phenothiazine, was first synthesized in 1883 in Germany. In 1894 it was first applied pharmaceutically as an antihelminthic agent. In 1932 its first derivative, promethazine, was applied as an antihistamine and soporific. Because of previous attempts by multiple French and German teams to treat schizophrenia with antihistamines, the French surgeon, Jacques Laborit, used promethazine as an anesthetic. He later used another phenothiazine compound, chlorpromazine, for the same purpose. Because of Laborit's early work and Jean Courvoisier's later work in the post World War II period on the neurophysiological effects of chlorpromazine, it was then intensively studied for antipsychotic potential. Delay and Deniker (1952) first applied it to schizophrenia. Since then, a variety of phenothiazine derivatives have been adapted for the treatment of schizophrenia and other related psychoses.

All phenothiazines are three-ring structures in which two benzine rings are connected by a sulfur and a nitrogen atom. Phenothiazines act as postsynaptic dopamine blockers, alpha adrenergic blockers, histamine-one and to a lesser degree histamine-two blockers, and, in some derivatives, anticholinergic agents. Although phenothiazines are quite sedating, overdoses can otherwise be treated simply by supporting respiration until the compound is metabolized.

Chlorpromazine and thioridazine have prominent anticholinergic activity. Up to 2000 mg of chlorpromazine have been used on a daily basis without lethality. However, death has occurred in the 1600–1800 mg range with a single dose of thioridazine. The other antipsychotic derivatives—including triflupromazine, perphenazine, fluphenazine, trifluoperazine, thiothixene, and chlorprothixene—are relatively safe.

Absorption of phenothiazines is dependent on the mode of administration. Intravenous injections, which are not usually recommended, achieve peak plasma levels in less than 20 minutes. Intramuscular injection brings peak plasma levels in less than 1 hour. Ingestion of an elixir or tablet gives peak levels in 2 or 3 hours. However, elixirs tend to give a higher concentration than tablets. The half-life of all phenothiazines regardless of mode of administration is about 4 to 6 hours for the distribution phase. The drug is 90% protein-bound in the plasma. The CSF: peripheral ratio is approximately 4:1 to 5:1 (Giannini, 1986; Tune, Creese, DePaulo, Coyle, & Snyder, 1980).

Metabolism is hepatic, whereas excretion occurs via the fecal-biliary route and urinary tract. Over 90% clearance of phenothiazines and their metabolites occurs within 2 to 6 weeks after the overdose. It has been reported that patients who have been maintained on phenothiazines have less catastrophic effects during an overdose than those persons who have not previously take any phenothiazine on a regular basis. This probably results from the fact that the phenothiazines induce hepatic microsomal enzymes. Thus, chronic usage of phenothiazines before the overdose may accelerate the metabolism of an otherwise lethal dosage. Conversely, the effects of an overdose may be enhanced by patients using meperidine. The meperidine/phenothiazine combination tends to enhance respiratory depression. Other drugs such as the sedative hypnotics, when used in combination with phenothiazines, may further exacerbate the depth of respiratory depression. Anticholinergic compounds such as diphenhydramine may increase the likelihood of a potentially fatal outcome.

Clinical Features of Toxicity

In the case of overdose, the patient may present with drowsiness, severe hypotension, hyperthermia, tachycardia, supraventricular arrythmias or ventricular arrythmias, convulsions, and very severe dystonic reactions. Antipsychotic agents ingested alone in an overdose rarely, if ever, cause death since they have a relatively high therapeutic index.

Treatment

Gastric lavage should always be performed even if several hours have lapsed after overdose, since the anticholinergic effects of those drugs may delay gastric emptying. This should then be followed by instillation of activated charcoal. Respiration should be supported throughout the period of risk from 12–72 hours. Since the anticholinergic property of particular phenothiazines could contribute to cardiac arrythmias, anticholinergics are better avoided in treating dystonic reactions. Diazepam 2–5 mg intravenously may be safer.

Neuroleptic malignant syndrome, which is reported to occur during chronic or acute phenothiazine therapy, may also be a component of antipsychotic overdose. For the details of this condition, the reader is referred to Chapter 11.

In antipsychotic overdose, dialysis is ineffective because the phenothiazines, butyrophenones, and thioxanthenes are highly protein-bound. Because of enterohepatic circulation, storage, in lipid tissue and the delayed appearance of hyperthermia and cardiac arrhythmias, the patient may remain in danger for up to 72 hours. Under no circumstance should a patient with an anticholinergic phenothiazine overdose be transferred directly from the emergency room to the psychiatric unit. Cardiac monitoring and frequent vital sign checks should be maintained for at least 24 hours. In many cases, close supervision should be maintained for a complete 72-hour period. Input, output, and electrolytes need to be monitored and any imbalances corrected.

HETEROCYCLIC ANTIDEPRESSANTS

Pharmacology

Tricyclic and tetracyclic antidepressants are among the most lethal compounds in overdose. As little as a 7-day supply of amitriptyline has been reported to cause death. The first tricyclic compound, iminodibenzyl, was synthesized in the late 1800s. Its derivative, imipramine, was studied from the 1940s and 1950s as an antipsychotic. In 1957 it was discovered to be an effective treatment for major depressive disorder. By 1959, however, the first overdose fatalities were reported. Today, the tricyclics alone account for about 15% of all hospitalized overdoses. This amounts to nearly 10,000 overdoses per year and makes the tricyclics, after heroin, the most common source of all overdoses.

The minimum lethal dose of tricyclics varies. Deaths have been reported for doses as low as 500 mg, whereas other patients have been reported to survive after ingesting 10,000 mg. Of all hospitalized patients, the death rate is between 2.5–55%. Severity of tricyclic antidepressant toxicity correlates well with a QRS complex of > 100 msec in the first 24 hours and/or a plasma tricyclic level of over 1000 ng/ml (Spiker & Biggs, 1976). Although depression is the major indication for tricyclic therapy, a large study of drug overdoses over a 2-year period revealed that only one fourth of all patients hospitalized with tricyclic overdoses actually had a major depression. Of the remainder, one half of the patients had some psychiatric disorder other than depression and one fourth had no psychiatric disorder whatsoever (Frommer, Kuling, Marx, & Rumack, 1987; Kathol & Henn, 1983).

To further complicate the issue, over one third of all antidepressant overdoses are associated with multiple substances. The key actions of the tricyclic and tetracyclic antidepressants associated with mortality include their anticholinergic and quinidine-like effects. These anticholinergic properties are a composite function of double phenyl groups and a cationic head. Because their anticholinergic effects slow peristalsis, large amounts of tricyclics are absorbed somewhat slowly. However, as a result of high lipid solubility, there is still a rapid uptake with a large volume of distribution of about 10–15 liters per kg. After tricyclics and tetracyclics enter circulation, a large percentage is quickly protein-bound. The percentage varies by nearly ten-fold because of such variables as pH, albumin levels, as well as variability in renal function and hepatic function. Generally, low pH and low albumin increase the amount of unbound antidepressant. It is this unbound tricyclic that is pharmacologically active. Unbound tricyclics and tetracyclics are preferentially taken up by heart tissue at a 5:1 ratio, hepatic tissue at a 30:1 ratio, and central nervous tissue at a 40:1 ratio (Grunthal, 1958; Ware, 1987; Wedin, Odera, & Gurman, 1986).

Heterocyclic antidepressants are mainly metabolized in the liver (66–80%) and also to some extent in the kidney (20–30%). Metabolism occurs by either demethylation or hydroxylation followed by glucuronide conjugation. Demethylation tends not to deactivate the tricyclics, whereas hydroxylation does. Hydroxylation is the key step in deactivating antidepressants and is performed by hepatic microsomal enzymes. Hydroxylation can be accelerated by tobacco, barbiturates, birth control pills, ethanol, methylphenidate, and trihexyphenidyl hydrochloride. It is impaired by disulfiram, morphine, and haloperidol. The presence of any of these substances tends to complicate the treatment of the overdose.

Clinical Features of Toxicity

Symptoms of toxicity occur at approximately 1200–1800 mg of most tricyclics and about 2000 mg for the tetracyclics. On the other hand, lethality occurs at around 1800 mg for tricyclics and about 2500–3000 mg for tetracyclics. Overdose effects are predominantly anticholinergic especially at the early phases. They include mydriasis, blurred vision, extreme dryness in mouth, tachycardia, dry skin, hyperpyrexia (although hypopyrexia has also been noted), urinary retention, decreased peristalsis, and excitability. Nonanticholinergic effects tend to occur later. These include convulsions, coma, hypotension, cardiac arrythmias, congestive heart failure, renal failure, pulmonary edema, and aspiration pneumonia. Some unusual manifestations include acute polyradiculoneuropathy, rhabdomyolysis, dysarthria, dysphagia, and intense visual hallucinations. Babinski reflexes are often positive. A large tricyclic overdose may also result in absent and decreased brain stem reflexes (i.e., the corneal reflex, pupillary response to light, oculocephalic reflex, and oculovestibular reflex) and ophthalmoplegia (Cassidy & Henry, 1987; Rosen, 1983).

Stat laboratory tests usually reveal metabolic acidosis and hypocalcemia. The electrocardiogram (ECG) shows very wide QRS complexes and heart block. On some occasions, circus rhythms, ventricular ectopic beats, and ventricular tachycardia can occur (Boehnert & Lovejoy, 1985; Goldberg, Capone, & Hurt, 1985).

Treatment

The initial step in the treatment of overdose is gastric lavage (see Schoonover, 1987, for a review). Ipecac is not recommended because of the risk of aspiration. Magnesium citrate with activated charcoal has been used to induce catharsis and reduce absorption of the antidepressant. However, this combination is not without risk. Because of decreased peristalsis from anticholinergic effects, charcoal bezoars have resulted in small bowel obstructions (Ray, Padin, Contie, & Halls, 1988). Magnesium citrate may also produce magnesium toxicity. This toxicity has been associated with acute neuromuscular deterioration followed by respiratory depression (Jones, Heiselman, Dougherty, & Eddy, 1986).

The next steps in the management include starting a temporary transvenous pacemaker, instituting monitoring, ensuring good ventilation, obtaining an antidepressant blood level, performing basic blood biochemistry studies, and inserting a routine pulmonary artery catheter to monitor blood gases, pulmonary artery, left atrial wedge pressures, and cardiac output. Central anticholinergic syndrome responds well to physostigmine 1–2 mg I.V. q 30 or 60 minutes; however, the use of physostigmine is associated with potentially serious cardiovascular side effects and should be avoided. Seizures can be managed by diazepam 5–10 mg intramuscularly or intravenously as necessary. Barbiturates should be avoided because of the possible risk of respiratory depression (Giannini & Miller, 1989). Hyperpyrexia is best treated with ice packs or cold sponges. Orthostatic hypotension is treated with leg elevation and vigorous hydration.

Cardiac arrythmias induced by the tricyclics and tetracyclics can be adjunctively treated with sodium bicarbonate. Bicarbonate seems to act by increasing the proportion of antidepressant bound to plasma albumin. Generally, sodium bicarbonate administered in volumes of 50 mmol together with ventilation by 100% oxygen can reduce the metabolic acidosis and result in a faster appearance of normal sinus rhythm (Molloy, Penner, Rabson, & Hall, 1984). Other experimental therapeutic modalities not yet applied for clinical treatment include the use of calcium-channel blockers (Trouve & Nahas, 1987), phenytoin (Mayron & Riviz, 1986), and antigen-binding fragments specific for the antidepressant (Hursting, Raisys, & Ophein, 1987). For details of treatment of the cardiovascular complications of heterocyclic agents, see Chapter 23.

Although most fatalities occur within 24 hours of overdose, the patient should be monitored for at least 72 hours. Several cases in the literature have reported patients who have died suddenly up to 6 days after acute overdose of tricyclic antidepressants. In some of these cases, it was hypothesized that myocardial necrosis occurred. Amitriptyline and its metabolites especially tend to have strong affinity for myocardial tissues. They cause changes in membrane permeability. All the tricyclics tend to inhibit adenosine triphosphate phosphohydralase resulting in a loss of the sodium-potassium transmembranal balance (Henry & Cassidy, 1986). When this is disturbed, necrosis can be the result.

Acute renal failure has also been observed (Jennings, Zlevey, & Harrington, 1983). This has been invariably due to rhabdomyolsis secondary to muscle necrosis caused by prolonged inactivity (Frenden & Swainson, 1985). Forced diuresis is the treatment of choice. Infusion of intravenous saline and repetitive intravenous dosages of furosemide up to 250 mg should be titrated to produce a urinary output of 100 ml/hr. If this fails, hemodialysis must be instituted.

REFERENCES

Andisen A, Skjolbberg H, 1969: Hemodialysis for lithium poisoning. *Lancet, 2*(613), 213–221.
Baldessarini RJ, Gelenberg AJ, 1979: Using physostigmine safely. *American Journal of Psychiatry, 136,* 1608–1609.

Boehnert MT, Lovejoy FH, 1985. Value of QRS duration after acute overdose of tricyclic antidepressant. *New England Journal of Medicine, 313*, 474–479.

Cassidy S, Henry J, 1987: Fatal toxicity of antidepressant drugs in overdose. *British Medical Journal, 295*, 1021–1024.

Delay J, Deniker P, 1952: Trente-buit case de psychoses traitees par la cur prolongee continue. In: *Compute Rendu du Congress*, edited by JR Landau. Paris: Mason et cie.

DiPalma JR, 1987: Lithium toxicity. *American Family Physician, 36*, 225–231.

El-Mallakh R, Lee RH, 1987: Seizures and transient cognitive deterioration as sequelae of acute lithium intoxication. *Veterinary Human Toxicology, 29*, 143–145.

Frenden TJ, Swaisen CP, 1985: Acute renal failure secondary to nontraumatic rhabdomyolysis following amoxepine overdose. *New Zealand Medical Journal, 98*, 690–691.

Frommer DA, Kuling KW, Marx JA, Rumack B, 1987: Tricyclic antidepressant overdose. *Journal of the American Medical Association, 257*, 521–526.

Giannini AJ, 1986: *Biological foundation of clinical psychiatry.* New York: Elsevier/Medical Examination.

Giannini AJ, Price WA, 1986: Neurotoxicity caused by lithium-verapamil synergism. *Journal of Clinical Pharmacology, 26*, 717–718.

Giannini AJ, Miller NS, 1989: Drug abuse: A biopsychiatric model. *American Family Physician, 40*(5), 173–181.

Goldberg RJ, Capone RJ, Hurt JD, 1985: Cardiac complications following tricyclic antidepressant overdose. *Journal of the American Medical Association, 254*, 1772–1775.

Grunthal E, 1958: Untersuchungen uber die besondere psychologishe wirkung des thymolepticums. *Psychiatr Neurol Wischr, 136* 402–407.

Hansen HE, Amdisen A, 1978: Lithium intoxication (report of 23 cases and review of 200 cases from the literature). *Quarterly Journal of Medicine, 186*, 123–144.

Henry JA, Cassidy SC, 1986: Membrane stabilizing activity: A major cause of fatal poisoning. *Lancet, 281*, 1414–1417.

Hursting MJ, Raisys VA, Ophein KG, 1987: Drug specific Fab therapy in drug overdose. *Archives of Pathology and Laboratory Medicine, 11*, 693–697.

Jennings AE, Zlevey AS, Harrington JT, 1983: Amoxepine induced renal failure. *Archives of Internal Medicine, 143*, 1525–1529.

Jones J, Heiselman D, Dougherty J, Eddy A, 1986: Cathartic induced magnesium toxicity during overdose management. *Annals of Emergency Medicine, 15*, 1214–1218.

Kathol RG, Henn FA, 1983: Tricyclics—the most common agents used in potentially lethal overdoses. *Journal of Nervous and Mental Disorders, 171*, 250–253.

Klenfuss H, Kripke DF, 1987: Potassium reduces lithium toxicity. *Life Sciences 40*, 2531–2538.

Mayron R, Rviz E, 1986: Phenytoin: Does it reverse antidepressant induced cardiac conduction abnormalities? *Annals of Emergency Medicine, 15*, 876–880.

Molloy JDW, Penner SB, Rabson J, Hall KW, 1984: Use of sodium bicarbonate to treat tricyclic antidepressant-induced arrythmias in a patient with alkalosis. *Canadian Medical Association Journal, 130*, 1457–1459.

Ravaris CL, Nies A, Robinson DS, Gropetti A, 1978: Clinical pharmacology of phenelzine. *Archives of General Psychiatry, 35*, 629–635.

Ray MS, Padin R, Contie JD, Halls JM, 1988: Charcoal bezoar: Small bowel obstruction secondary to amitryptiline overdose therapy. *Digestive Diseases and Sciences, 33*, 106–107.

Reme C, Federspiel E, Pfeilschfter J, Justice AW, 1987: Potentiation by light of lithium induced retinal injury. *New England Journal of Medicine, 281*, 1478.

Rosen M, 1983: Tricyclic antidepressant overdose: Clinical features and management. *Heart and Lung, 12*, 222–225.

Schoonover SC, 1987: Depression. In: *The practitioner's guide to psychotropic drugs*, edited by EL Bassuk, SC Schoonover and AJ Gelenberg. New York: Plenum.

Spiker D, Biggs J, 1976: Tricyclic antidepressant—prolonged plasma levels after overdose. *Journal of the American Medical Association, 236*, 1711–1712.

Steinhart CM, Peason-Shaver AL, 1988: Poisoning. *Critical Care Clinics, 4*, 845–871.

Stern TA, 1983: Continuous infusion of physostigmine in anticholinergic delirium. *Journal of Clinical Psychiatry, 44*, 463–464.

Susman VL, Addonizio G, 1987: Reinduction of neuroleptic malignant syndrome by lithium. *Journal of Clinical Psychopharmacology, 5*, 339–342.

Trouve R, Nahas G, 1987: Ca-2 modulators as antidotes to imipramine toxicity. *Proceedings of the Society of Experimental Biology and Medicine, 185,* 498–503.

Tune LE, Creese I, DePaulo JR, Coyle JT, Snyder SH, 1980: Clinical state and serum neuroleptic levels measured by radioreceptor assay in schizophrenia. *American Journal of Psychiatry, 137,* 187–190.

Turner P, Young JH, Paterson J, 1967: Influence of urinary pH on the excretion of tranylcypromine sulfate. *Nature, 215,* 881–882.

Ware MR, 1987: Tricyclic antidepressants overdose. *Southern Medical Journal, 80,* 1410–1415.

Wedin GP, Odera GM, Gurman R, 1986: Relative toxicity of cyclic antidepressants. *Annals of Clinical Psychiatry, 15,* 747–802.

5

Psychotropic Drugs and Teratogenicity

Kathleen A. Pajer

In the early 1960s, two investigators independently reported an unusually high rate of phocomelia, a previously rare birth defect (Lenz, 1962; McBride, 1961). Within 6 months, it became clear that there was a relative epidemic of phocomelia and related limb defects, eventually traced to prenatal thalidomide exposure at 4–7 weeks of gestation. The thalidomide tragedy radically altered the way pregnancy was viewed. Previously, it was assumed that the placenta acted as a filter, protecting the fetus from potential environmental toxins such as drugs. The thalidomide experience made it apparent, however, that the placenta functions more as a diffusion medium and that all drugs are potential teratogens.

In the last two decades, a number of studies have attempted to estimate the teratogenic risk associated with psychotropic drugs other than thalidomide. Much of the data come from case reports or studies in which the subjects are not psychiatric patients. These studies are useful in suggesting possible risk or safety, but cannot fully answer the question of interest to the psychiatrist: Do psychiatrically ill pregnant women who take a particular psychotropic medication have a higher risk of having infants with birth defects?

In an effort to answer this question, a comprehensive review has been done of all the human data found in a search of the literature on the teratogenicity of antipsychotics, benzodiazepines, antidepressants, lithium, and carbamazepine. The review concludes with clinical guidelines, based on interpretation of the data. Animal data, although provocative, are often conflicting, and therefore will not be discussed. The reader is referred to several excellent reviews on this topic (Schardein, 1985; Schardein & Keller, 1989).

PRINCIPLES OF TERATOLOGY

Before evaluating the data on each drug category, it is important to understand the criteria used to classify a drug as a teratogen. Teratology is the study of abnormal fetal development. The identification of teratogens is complicated by the developmental process of gestation; the complex relationships between the pharmacokinetics in the mother, fetus, and placenta; and the modulating effects of various environmental factors such as alcohol consumption, nutrition, exposure to pollutants, and so on. As a result, teratologists have proposed the following criteria for the recognition of a new teratogenic agent in humans (paraphrased from Wilson, 1973):

1. An abrupt increase in the incidence of a particular defect or unusual constellation of defects.

2. Temporally associated known environmental change.

3. Known exposure to the putative teratogen at a critical time during gestation, and the timing of the exposure must be consistent with the type of defect produced.

4. Absence of other risk factors for the defect(s) in women exposed to the putative teratogen.

The classic teratogen is thalidomide. Investigations were conducted in response to the epidemic of phocomelia, and thalidomide was new and widely prescribed before the epidemic. All cases had been exposed on days 20–36 of gestation and were consistent with the critical time for limb development; no other consistent risk factor could be identified in the cases.

Unfortunately, the teratogenic risk of other psychotropic medications is not as easily determined. The defects that have been reported are not as rare or obvious as phocomelia, the prevalence of drug exposure in the general population may be quite low, and it is often impossible to rule out other risk factors in this population. These problems raise important methodological issues in the interpretation of these data.

METHODOLOGICAL ISSUES

Additional Risk Factors

One of the most difficult factors involved in answering the question of interest is the role that other risk factors may have in producing the birth defects of interest. Additional risk factors fall into two categories: risk factors present before the fetus is exposed to the psychotropic drug and risk factors to which a fetus may be exposed coincident with exposure to the medication. Some data suggest that severe psychiatric disorders alone (e.g., schizophrenia or bipolar disorder) carry teratogenic risks independent of psychotropic medication (Rieder, Rosenthal, Wender, & Blumenthal, 1975; Sobel, 1961). In addition, there are many studies demonstrating that a family history of birth defects is a significant risk factor for congenital malformations. It is therefore also important to elicit any past history of spontaneous abortions, since this may be an indirect indication of genetic abnormalities.

The second type of risk factor is one that accompanies the exposure to the medication. These coexposures are especially problematic in the psychiatrically ill woman who may take more than one medication, use or abuse drugs (including alcohol), smoke heavily, and have little prenatal care resulting in poor nutrition and medical complications of pregnancy. Any study of the teratogenicity of a psychiatric medication should account for these possible additional determinants of the defect.

Definition of Defects

The comparison of studies is also complicated by interstudy differences in the definition of defects and the length of follow-up. These have been shown to directly influence the incidence rates reported. A related issue is behavioral teratogenicity. Investigators have hypothesized that teratogens produce defects on a continuum, ranging from behavioral defects (presumed subanatomic central nervous system defects) to gross physical defects incompatible with survival (Ornoy & Yanai, 1980; Wilson, 1973). There are animal data to suggest that psychotropic drugs are associated with permanent neurochemical changes expressed as hyperactivity, learning difficulties, mental retardation, mood instability, and so on (Coyle, Wayner, & Singer, 1975; Voorhees & Butcher, 1982). There are few human studies on this topic, but it is an important clinical and research consideration.

Research Design

In addition to taking into account these issues, it is important to evaluate the research design. Certain designs are more appropriate than others, given certain characteristics of the population studied. The follow-up design (ideally, with a control group) might appear to be the best choice, but may provide a false sense of security if the outcome of interest has a low incidence rate, as do most of the birth defects. In this case, it takes a great many subjects to detect a significant difference between exposed and nonexposed groups. Most of the evidence on psychiatric drug teratogenicity comes from case reports, case series, uncontrolled retrospective studies, case-control studies, registries, and large cohort studies of pregnant women, a small number of whom are exposed to psychiatric medications.

Case reports and case series suffer from problems in generalizability, but can be useful as evidence of a causal association if they rule out other putative causes for the defect and/or describe similar defects (e.g., the first reports of fetal alcohol syndrome). Most reports regarding psychotropic medications do neither.

Uncontrolled retrospective studies often follow case reports, but may be quite misleading. Such studies rely on maternal recall and/or medical chart information, both of which may contain errors of overinclusion, or omission. The retrospective nature of the design makes it impossible to rule out baseline risk factors or coexposures. Furthermore, many women in the general population are never exposed to some drugs (e.g., antidepressants), and the etiologies of the defects are multifactorial. A retrospective study may thus report a nonsignificant level of exposure to the drug compared to other etiologies, but this may result from the low exposure rate in the general population, not an absence of effect.

Case-control design is an improvement over the retrospective study in that it provides an unaffected control group. Additionally, if one wants to study an outcome that normally has a low incidence rate (as is the case with birth defects), beginning with the defect and working backward eliminates the problem of following large numbers of subjects prospectively, most of whom will not produce the outcome of interest. Unfortunately, the case-control method does not eliminate the problems of recall bias or the low level of exposed women in the general population. Both types of studies, however, may provide important information regarding teratogenicity if the medication is widely used, as is the case with benzodiazepines.

Voluntary registries suffer from reporting bias (i.e., the cases in which there is an adverse outcome are more likely to be reported than those in which there is a normal outcome). If, however, a registry receives a large number of reports of a relatively rare defect, this can indicate that the drug may have teratogenic effects.

Cohort studies of pregnant women have the advantages of prospective design, but usually have small numbers of medicated psychiatrically ill women. Study of

these medications is therefore difficult. If the drugs are widely used (e.g., benzodiazepines or antipsychotics as antiemetics), this design is appropriate.

There is no one research design that can best estimate the teratogenic risk of the
psychiatric drugs. Depending on the characteristics of each medication category,
certain designs may be better suited to answering the question of causality than
others.

DRUG DATA

With these caveats in mind, let us turn to the drugs themselves. Tables 1–5 list
the systematic studies for each category. Case reports are not included in the tables
but are summarized in the text. Any trends that emerge from these summaries
must be interpreted cautiously, as the reports are nonuniform in ruling out other
possible risk factors. Since design issues are important in evaluating causality, the
studies have been classified by design. The trimester of exposure is indicated, and
if the study has attempted to account for other risk factors, this is also noted. An
asterisk indicates any study in which an effort was made to assess behavioral
teratogenicity.

Antipsychotics

The psychiatric disorders normally treated with antipsychotics (e.g., psychoses)
have a relatively low prevalence in the general population. However, there are
nonpsychiatric indications for the use of antipsychotics, including nausea associated with pregnancy and hyperemesis gravidarum. The doses for these illnesses
are lower than those used in treating psychiatric disorders. The widespread use of
these medications as antiemetics make both prospective and case-control studies
useful in estimating risks for common or uncommon birth defects, respectively.
Population-based cohort studies also are appropriate, since large numbers of
women may be exposed.

The main difficulty in using these types of studies is that if an antipsychotic is
implicated as teratogenic in these types of women, it would be necessary to demonstrate that the medical condition itself was not the primary factor. If low dosages
are not shown to be teratogenic, generalizability to safety at higher doses remains
tenuous. Nonetheless, if the drugs emerge as safe at lower doses, there is some
valid basis on which to use low doses in psychiatric illness.

Phenothiazines

The majority of the data on antipsychotics is from studies of the phenothiazines
(Table 1). Chlorpromazine is the most well-studied medication, but interpretation
of the data suffers from several methodological problems. The work of Kris (1962,
1965) is often cited as evidence of the safety of chlorpromazine but provides only
several repeated case reports. Sobel (1960) followed pregnant, psychiatrically ill
women on chlorpromazine, comparing them to a control group of psychiatrically
ill, institutionalized women who had received other treatments (e.g., insulin
shock, electroconvulsive therapy, and reserpine) or no treatment. This study reported no significant difference between the chlorpromazine and nontreated
groups, but the overall rate of defects in both groups was higher (7.7%) than in

Table 1 Teratogenicity of antipsychotics

Study	Design	N	Medication	Tri-mester	Outcomes	Other risk factors
Kris, 1962; Kris, 1965; Kris & Carmichael, 1957	Follow-up	52	Chlorpromazine	1–3	No abnormalities	—
Sobel, 1960	Controlled follow-up (controls = other treatments)	275	Chlorpromazine (n = 74)	1–3	7.7% exposed had some abnormality vs. 7% unexposed	—
Ayd, 1964	Follow-up	27	Chlorpromazine (n = 16) Chlorpromazine (n = 11)	1 2–3	No abnormalities at birth; WNL at 2–7 YOA	—
Rumeau-Rouquette et al., 1976	Cohort	12,764	All phenothiazines (n = 315)	1	3.5% exposed had some anomaly vs. 1.6% unexposed	Other risk factors did not ↑ risk
Scanlon, 1972	Follow-up	23	Thioridazine	1–2	Normal infants	—
Moriarty & Nance, 1963	Controlled follow-up	9,952	Trifluoperazine	1	2.1% exposed had stillbirths/deformities vs. 2.6% unexposed	—
Schrire, 1963	Follow-up	478	Trifluoperazine	1	.4% abortions; no deformities in remaining pregnancies	—

(See footnote on next page)

(Table continues on next page)

Table 1 Teratogenicity of antipsychotics (*Continued*)

Study	Design	N	Medication	Tri-mester	Outcomes	Other risk factors
Rawlings et al., 1963	Follow-up	341	Trifluoperazine	1	Abortions 23% Perinatal deaths 3.3% Malformations 1.5%	All Ss were "abortion prone"
Milkovich & van den Berg, 1976	Cohort	11,481	Phenothiazine (n = 543)	1	4.2% exposed were severe defects vs. 3.2% N/V but no drug vs. 3.7% no N/V	—
Sloane et al., 1977	Cohort	50,282	All phenothiazines (n = 1,309)	1	7.2% exposed had some malformation vs. 6.4% unexposed; adjusted mean IQ scores exposed = 96.5% vs. 96.9% unexposed at 4 YOA	IQ adjusted for SES + race
General Practitioner Research Group, 1963; Wheatley, 1964	Follow-up	164	Phenothiazines		6.1% exposed had deformities stillbirths, miscarriages	—
Van Waes & de Velde, 1969	Controlled follow-up (haloperidol exposure vs. no exposure)	1,830	Haloperidol (n = 92)	1	3.0% exposed had stillbirths, deformities, or neonatal deaths vs. 3.1% unexposed	All Ss = hyperemesis
Hanson & Oakley, 1975	Retrospective (cases = deformities)	31	Haloperidol	1–3	0% recalled exposure	—

YOA, years of age; Ss, subjects; N/V, nausea/vomiting; SES, socioeconomic status; ↑, increased; WNL, within normal limits.

the general population (3–5%). These findings do not necessarily indicate that chlorpromazine is "safe," but rather are interpretable as indicating that the treated and untreated psychiatrically ill women may have equal levels of risk. Ayd (1964) described a follow-up of 27 women exposed to chlorpromazine and concluded that all the children were normal, as judged by reports of parents and pediatricians.

In contrast to these data from small follow-up studies, the one large cohort study to give data on individual phenothiazines reported that the highest rate of birth defects was found with chlorpromazine (7.0%) compared to the rate in the unexposed group (1.6%) (Rumeau-Rouquette, Goujard, & Huel, 1976). This rate of defects is similar to that reported by Sobel (1960). The majority of women who produced malformed infants had received the drug for psychiatric symptoms. Seventy-five percent of the subjects also took other psychotropic medications, and most of the group had histories of multiple miscarriages or previous births of abnormal infants.

There are a total of 12 case reports (15 infants) of the use of chlorpromazine in the first trimester. Eight were normal (Gross, 1962); four had transient extra-pyramidal symptoms (EPS), but were developmentally normal at follow-ups ranging from 6 months to 6 years (Hill, Desmond, & Kay, 1966; Levy & Wisniewski, 1974; O'Connor, Johnson & James, 1981); one died in utero with a ruptured omphalocele and with ectromelia (O'Leary & O'Leary, 1964); and one had anky-loglossum superius syndrome and iliac atresia (Nevin, Kernohan, & Ross, 1980). This last case was also exposed to imipramine, diazepam, and meclizine throughout the pregnancy, so it is difficult to implicate one drug.

There are five case reports of women using the drug in the second and/or third trimesters. Three infants experienced transient sedation and/or EPS (two were developmentally normal at 6 and 18 months, and one was mentally retarded at 4 years) (Hammond & Toseland, 1970; Tamer, McKey, Arias, Worley, & Fogel, 1969); and two had congential small left colon syndrome (Falterman & Richardson, 1980). The infants with the best outcomes were exposed to chlorpromazine alone.

Thioridazine has been studied in one uncontrolled follow-up of 23 psychiatrically ill pregnant women (Scanlon, 1972). Although there were no abnormalities, follow-up time and methods were not specified. One case report presented a woman treated with thioridazine and benztropine who had a normal infant (Hill, Desmond, & Kay, 1966). Another report of thioridazine and trifluoperazine treatment was associated with the birth of an infant with transposition of the great vessels and a patent foramen ovale (Vince, 1969). The dosages were in the range necessary for treatment of a moderately severe psychosis.

The remaining commonly used phenothiazines (trifluoperazine and fluphenazine) have not been studied in psychiatrically ill women, with the exception of case reports. The data on trifluoperazine come from one controlled and two uncontroled follow-up studies. Moriarty and Nance (1963) compared the pregnancy outcomes of 480 pregnant women who participated in the original clinical trials using trifluoperazine with an historical nonexposed control group of 8,472 subjects. Of the subjects 87% received the drug for nausea and vomiting, and the remainder received it for "mild mental and emotional disturbances," but the data were not analyzed separately. There was no difference between the two groups in the incidence of congenital malformations or still births.

Schrire (1963) traced the women participating in the original British clinical trials of trifluoperazine. He examined the infants or obtained information from attending pediatricians. Most women received the drug for nausea and vomiting, and the outcomes studied were abortion rate and the incidence of skeletal deformities. There was no control group, but the rates of both outcomes were much lower than in the general population. Rawlings, Ferguson, and Maddison (1963) reported that trifluoperazine was used in 341 abortion-prone patients, with a malformation rate of 1.5%, although they did not specify dosages and there was no control group. There are also 4 case reports (5 infants) regarding the use of this drug. Three (including twins) were born with phocomelia (Corner, 1962; Hall, 1963); one had anencephaly (New Zealand Committee on Adverse Drug Reactions, 1968); and one had transient EPS (James, 1988). The most benign outcome was associated with the most polypharmacy.

The only data about fluphenazine are from two case reports. Both mothers took additional drugs. Fluphenazine and benztropine use resulted in a normal infant with transient EPS (Cleary, 1977). Fluphenazine and Debendox (an antiemetic, possibly teratogenic) throughout pregnancy was associated with an infant with multiple craniofacial and genitourinary deformities, but with normal cognitive development at 1 year (Donaldson & Bury, 1982). Other possible causes were ruled out, except for the fact that the mother was a slightly dysmorphic chronic schizophrenic.

There are also several studies that investigated a general category of "phenothiazines," without information on specific drugs (Table 1). In a large cohort study, Milkovich and van den Berg (1976) reported no statistically significant difference in birth defects between the exposed and unexposed groups. Sloane et al. (1977) report similar results, and followed approximately 80% of their cohort for 4 years, measuring IQ at this time. There was no difference between the mean IQ scores of the exposed and nonexposed groups. It is also of interest that Platt et al. (1988) measured the growth of the antipsychotic-exposed children and reported that they were taller than normal controls at 4 months, 1 year, and 7 years. The results of these last two studies are at odds with those reported by Rumeau-Rouquette et al. (1976), but it is important to note that rate of defects in the control groups for these latter studies was higher than the control group rate in the Rumeau-Rouquette study (Milkovich & van den Berg: 3.7%, Sloane et al.: 6.4% vs. Rumeau-Rouquette et al.: 1.6%). The difference between the exposed group rate from Rumeau-Roquette et al.'s study the control group rates in the other two studies may not have emerged as statistically significant. This implies either that the three studies were investigating populations characterized by different exposures (e.g., varying severities in the illnesses for which the drugs were given) or that there were other risk factors present, common to most of the women in each study (e.g., an environmental exposure that would have elevated the rate of defects in the controls). Unfortunately, there is no way to account for the differences in their studies.

Butyrophenones

The only butyrophenone studied is haloperidol, and there are no systematic investigations of psychiatrically ill women. Van Waes and van de Velde (1969) conducted a controlled follow-up of women given low-dose haloperidol for hyperemesis gravidarum. The rates of birth defects between exposed and nonexposed were similar and commensurate with population estimates. The second investigation was a retrospective study that investigated the use of haloperidol by mothers of 31 severely deformed infants (Hanson & Oakley, 1975). None recalled using the drug during pregnancy.

Two case reports describe first-trimester haloperidol use. Kopelman, McCullar, and Heggeness (1975) reported multiple limb deformities in an infant who had been exposed to haloperidol, but also to many other drugs, all suspected teratogens. Another report of haloperidol use alone was associated with anencephaly (New Zealand Committee on Adverse Drug Reactions, 1975).

Use of the drug in the second trimester has been reported in three cases. Two infants were normal (Donaldson, 1982; Patterson, 1979), and one described hypoplasia of several digits, and arthrogryposis (Meyer, 1984). This mother also used meprobamate, a drug with questionable teratogenicity.

The data on the antipsychotic medications are somewhat meager, especially with regards to use in pregnant, psychiatrically ill women. There does not seem to be a strong risk for obvious birth defects with any of the antipsychotics, although the incidence rate across studies for chlorpromazine is consistently higher than most population estimates, indicating that this drug is best avoided. It is not possible to draw conclusions regarding behavioral effects. There is fairly solid evidence that the other antipsychotics in low doses and administered alone to women with few other baseline risk factors are safe. This does not characterize many of the psychiatrically ill women who would be in need of treatment, but does allow some rational basis for treatment with low doses of the medications.

It is also important to point out that women using antipsychotics are clearly at increased risk for having infants with EPS. In all cases, this was associated with use of the antipsychotic medication near delivery. It appears to be a transient, benign problem (there are no long-term data available), but it can be minimized by lowering the dose of medication or discontinuing it entirely 2–3 weeks before delivery. Affected infants may be treated with diphenhydramine or benztropine mesylate.

Anxiolytics

In contrast to the antipsychotics, the anxiolytics have been widely prescribed and are relatively well studied (Table 2). The medications most studied are chlordiazepoxide (CDZ) and diazepam (DZ), although there are case reports on several other individual anxiolytics. Several studies have also implicated meprobamate as a teratogen (Crombie et al., 1975; Hartz, Heinonen, Shapiro, Siskind, & Sloane, 1975; Milkovich & van den Berg, 1974). Since this drug is rarely used today, these data will not be reviewed.

Chlordiazepoxide

CDZ has been studied in eight major investigations. All except one indicate a higher rate of malformation in infants from exposed mothers, although the rates are not always quantitatively or stochastically significant. Milkovich and van den Berg (1974) studied all the women in a large cohort study who had received CDZ for minor psychiatric symptoms, comparing them to women who had received other drugs for similar indications and to symptomatic women who had received no drugs. This design was controlled for possible risk associated with the symp-

Table 2 Teratogenicity of antiolytics

Study	Design	N	Medication	Tri-mester	Outcomes	Other risk factors
Milkovich & van den Berg, 1974	Cohort; subsample all anxious Ss	1,904	Chlordiazepoxide (*n* = 175)	1	11.4% exposed had severe congenital anomalies vs. 4.6% other drugs (except meprobamate) vs. 2.6% no drugs	—
Crombie et al., 1975	Cohort	9,147	Chlordiazepoxide (*n* = 38) Diazepam (*n* = 4)	1 1	2.6% exposed had malformation vs. 1.6% unexposed	Medicated women had ↑ rate of previous problem pregnancies
Rumeau-Roquette et al., 1975	Cohort	12,764	Chlordiazepoxide (*n* = 98) Diazepam (*n* = 60)	1 1	2% exposed had malformation 0% exposed had malformation vs. 1.8% unexposed	—
Hartz et al., 1975	Cohort	50,282	Chlordiazepoxide (*n* = 257)	1	4.3% exposed had some malformation vs. 4.5% unexposed; mean IQ exposed = 96.7% vs. 96.9% at 4 YOA	SES, ethnic group, hospital did not change results
Kullander & Källén, 1976	Cohort	6,376	Chlordiazepoxide (*n* = 90)	1	9% exposed had some malformation or stillbirth vs. 13% unexposed	—
Rothman et al., 1979	Case-control (cases = CHD)	1,826	Chlordiazepoxide Diazepam	1	1.0% cases had exposure vs. .3% controls 3.8% cases had exposure vs. 1.8% controls	—
Bracken & Holford, 1981	Case-control (cases = any malformations)	4,428	Chlordiazepoxide Diazepam	1	.36% cases had exposure vs. .20% (controls) 2.5% cases had exposure vs. .91% controls	—
Safra & Oakley, 1975	Retrospective, all severe congenital anomalies	278	Diazepam	1	14.3% cleft lip ± cleft palate babies had exposure	—
Aarskog, 1975	Case-control (cases = all oral clefts)	469	Diazepam	1	6.3% clefts had exposure vs. 1.1% controls	FH (+) clefts in 46.8% cases; other possible risk factors in 54.1% cases

Study	Study type	n	Drug		Results	Comments
Zierler & Rothman, 1985	Case-control (cases = CHD)	1,036	Diazepam	↑	1.3% cases had exposure vs. 1.4% controls	—
Czeizel, 1983	Case-control (cases = oral clefts; controls = anencephaly/spina bifida)	1,377	Diazepam	↑	4.1% cases had exposure vs. 4.4% controls	—
Rosenberg et al., 1983	Case-control (cases = oral all other malformations)	3,109	Diazepam	↑	2.1% cases had exposure to diazepam vs. 2.2% controls .81% cases had exposure to other benzodiazepines vs. .48% controls	Stratification by FH (+) maternal DM infection, or seizure disorder did not change results
Shiono & Mills, 1984	Cohort	33,249	Diazepam	↑	.1% exposed had oral cleft vs. .1% unexposed	—
Saxén & Saxén, 1975	Case-control (cases = oral clefts)	1,189	Benzodiazepines (primarily diazepam)	↑	5.4% clefts had exposure vs. 2.5% normal controls	—
Saxén, 1975	Case-control (cases = oral clefts)	388	Antineurotics (primarily diazepam)	↑	3.7% clefts had exposure vs. 2.1% normal controls	—
Greenberg et al., 1977	Case-control (cases = any malformations)	1,672	Benzodiazepines	↑	4.3% cases had exposure vs. 2.9% controls	Proportions of cases = controls when stratified by FH malformations
Winship et al., 1984	Case-control (cases = CNS deformities)	1,528	Benzodiazepines	↑	1.8% cases had exposure vs. 1% normal controls	—
Laegrid et al., 1989, 1989	Follow-up	40 (41 infants)	Benzodiazepines (oxazepam or diazepam)	↑, or 1–3	20% had multiple similar dysmorphic craniofacial features ± other abnormalities; 14% had some behavioral effects in childhood	ETOH + drug use/abuse denied
Barry & St. Clair, 1987	Case series from Upjohn	441	Alprazolam, triazolam	↑, or 1–3	No defects	—

CHD, congenital heart disease; SES, socioeconomic status; FH, family history; DM, diabetes mellitus; ↑, increased; YOA, years of age.

toms themselves. They reported a nonsignificant trend for a three-fold increase in the incidence of defects with CDZ, compared to the other two groups. The number of subjects in the CDZ group was much less than in the other groups, and the trend may have been significant if there had been a larger subsample.

Crombie et al. (1975) reported that 2.6% of women exposed to CDZ in a large cohort study had infants with defects, compared with a rate of 1.5% for the unexposed. Rumeau-Rouquette et al. (cited by Crombie et al., 1975) reported similar rates, with 2% of the exposed women producing infants with birth defects versus 1.8% of the unexposed. In yet another cohort study, the malformation rate was 4.3% for exposure in the first trimester, compared with 4.5% in the unexposed (Hartz et al., 1975). These authors reported no significant differences in IQ scores at 4 years of age in the exposed children. The final cohort data come from Kullander and Källén (1976) who reported that out of 90 women exposed to CDZ, 9% had infants with some type of defect, versus 13% of the controls. None of these studies provided evidence for a consistent defect or syndrome.

One case-control study reported that 1% of cases of congenital heart disease had prenatal exposure to CDZ, compared with 0.3% of controls, a nonsignificant difference (Rothman, Fyler, Goldblatt, & Kreidberg, 1979). Another case-control study of infants and children with any type of malformation reported that .36% of the cases had exposure to CDZ, compared with .20% of the controls (Bracken & Holford, 1981).

In contrast to the large numbers of women systematically studied, there are only two case reports (three infants) of adverse effects with CDZ. Two (twins) exposed throughout all three trimesters were born with mild, transient withdrawal symptoms (Athinarayanan, Pierog, Nigam, & Glass, 1976); and one resulted in a transiently sedated infant, who seemed "tense and hypertonic" at all follow-ups (Bitnun, 1969).

Diazepam

The data regarding DZ are somewhat contradictory. Crombie et al. and Rumeau-Rouquette et al. both reported no malformations in DZ-exposed offspring (both reported in Crombie et al., 1975). One retrospective study reported high rates of DZ exposure in infants who had severe anomalies (14.3%) and all types of oral clefts (6.3%) (Safra & Oakley, 1975). A case-control study found that the exposure rate in oral clefts was 6.3%, compared with 1.1% in normal controls (Aarskog, 1975). However, a family history of oral clefts was present in nearly 50% of these subjects.

Two case-control studies have investigated DZ exposure in congenital heart disease. Rothman et al. (1979) found that 3.8% of the cases had been exposed to DZ, compared with 1.8% of the controls. Another reported no differences between the cases and controls (Zierler & Rothman, 1985).

In a case-control study of cases of any type of malformation, 2.5% of the cases had exposure to DZ, versus 0.91% of the controls (Bracken & Holford, 1981). Another case-control study of this drug did not demonstrate any quantitiative or stochastic differences in the rates of exposure between cases of oral clefts and controls with central nervous system (CNS) defects (Czeizel, Pazsy, Pusztai, & Nagy, 1983). This conclusion is less convincing than others, because there is no guarantee that DZ does not produce CNS defects. A similar result was reported by

Rosenberg et al. (1983) comparing oral clefts and all other types of malformations, but the same criticism applies to the choice of the control group.

There is only one cohort study that specifically investigated DZ use. Shiono and Mills (1984) studied 854 pregnant women exposed to DZ and found no difference in the incidence of oral clefts between the exposed and nonexposed groups.

Several studies have studied benzodiazepines or "benzodiazepines (primarily diazepam)," most using the case-control design. Saxén and Saxén (1975) compared cases of oral clefts with normal controls and reported a benzodiazepine exposure rate in the cases as 5.4%, compared with 2.0% in the controls. Saxen (1975) in another study with a new group of subjects reported that 3.7% of the cases (mothers of babies with oral clefts) had been exposed, versus 2.1% of the mothers of healthy babies. Greenberg, Inman, Weatherall, Adelstein, & Haskey (1977) reported that 4.3% of the cases of any type of malformation had been exposed to benzodiazepines, compared with 2.9% of the controls. Information on family histories of birth defects was elicited, and when the data were stratified by this variable, the two groups had equal rates. Winship, Cahal, Weber, & Griffin (1984) found that 1.8% of the cases of CNS defects had exposure to benzodiazepines, compared to 1% of the controls.

The most indicting evidence against DZ comes from Laegrid, Olegard, Wahlstrom, and Conradi (1987, 1989). They report a follow-up study of 36 women exposed to benzodiazepines, primarily DZ: 20% gave birth to infants with similar dysmorphic facies, and 14% developed moderate to severe cognitive and behavioral disorders. All women denied other drug or alcohol exposure.

There are seven case reports (eight infants) regarding DZ. In one, DZ used with an antidepressant produced a nonviable infant with malformation of the body stalk (New Zealand Committee on Adverse Drug Reactions, 1968); two produced multiple skeletal defects (both with coexposure to other possible teratogens) (Istvan, 1970; Ringrose, 1972); one was associated with cataracts; two (same mother, different pregnancies) resulted in transient sedation, but normal development at 2 and 5 years (Haram, 1977); and one had "floppy infant syndrome" (severe hypotonia, possibly apnea, hypothermia, and poor suck reflex) (Speight, 1977). In one exposed to a large dose of DZ (580 mg in a suicide attempt) on the 43rd day of gestation, there were multiple musculoskeletal deformities (normal genotype) (Rivas, Hernandez, & Cantu, 1984).

DZ use beyond the first trimester has been associated with either "floppy infant syndrome" (Gillberg, 1977) or symptoms of sedative withdrawal (Mazzi, 1977; Rementeria & Bhatt, 1977).

There are also several reports regarding the use of other anxiolytics. Exposure to alprazolam or triazolam was reported to UpJohn in a voluntary registry fashion on 441 women (Barry & St. Clair, 1987). The data is not precisely reported, but no pattern of malformations or excessive rate of defects appears to be associated with either drug. Nitrazepam exposure has been reported in twins and was associated only with transient sedation (Speight, 1977). Chlorazepate exposure was associated with multisystem deformities when used by an adolescent mother (Patel & Patel, 1980); one case of clonazepam use throughout pregnancy was associated with mild transient sedation (Kriel & Cloyd, 1982), but another case was associated with "floppy infant syndrome" (Fisher, Edgren, Mammel, & Coleman 1985).

The anxiolytics are well studied, but the major problems in interpreting these data are that the definitions of birth defects varied between studies, the indications for the medications were only described in one study, and the control of other risk factors was only done in one study. The one study that did not control for additional risk factors reported no difference between the groups, and this negative finding could be explained on the basis of insufficient sample size. This indicates that previous reports of differences may have been a result of factors other than the CDZ. The retrospective data on oral clefts and congenital heart disease raised concern about DZ exposure, but this has not been supported by data from other types of studies. There have been no other reports in the literature on a constellation of defects, such as the syndrome reported above by Laegrid et al. (1987, 1989), and the case report literature on both drugs does not indicate a trend toward such. There are insufficient data on any of the other anxiolytics to speculate on their teratogenic potential.

Antidepressants

The bulk of the data on antidepressants comes from investigations of imipramine and amitriptyline (Table 3). These medications are largely given only for psychiatric symptoms, so the rate of exposure in the general population is low. This indicates that caution should be used in interpreting retrospective studies.

It is of historical interest to note that the first report of possible antidepressant-associated limb defects was by McBride (1972), one of the first investigators to report thalidomide-related phocomelia. He reported three cases of imipramine associated with limb reduction defects, but further examination of the data revealed that only one of the cases had been exposed to imipramine, and the other two had been exposed to amitriptyline. There were no data collected to rule out other possible risk factors (Morrow, 1972).

This sparked a flurry of retrospective studies (see Table 3), searching for an association between limb reduction defects and antidepressant exposure. Morrow (1972) described two such studies. Searching the records of 53 mothers of infants with limb deformities, he found that none had used imipramine. He then selected another 169 cases of the defect, and again could find no associated imipramine use. A number of other retrospective studies were done, unsuccessfully attempting to link tricyclic antidepressants (CAs) (primarily imipramine and amitriptyline) with limb malformations (Banister, DaFoe, Smith, & Miller, 1972; Rachedefsky, Flynt, Ebbin, & Wilson, 1972).

Several uncontrolled follow-up studies have also been done. One reported the use of a variety of TCAs, all associated with normal outcomes (Scanlon, 1969). Two reported no abnormalities associated with imipramine use, but one infant exposed to amitriptyline had transient bilateral edema of hands and feet (Crombie, Pinsent, & Fleming, 1972; Sim, 1972). Another such study, however, reported that imipramine use was associated with a spontaneous abortion rate of 5.6% ($n = 1$), and 11.8% ($n = 2$) of the infants had gastrointestinal deformities. This same study reported that 6% ($n = 2$) of the amitriptyline pregnancies resulted in stillbirth or miscarriage, and 3% ($n = 1$) of the infants had hypospadias (Kuenssberg & Knox, 1972). The lack of control groups and lack of information regarding other risk factors makes interpretation of these data tenuous.

There are three case-control studies that address the question. Idanpaan-

Table 3 Teratogenicity of antidepressants

Study	Design	N	Medication	Tri-mester	Outcomes	Other risk factors
Morrow, 1972	Restrospective (Australian registry; specifically studied limb reduction data	53	Imipramine	1	0% cases had exposure	—
	Retrospective (cases = limb deformities)	169/43,000 delivery records	Imipramine	1	0% cases had exposure	
Rachelefsky et al., 1972	Retrospective (Atlanta and Los Angeles registries; severe limb anomalies)	48	Any tricyclic antidepressant (TCA)	1	0% cases had exposure	—
Banister et al., 1972	Retrospective (multisite Canadian registries; reduction deformities)	143	Any TCA	1	.6% cases had exposure to amitriptyline	—
Sim, 1972	Follow-up		Imipramine	?	Normal infants	—
Crombie et al., 1972	Follow-up		Imipramine ($n = 19$)	1–2	Normal infants	—
			Amitriptyline ($n = 28$)	1–2	3.6% ($n = 1$) exposed had transient "swelling hands and feet"	—
Kuenssberg & Knox, 1972	Follow-up	48	Imipramine ($n = 17$)	1	5.9% spontaneous abortion; 11.8% had gastrointestinal deformities	
			Amitriptyline ($n = 31$)	1	3.2% spontaneous abortion; 9.8% hypospadias	
Idänpään-Heikkilä & Saxén, 1973	Case-control (cases = CNS, skeletal, craniofacial defects)	5,568	Any TCA	1	.18% cases were exposed vs. .04% controls	—
Bracken & Holford, 1981	Case-control (cases = any malformations)	4,428	Antidepressants	1	Odds ratio = 7.6	—
Winship et al., 1984	Case-control (cases = CNS defects)	1,528	Any type of antidepressant	1	1.0% cases had exposure vs. .9% controls	—
Kullander & Källén, 1976	Cohort	6,376	Antidepressants (primarily imipramine, $n = 29$)	1	17.2% exposed had stillbirth or some malformation vs. 13% unexposed	—
Heinonen et al., 1977	Cohort	50,282	Amitriptyline ($n = 21$)	1	0% exposed had malformation	Risk ↑ when adjusted for hospital and race
			MAOIs ($n = 21$)		14.3% exposed had malformation	
			Imipramine ($n = 19$), nortriptyline ($n = 1$)		10% exposed had malformation vs. 6.5% unexposed	

↑, increased.

63

Heikkila and Saxen (1973) studied cases of CNS, skeletal, and craniofacial defects, and reported that 0.18% of the cases were exposed to a TCA versus 0.04% of the controls. Bracken and Holford (1981) defined cases as any type of malformation, and reported nearly an 8-fold increase in risk of malformations in the antidepressant group, compared with controls (dosage, drugs, and specific proportions of sample exposed were not given). Winship, Cahal, Weber, & Griffin (1984) reported that 1.0% of the CNS defects were exposed to some type of antidepressant, compared to 0.9% of the controls.

There are two cohort studies available on this drug category. Kullander and Kallõn (1976) reported that 17.2% of women exposed to an antidepressant (N = 29) had a stillbirth or some other type of malformation (loosely defined), compared to 13% of the nonexposed. Heinonen, Sloane, & Shapiro (1977) reported that amitriptyline-exposed infants had no deformities, but that 10% of the imipramine-exposed group was malformed, compared with 6.5% of the control group.

There are 11 case reports on first-trimester TCA use. One infant was normal, after exposure to both amitriptyline and imipramine throughout pregnancy (Goldfarb & Keating, 1981); two had CNS defeats (Barson, 1972; New Zealand Committee on Adverse Drug Reactions, 1971); three had multiple musculoskeletal defects (Bourke, 1974; Freeman, 1972; Wertelecki, Purvis-Smith, & Blackburn, 1981); two developed transient sedation and withdrawal (one also had urinary retention) (Shearer, Schreiner, & Marshall, 1972; Webster, 1973); one experienced cardiac problems (Abramovici, Abramovici, Kalman, & Liban, 1981); one had bilateral anophthalmia (Golden & Perman, 1980); and one had cleft palate (New Zealand Committee on Adverse Drug Reactions, 1971).

Three infants exposed after the first trimester to amitriptyline, nortriptyline, or imipramine had pulmonary hypertension (and death) (Teisberg & Hognestad, 1973), sedation and ECG changes (Sjöqvist, Bergfors, Borga, Lind, & Ygge, 1972), and transient left bundle branch block (Singh & Tandon, 1977), respectively.

There is only one study that gives data regarding the use of monoamine oxidase inhibitors (MAOI). In this cohort study, 14.3% of the MAOI-exposed infants had malformations, compared with 6.5% of the controls (Heinonen et al., 1977). There is one case report of tranylcypromine and trifluoperazine use associated with a large sacrococcygeal teratoma (Bergamaschi & Berlingieri, 1968).

There is little information on the newer antidepressants. Seventeen women became pregnant during the clinical trials of fluoxetine and all produced healthy infants (Cooper, 1988). Dothiepin use throughout pregnancy was associated with reversible fetal tachyarrhythmia (Prentice & Brown, 1989). There are no data about the behavioral teratogenicity of the antidepressants.

The earlier concern about antidepressants producing limb reduction defects has not been substantiated by later research. Although some studies reported no increased risk with these drugs, others did report an increased risk that did not reach statistical significance, probably resulting from small sample sizes. Interpretation of the research is restricted by small sample sizes, the absence of control groups, and lack of consideration of other risk factors. It is difficult to assert with confidence that the antidepressants as a group are safe to administer during the first trimester, but there is no clear evidence of teratogenic risk. Therefore, a clinical risk/benefit analysis needs to be done with each patient.

Lithium

In contrast to the medications described, information on lithium has come from registry data and case reports (Table 4). Half of these case reports included exposure to other drugs, whereas the rate of exposure to other medications in the registry data is unknown.

There have been four studies of lithium. Two of these are reports from the Register of Lithium Babies, a voluntary international registry formed in 1968. The registry published initial conclusions (based on 118 cases) that lithium did not present a teratogenic risk (Schou, Goldfield, Weinstein, & Villenuve, 1973). The American portion of the registry, however, continued to collect data. The registry has since retracted its position on the safety of lithium, based on a total of 225 cases (Weinstein, 1980). Of these cases 11.1% had some congenital defect; 72% had Ebstein's anomaly or some other cardiac defect. This rate is clearly higher than the general population rate of congenital heart disease.

In one of the few studies investigating behavioral teratogenicity, Schou (1976) followed 117 "nondeformed" lithium babies from the registry, comparing them with their nonexposed siblings on the basis of neurodevelopment. Of the exposed children, 16.6% were neurodevelopmentally delayed versus 10.5% of the siblings. He concluded that lithium was not a behavioral teratogen, based on these data.

The only other formal study of lithium matched three mandatory registries (Källén & Tandberg, 1983). A discharge diagnosis registry was linked with a medical birth registry, identifying 350 bipolar women who had given birth. These cases were then linked with a congenital defect registry, enabling the investigators to estimate the incidence of birth defects in bipolar women who were and were not medicated. They also could construct a group of women who were not bipolar until after pregnancy began, and controlled for maternal age, parity, and cigarette use. Of the mothers using lithium, 35.6% had miscarriages, stillbirths, or infants with congenital defects, compared with 7.5% of the nonexposed. Of the infants exposed to lithium, 7% had cardiac defects.

There are 13 case reports of exposure to lithium alone in the first trimester. One infant was normal (Fries, 1970); one had congenital diabetes insipidus, respiratory distress, and hypotonia (Belik, Yoder, & Pereira, 1982); one was stillborn (Khandelwal, Sagar, & Saxena, 1989); two developed transient hypotonia, one with respiratory depression (Silverman, Winters, & Strande, 1971; Stothers, Wilson, & Royston, 1973); two had transient hypothyroidism (Karlsson, Lindstedt, Lundberg, & Selstam, 1975; Nars & Girard, 1977); and six presented with a variety of cardiac defects, three of whom included Ebstein's anomaly (Allan, Desai, & Tynan, 1982; Arnon, Marin-Garcia, & Peeden, 1981; Long & Willis, 1984; O'Donovan, O'Herlihy, & Roystan, 1984; Park, Sridaromont, Ledbetter, & Terry, 1980; Wilson, Forfar, & Godman, 1983). Six case reports describe first-trimester lithium use with other psychotropic drugs. One infant was normal (Long & Willis, 1984); one had transient cyanosis and hypotonia (Tunnessen & Hertz, 1972); one had congenital diabetes insipidus and goiter (Mizrahi, Hobbs, & Goldsmith, 1979); and three had cardiac problems, one of whom had persistent motor delay (Morrel, Sutherland, Buamah, Oo, & Pain, 1983; Rane, Tomson, & Bjarke, 1978; Stevens, Burman, & Midwinter, 1974)

Lithium alone after the first trimester has been associated with a normal infant

Table 4 Teratogenicity of lithium carbonate

Study	Design	N	Medication	Tri-mester	Outcomes	Other risk factors
Nora et al., 1974; Lewis & Suris, 1970; Vacaflor et al., 1970; Schou et al., 1973; Weinstein & Garfield, 1975; Weinstein, 1980	Register of lithium babies	225	Lithium	1 or 1–3	11.1% congenital deformities 72% of these had Ebstein's anomaly or other CHD	—
Schou, 1976	Controlled follow-up (cases = nondeformed "lithium babies"; controls = nonexposed sibs)	117	Lithium	1–3	16.6% exposed had developmental abnormalities vs. 10.5% unexposed	—
Källén & Tandberg, 1983	Historical controlled follow-up	350	Lithium alone (n = 41) Lithium + other meds (n = 18)	1	35.6% exposed had perinatal deaths/malformations vs. 7.5% unexposed	All Ss had bipolar affective disorder; cigarette use and maternal age ↑ effect

↑, increased; Ss, subjects.

(Mallinger et al., 1984). The use of lithium with other drugs after the first trimester has been associated with transient cyanosis, hypotonia, and systolic murmurs (Mackay, Loose, & Glen, 1976; Willbanks, Bressler, Peete, Cherny, & London, 1970).

Although most of the data about lithium come from case reports and the registry, the frequent appearance of cardiac abnormalities is unmistakable. In addition, the one systematic study by Källén and Tandeberg (1983) confirms the increased teratogenic risk with controlled data. The consistent reports of abnormalities even when lithium is used alone provides support to the theory that lithium itself is teratogenic. Therefore, avoidance of lithium during the first trimester is recommended, although avoidance during the remaining trimesters is not as clearly indicated.

Carbamazepine

Carbamazepine is increasingly used as an alternative to lithium in the treatment of bipolar patients (Table 5). This medication appeared to be the least teratogenic anticonvulsant (Nakane et al., 1980; Neibyl, Blake, Freeman, & Luff, 1979), but several recent studies have raised doubts about its safety. In brief, there are three major controlled follow-up studies, with substantial numbers of women exposed to carbamazepine alone. These investigations all report evidence of intrauterine growth retardation (Hiilesmaa, Teramok, & Granstrom, 1981; Bertollini, Kallen, Mastroiacovo, & Robert, 1987); and there are data suggesting a syndrome of craniofacial defects, fingernail hypoplasia, and developmental delay in addition to the intrauterine growth retardation (Jones, Lacro, Johnson, & Adams 1989). This occurred in nearly a quarter of the children exposed. Thus, it appears that carbamazepine is not a good alternative to lithium in the pregnant woman.

CLINICAL GUIDELINES

In general, none of the psychotropic drugs except lithium and carbamazepine uniformly should be avoided during the first trimester, or in the case of carbamazepine, throughout pregnancy. It is important in deciding whether to treat a woman pharmacologically, that all data about her case be assessed, and a full risk/benefit analysis be done. The teratogenic risks of medications may be minor when compared to the effects of malnutrition and dehydration that may result from severe depression or psychosis. The following guidelines are recommended in a general way, but each case must be evaluated individually.

Evaluation of the Pregnant, Psychiatrically Ill Woman

1. Past obstetrical history: spontaneous abortions, stillbirths, or previous births of abnormal infants.

2. Family history: psychiatric history of patient and family; history of congenital defects or problems in patient and family (include father of the baby and his family).

3. Data regarding nutrition, cigarette use and alcohol use, occupational exposures.

Table 5 Teratogenicity of carbamazepine

Study	Design	N	Medication	Tri-mester	Outcomes	Other risk factors
Nakane et al., 1980	Follow-up	453 (total number of infants = 902)	Carbamazepine (n = 129)	1	8.5% exposed = some type malformation vs. 7.1% unexposed	All Ss had epilepsy, polytherapy had greater risk than monotherapy
Hiilesmaa et al., 1981	Controlled follow-up	133 (total number of infants = 143)	Carbamazepine alone (n = 20)	1–3	↓ head circumference at birth + 18 months	All Ss had epilepsy
			Carbamazepine in combination (n = 21)	1–3	↓ head circumference at 18 months compared with unmedicated epileptics and controls	
Bertollini et al., 1987	Follow-up	557	Carbamazepine (n = 70)	1–3	1.4% exposed had hypospadias; ↓ mean body weight, length, head circumference	Cigarette use did not explain ↑ risk
Jones et al., 1989	Controlled follow-up (cases = carbamazepine contacts to California Teratogen Registry; low-dose controls = alcohol contacts to registry)	145	Carbamazepine only (n = 50) Carbamazepine + other anticonvulsants (n = 22)		70% exposed had some malformation vs. 26% controls; 20% exposed to carbamazepine alone had developmental delays	All cases but 1 had epilepsy

↓, decreased; Ss, subjects; ↑, increased.

4. History of current medication/street drug use (if any); attempt to correlate times of medication use and dosages with approximate gestational ages of the fetus. There are no psychiatric medications with such a clearly increased risk of a severe congenital defect that abortion is automatically indicated.

5. Assessment for current need for medications in routine psychiatric examination.

Recommendations for Care

If medications are deemed necessary for the health and well-being of the mother and fetus, the following general guidelines may be used. Drugs should be administered in divided doses throughout the day if possible, to avoid giving drug boluses to the fetus. Dosages should be decreased as low as possible 1–3 weeks before delivery to minimize direct effects on the fetus.

1. *Psychosis:* Chlorpromazine is best avoided; the best alternative appears to be haloperidol or trifluoperazine. Dosages should be kept as low as possible, but adequate treatment of symptoms is the primary goal and this should not be compromised. EPS may be managed with benztropine.

2. *Mania:* Lithium should be avoided in the first trimester, and acute mania managed with antipsychotics. In severe cases, electroconvulsive therapy (ECT) may be used (see next list item). If lithium exposure has occurred in the first trimester, serial sonograms can help identify cardiac defects prenatally, preparing parents and the treatment team for intervention at birth, if necessary. Lithium may be used if absolutely necessary during the second and third trimesters, although transient diabetes insipidus and thyroid problems in the infant appear to be a problem. Serum levels should be used to dictate dosages, because of altered maternal pharmacokinetics. Carbamazepine should be avoided entirely.

3. *Depression:* ECT is the preferred treatment for severe major depressions during the first trimester (Forssman, 1955; Remick & Maurice, 1978: Repke & Berger, 1984; Varan, Gillieson, Skener, & Sarwar-Foncer, 1985; Wise, Ward, Townsend-Parchman, Gillstrap, & Hauth, 1984). If ECT is contraindicated or unacceptable to the patient, then until further information is available on the newer antidepressants, such as fluoxetine, a tricyclic antidepressant should be used. The most extensive positive experience has been with imipramine, but the side effects may be difficult for the pregnant patient to tolerate. Unpublished data from Pittsburgh (K. Wisner, M.D., personal communication) indicate that nortriptyline may be a good alternative, but there are not enough data on any of the other medications to draw conclusions about teratogenic risks. As with lithium, drug levels where indicated and clinical response should determine the dosages, not a priori ideas about appropriate dose.

4. *Anxiety disorders:* These are rarely life-threatening, and since the data on some of the benzodiazepines are contradictory, these drugs are best avoided in the first trimester. When severe panic disorder is present, a tricyclic such as imipramine may be helpful, but should only be provided in concert with a fully informed consent concerning fetal risk. Behavioral therapy is often a good alternative to medications; if the condition becomes severe in the later trimesters, management with benzodiazepines should be safe.

5. *General advice:* Encourage cessation of cigarette smoking, alcohol use, and the use of any other drugs. Ensure that the patient has good nutrition, obtains prenatal care, and takes prenatal vitamins, which may have a protective effect against some types of defects (Winship et al., 1984).

REFERENCES

Aarskog D, 1975: Association between maternal intake of diazepam and oral clefts. *Lancet, 2,* 921.

Abramovici A, Abramovici I, Kalman G, Liban E, 1981: Teratogenic effect of chlorimipramine in a young human embryo. *Teratology, 24,* 42A.

Allan ID, Desai G, Tynan MJ, 1982: Prenatal echocardiographic screening for Ebstein's anomaly for mothers on lithium therapy. *Lancet, 2,* 875–876.

Arnon RG, Marin-Garcia J, Peeden JN, 1981: Tricuspid valve regurgitation and lithium carbonate toxicity in a newborn infant. *American Journal of Diseases of Children, 135,* 941–943.

Athinarayanan P, Pierog SH Nigam SK, Glass L, 1976: Chlordiazepoxide withdrawal in the neonate. *American Journal of Obstetrics and Gynecology, 124,* 212–213.

Ayd FJ, 1964: Children born of mothers treated with chlorpromazine during pregnancy. *Clinical Medicine, 71,* 1758–1763.

Banister P, DaFoe C, Smith ESO, Miller J, 1972: Possible teratogenicity of tricyclic antidepressants. *Lancet, 1,* 838–839.

Barry WS, St. Clair S, 1987: Exposure to benzodiazepines in utero. *Lancet, 1,* 1436–1437.

Barson AJ, 1972: Malformed infant. *British Medical Journal, 1,* 1945.

Belik J, Yoder M, Pereira GR, 1982: Fetal macrosomia: An unrecognized adverse effect of maternal lithium therapy. *Neonatology, 59,* 304A.

Bergamaschi MMP, Berlingieri D, 1968: Traitement neuroleptique au dōbut de la grossesse et teratone sacrococcygien du foetus. *Bulletin Federale Societe Gynecologie et Obstetrica, 20,* 316–318.

Bertolini R, Källén B, Mastroiacovo P, Robert E, 1987: Anticonvulsant drugs in monotherapy: Effect on the fetus. *European Journal of Epidemiolgy, 3,* 164–171.

Bitnun S, 1969: Possible effect of chlordiazepoxide on the fetus. *Canadian Medical Association Journal, 100,* 351.

Bourke GM, 1974: Antidepressant teratogenicity. *Lancet, 1,* 98.

Bracken MB, Holford TR, 1981: Exposure to prescribed drugs in pregnancy and association with congenital malformations. *Obstetrics and Gynecology, 58,* 336–344.

Cleary MF, 1977: Fluphenazine decanoate during pregnancy. *American Journal of Psychiatry, 134,* 815–816.

Cooper GI, 1988: The safety of fluoxetine—An update. *British Journal of Psychiatry, 153,* 77–86.

Corner BD, 1962: Congenital malformations—Clinical considerations. *Medical Journal of the Southwest, 77,* 46–52.

Coyle I, Wayner MJ, Singer G, 1975: Behavioral teratogenesis: A critical review. *Pharmacology Biochemistry and Behavior, 4,* 191–200.

Crombie DL, Pinsent RJ, Fleming D, 1972: Imipramine in pregnancy. *British Medical Journal, 1,* 745.

Crombie DL, Pinsent RJ, Fleming DM, Rumeau-Rouquette C, Goujard J, Huel G, 1975: Fetal effects of tranquilizers in pregnancy. *New England Journal of Medicine, 293,* 198–199.

Czeizel A, Pazsy A, Pusztai J, Nagy M, 1983: Aetiological monitor of congenital abnormalities: A case-control surveillance system. *Acta Pediatrica Hungarica, 24,* 91–99.

Donaldson GL, Bury RG, 1982: Multiple congenital abnormalities in a newborn boy associated with maternal use of fluphenazine enanthate and other drugs during pregnancy. *Acta Paediactrica Scandinavica, 71,* 335–338.

Donaldson JO, 1982: Control of chorea gravidarum with haloperidol. *Obstetrics and Gynecology, 59,* 381–382.

Falterman CG, Richardson CJ, 1980: Small left colon syndrome associated with maternal ingestion of psychotropic drugs. *Journal of Pediatrics, 97,* 308–310.

Fisher JB, Edgren BE, Mammel MC, Coleman JM, 1985: Neonatal apnea associated with maternal clonazepam therapy: A case report. *Obstetrics and Gynecology, 66,* 34S–35S.

Forssman H, 1955: Follow-up study of sixteen children whose mothers were given electric convulsive therapy during gestation. *Acta Psychiatrica and Neurologica Scandinavica, 30,* 437–441.

Freeman R, 1972: Limb deformities: Possible association with drugs. *Medical Journal of Australia, 1,* 606–607.

Fries H, 1970: Lithium in pregnancy. *Lancet, 1,* 1233.

General Practitioner Clinical Trials, 1963: Drugs in pregnancy survey. *The Practitioner, 191,* 775–780.

Gillberg C, 1977: "Floppy infant syndrome" and maternal diazepam. *Lancet, 2,* 244.

Golden SM, Perman KI, 1980: Bilateral clinical ophthalmia: Drugs as potential factors. *Southern Medical Journal, 73,* 1404–1407.

Goldfarb C, Keating G, 1981: Use of antidepressants from conception to delivery. *Journal of the Medical Society of New Jersey, 78,* 357–360.

Greenberg G, Inman WH, Weatherall JA, Adelstein AM, Haskey J, 1977: Maternal drug histories and congenital abnormalities. *British Medical Journal, 2,* 853–856.

Gross M, 1962: Discussion of Dr. Kris' report. *Recent Advances in Biological Psychiatry, 4,* 186–187.

Hall G, 1963: A case of phocomelia of the upper limbs. *Medical Journal of Australia, 1,* 449–450.

Hammond JE, Toseland PA, 1970: Placental transfer of chlorpromazine. *Archives of Disease in Childhood, 45,* 139–140.

Hanson JW, Oakley GP, 1975: Haloperidol and limb deformity. *Journal of the American Medical Association, 231,* 26.

Haram K, 1977: "Floppy infant syndrome" and maternal diazepam. *Lancet, 2,* 612–613.

Hartz SC, Heinonen OP, Shapiro S, Siskind V, Sloane D, 1975: Antenatal exposure to meprobamate and chlordiazepoxide in relation to malformations, mental, development, and childhood mortality. *New England Journal of Medicine, 292,* 726–728.

Heinonen OP, Sloane D, Shapiro S, 1977: Birth defects and drugs in pregnancy. Littleton: Publishing Sciences Group.

Hiilesmaa VK, Teramok, Granstr-m M-L, 1981: Fetal head growth retardation associated with maternal antiepileptic drugs. *Lancet, 2,* 165–167.

Hill RM, Desmond MM, Kay JL, 1966: Extrapyramidal dysfunction in an infant of a schzophrenic mother. *Journal of Pediatrics, 64,* 589–595.

Idanpaan-Heikkila J, Saxen L, 1973: Possible teratogenicity of imipramine/chloropyramine. *Lancet, 2,* 282–283.

Istvan EJ, 1970: Drug-associated congenital abnormalities? *Canadian Medical Association Journal, 103,* 1394.

James ME, 1988: Neuroleptic malignant syndrome in pregnancy. *Psychosomatics, 29,* 119–122.

Jones KL, Lacro RV, Johnson KA, Adams J, 1989: Pattern of malformations in the children of women treated with carbamazepine during pregnancy. *New England Journal of Medicine, 320,* 1661–1666.

Källén B, Tandberg A, 1983: Lithium and pregnancy. *Acta Psychiatrica Scandinavica, 68,* 134–139.

Karlsson K, Lindstedt G, Lundberg PA, Selstam U, 1975: Transplacental lithium poisoning: Reversible inhibition of fetal thyroid. *Lancet, 1,* 1295.

Khandelwal SK, Sagar RS, Saxena S, 1989: Lithium in pregnancy and still birth: A case report. *British Journal of Psychiatry, 154,* 114–116.

Kopelman AE, McCullar FW, Heggeness L, 1975: Limb malformations following maternal use of haloperidol. *Journal of the American Medical Association, 231,* 62–64.

Kriel RL, Cloyd J, 1982: Clonazepam and pregnancy. *Annals of Neurology, 11,* 544.

Kris EB, 1962: Children born to mothers maintained on pharmacotheapy during pregnancy and postpartum. *Recent Advances in Biological Psychiatry, 4,* 180–186.

Kris EB, 1965: Children of mothers maintained on pharmacotherapy during pregnancy and postpartum. *Current Therapeutic Research, 7,* 785–789.

Kuenssberg EV, Knox JDE, 1972: Imipramine in pregnancy. *Lancet, 1,* 292.

Kullander S, Källén B, 1976: A prospective study of drugs and pregnancy. *Acta Obstetrica Scandinavica, 55,* 25–33.

Laegrid L, Olegard R, Wahlstrom J, Conradi N, 1987: Abnormalities in children exposed to benzodiazepines in utero. *Lancet, 1,* 108–109.

Laegrid L, Olegard R, Wahlstrom J, Conradi N, 1989: Teratogenic effects of benzodiazepine use during pregnancy. *Journal of Pediatrics, 114,* 126–131.

Lenz W, 1962: Thalidomide and congenital abnormalities. *Lancet, 1,* 271.

Levy W, Wisneiwski K, 1974: Chlorpromazine causing extrapyramidal dysfunction. *New York State Journal of Medicine, 74,* 684–685.

Long WA, Willis PN, 1984: Maternal lithium and neonatal Ebstein's anomaly. Evaluation of cross-sectional echocardiograpy. *American Journal of Perinatology, 1,* 182–184.

MacKay AVP, Loose R, Glen AIM, 1976: Labor on lithium. *British Medical Journal, 1,* 878.

Mallinger AG, Hanin I, Stumpf RL, Mallinger J, Kopp U, Erstling C, 1984: Lithium treatment during pregnancy: A case study of erythrocyte choline content and lithium transport. *American Journal of Clinical Psychiatry, 44*, 381–384.

Mazzi E, 1977: Possible neonatal diazepam withdrawal: A case report. *American Journal of Obstetrics and Gynecology, 129*, 586–587.

McBride, WG, 1961: Thalidomide and congenital abnormalities. *Lancet, 2*, 1358.

McBride WG, 1972: Limb deformities associated with iminodibenzyl hydrochloride. *Medical Journal of Australia, 2*, 492.

Meyer V, 1984: Unpublished letter to McNeil Pharmaceutical.

Milkovich L, van den Berg BJ, 1974: Effect of prenatal meprobamate and chlordiazepoxide hydrochloride on human embryonic and fetal development. *New England Journal of Medicine, 291*, 1268–1271.

Milkovich L, van den Berg BJ, 1976: An evaluation of the teratogenicity of certain anti-nauseant drugs. *American Journal of Obstetrics and Gynecology, 125*, 244–248.

Mizrahi EM, Hobbs JF, Goldsmith DI, 1979: Nephrogenic diabetes insipidus in transplacental lithium intoxication. *Journal of Pediatrics, 94*, 493–495.

Moriarty AJ, Nance MR, 1963: Trifluoperazine and pregnancy. *Canadian Medical Association Journal, 88*, 375–376.

Morrel P, Sutherland GR, Buamah PK, Oo M, Bain HH, 1983: Lithium toxicity in a neonate. *Archives of Diseases in Childhood, 58*, 539–541.

Morrow AW, 1972: Imipramine and congenital abnormalities. *New Zealand Medical Journal, 1*, 228–229.

Nakane Y, Okuma T, Takahashi R, Sato Y, Wada T, Sato T, Fukushima Y, Kumashiro H, Ono T, Takahashi T, Aoki Y, Kazamatsuri H, Inami M, Komai S, Seino M, Miyakoshi M, Tanimura T, Hazama H, Kawahara R, Otsuki S, Hosokawa K, Inanaga K, Nakazawa Y, Yamamoto K, 1980: Multi-institutional study on the teratogenicity and fetal toxicity of antiepileptic drugs: A report of a collaborative study group in Japan. *Epilepsia, 21*, 663–680.

Nars PW, Girard J, 1977: Lithium carbonate intake during pregnancy leading to large goiter in a premature infant. *American Journal of Diseases of Children, 131*, 924–925.

Neibyl JR, Blake DA, Freeman JM, Luff RD, 1979: Carbamazepine levels in pregnancy and lactation. *Obstetrics and Gynecology, 53*, 139–140.

Nevin NC, Kernohan DC, Ross AM, 1980: Ankyloglossum superious syndrome. *Oral Surgery, 50*, 254–256.

New Zealand Committee on Adverse Drug Reactions, 1968: *New Zealand Medical Journal, 67*, 635–641.

New Zealand Committee on Adverse Drug Reactions, 1971: *New Zealand Medical Journal, 74*, 184–191.

New Zealand Committee on Adverse Drug Reactions, 1973: *New Zealand Medical Journal, 78*, 309–316.

New Zealand Committee on Adverse Drug Reactions, 1975: *New Zealand Medical Journal, 82*, 308–310.

O'Connor M, Johnson GH, James DI, 1981: Intrauterine effect of phenothiazines. *Medical Journal of Australia, 1*, 416–417.

O'Donovan P, O'Herliky C, Roystan D, 1984: Hydrops fetalis and congenital mitral stenosis associated with maternal lithium treatment. *Journal of Obstetrics and Gynecology, 5*, 101–105.

O'Leary JL, O'Leary JA, 1964: Non-thalidomide ectromelia. *Obstetrics and Gynecology, 23*, 17–20.

Ornoy A, Yanai J, 1980: Central nervous system teratogenicity: Experimental models for human problems. *Advances in the Study of Birth Defects, 4*, 1–21.

Park JM, Sridaromont S, Ledbetter EO, Terry WM, 1980: Ebstein's anomaly of the tricuspid valve associated with prenatal exposure to lithium carbonate. *American Journal of Diseases of Children, 134*, 703–704.

Patel DA, Patel AR, 1980: Chlorazepate and congenital malformations. *Journal of the American Medical Association, 244*, 135–136.

Patterson JF, 1979: Treatment of chorea gravidarum with haloperidol. *Southern Medical Journal, 72*, 1220–1221.

Platt JE, Friedhoff AJ, Broman SH, Bond RN, Laska E, Lin SP, 1988: Effect of neuroleptic drugs on children's growth. *Neuropsychopharmacology, 3*, 205–212.

Prentice A, Brown R, 1989: Fetal tachyrhythmia and maternal antidepressant treatment. *British Medical Journal, 298*, 190.

Rachelefsky GS, Flynt JW, Ebbin AJ, Wilson MG, 1972: Possible teratogenicity of tricyclic antidepressants. *Lancet, 1,* 838.

Rane A, Tomson G, Bjarke B, 1978: Effects of maternal lithium therapy in a newborn infant. *Journal of Pediatrics, 93,* 296–297.

Rawlings WJ, Ferguson R, Maddison TG, 1963: Phenmetrazine and trifluoperazine. *Medical Journal of Australia, 1,* 370.

Rementeria JL, Bhatt K, 1977: Withdrawal symptoms in neonates from intrauterine exposure to diazepam. *Journal of Pediatrics, 90,* 123–126.

Remick RA, Maurice WM, 1978: ECT in pregnancy. *American Journal of Psychiatry, 135,* 761–762.

Repke JT, Berger NG, 1984: Electroconvulsive therapy in pregnancy. *Obstetrics and Gynecology, 63,* 395–415.

Rieder RO, Rosenthal D, Wender P, Blumenthal H, 1975: The offspring of schizophrenics. *Archives of General Psychiatry, 32,* 200–211.

Ringrose CAD, 1972: The hazard of neurotropic drugs in the fertile years. *Canadian Medical Association Journal, 106,* 1058.

Rivas F, Hernandez A, Cantu JM, 1984: Accentric craniofacial cleft in a newborn female prenatally exposed to a high dose of diazepam. *Teratology, 30,* 179–180.

Rosenberg L, Mitchell AA, Parsells JL, Pashayan H, Louik C, Shapiro S, 1983: Lack of relation of oral clefts to diazepam use during pregnancy. *New England Journal of Medicine, 309,* 1282–1285.

Rothman KJ, Fyler DC, Goldblatt A, Kreidberg MB, 1979: Exogenous hormones and other drug exposures of children with congenital heart disease. *American Journal of Epidemiology, 109,* 433–439.

Rumeau-Rouquette C, Goujard J, Huel G, 1976: Possible teratogenic effect of phenothiazines in human beings. *Teratology, 15,* 57–64.

Safra MJ, Oakley GP, 1975: Association between cleft lip with or without cleft palate and prenatal exposure to diazepam. *Lancet, 2,* 478–480.

Saxen I, 1975: Epidemiology of cleft lip and palate. *British Journal of Preventive and Social Medicine, 29,* 103–110.

Saxen I, Saxen L, 1975: Association between maternal intake of diazepam and oral clefts. *Lancet, 2,* 498.

Scanlon FJ, 1969: Use of antidepressant drugs during the first trimester. *Medical Journal of Australia, 2,* 1077.

Scanlon FJ, 1972: The use of thioridazine (Mellaril) during the first trimester. *Medical Journal of Australia, 1,* 1271–1272.

Schardein JL, 1985: *Chemical induction of birth defects.* New York: M. Dekker.

Schardein JL, Keller KA, 1989: Potential human developmental toxicants and the role of animal testing in their identification and characterization. *CRC Critical Reviews in Toxicology, 19,* 251–339.

Shearer WT, Schreiner RL, Marshall RE, 1972: Urinary retention in a neonate secondary to maternal ingestion of nortriptyline. *Journal of Pediatrics, 81,* 570–572.

Schou M, 1976: What happened later to lithium babies? *Acta Psychiatrica Scandinavica, 54,* 193–197.

Schou M, Goldfield MD, Weinstein MR, Villenuve A, 1973: Lithium and pregnancy. I. Report from the register of lithium babies. *British Medical Journal, 2,* 135–136.

Schrire I, 1963: Trifluoperazine and foetal abnormalities. *Lancet, 1,* 174.

Shiono PH, Mills JL, 1984: Oral clefts and diazepam use during pregnancy. *New England Journal of Medicine, 311,* 919–920.

Sim M, 1972: Imipramine and pregnancy. *British Medical Journal, 1,* 45.

Sjögvist F, Bergfors PG, Borga O, Lind M, Ygge H, 1972: Plasma disappearance of nortriptyline in a newborn infant following placental transfer from an intoxicated mother: Evidence for drug metabolism. *Journal of Pediatrics, 80,* 496–500.

Silverman JA, Winters RW, Strande C, 1971: Lithium carbonate therapy during pregnancy: Apparent lack of effect on the fetus. *American Journal of Obstetrics and Glynecology, 109,* 934–936.

Singh M, Tandon R, 1977: Transient left bundle branch block in a neonate. *Indian Pediatrics, 14,* 735–737.

Sloane D, Siskind V, Heinonen OP, Monson RR, Kaufman DW, Shipiro S, 1977: Antenatal exposure to the phenothiazines in relation to congenital malformations, perinatal mortality rate, birth weight, and intelligence quotient score. *American Journal of Obstetrics and Gynecology, 128,* 486–488.

Sobel DE, 1960: Fetal damage due to ECT, insulin coma, chlorpromazine or reserpine. *Archives of General Psychiatry, 2,* 606–611.

Sobel DE, 1961: Infant mortality and malformations in children of schizophrenic women. *Psychiatric Quarterly, 35*, 60–64.

Speight ANP, 1977: Floppy-infant syndrome and maternal diazepam and/or nitrazepam. *Lancet, 2*, 878.

Stevens D, Burman D, Midwinter A, 1974: Transplacental lithium poisoning. *Lancet, 2*, 595.

Stothers JK, Wilson DW, Royston N, 1973: Lithium toxicity in the newborn. *British Medical Journal, 2*, 233–234.

Tamer A, McKey R, Arias D, Worley L, Fogel BJ, 1969: Phenothiazine-induced extrapyramidal dysfunction in the neonate. *Journal of Pediatrics, 75*, 479–480.

Teisberg P, Hognestad J, 1973: Primary pulmonary hypertension in infancy. *Acta Paediatrica Scandinavica, 62*, 69–72.

Tunnessen WW, Hertz CG, 1972: Toxic effects of lithium in newborn infants: A commentary. *Journal of Pediatrics, 81*, 804–807.

Van Waes A, van de Velde E, 1969: Safety evaluation of haloperidol in the treatment of hyperemesis gravidarum. *Journal of Clinical Pharmacology, 9*, 224–227.

Varan LR, Gillieson MS, Skene DS, Sarwar-Foner GJ, 1985: ECT in an acutely psychotic pregnant woman with actively aggressive (homicidal) impulses. *Canadian Journal of Psychiatry, 30*, 363–366.

Vince DJ, 1969: Congenital malformations following phenothiazine administration during pregnancy. *Canadian Medical Association Journal, 100*, 223.

Voorhees CV, Butcher RE, 1982: Behavioral teratogenicity. In: *Developmental toxicology*, edited by K Snell. New York: Praeger.

Webster PAC, 1973: Withdrawal symptoms in neonates associated with antidepressant therapy. *Lancet, 2*, 318–319.

Weinstein MR. 1980: Lithium treatment of women during pregnancy and in the post-delivery period. In: *Handbook of lithium therapy*, edited by FN Johnson. Lancaster: MTP Press.

Wertelecki W, Purvis-Smith SG, Blackburn WR, 1981: Amitriptyline/perphenazine maternal overdose and birth defects. *Teratology, 21*, 74A.

Willbanks GD, Bressler B, Peete CH, Cherny WB, London WB, 1970: Toxic affects of lithium carbonate in a mother and newborn infant. *Journal of the American Medical Association, 213*, 865–867.

Wilson JG, 1973: *Environment and birth defects*. New York: Academic Press.

Wilson N, Forfar JC, Godman MJ, 1983: Atrial flutter in the newborn resulting from maternal lithium ingestion. *Archives of Diseases in Childhood, 58*, 538–549.

Winship KA, Cahal DA, Weber JCP, Griffin JP, 1984: Maternal drug histories and central nervous system anomalies. *Archives of Diseases in Childhood, 59*, 1052–1060.

Wise MG, Ward SC, Townsend-Parchman W, Gillstrap LC, Hauth JC, 1984: Case report of ECT during high-risk pregnancy. *American Journal of Psychiatry, 141*, 99–101.

Wisner K, August 1989: Personal communication.

Zierler S, Rothman KJ, 1985: Congenital heart disease in relation to maternal use of bendectin and other drugs in early pregnancy. *New England Journal of Medicine, 313*, 347–352.

6

Psychotropic Drug-Induced Dysfunction in Children

Michael D. Rancurello, Gary Vallano, and G. Scott Waterman

Virtually every psychotropic agent used in the treatment of adults with major psychiatric disorders has also been used in the treatment of child and adolescent patients. Although anecdotal and nonsystematic treatment trials, preconceptions about the nature of childhood, and historical biases concerning the etiology and classification of child psychiatric disorders represent obstacles to the accumulation of new knowledge, the field has advanced rapidly over the past 15 years. Specific guidelines do exist to assist the practitioner in making rational treatment decisions (Campbell & Spencer, 1988), and a great deal is known about the natural history, epidemiology, and comorbidity of psychiatric disorders in children and adolescents (Garfinkel, Carlson, & Weller, 1990; Last & Hersen, 1990).

This chapter is not meant to be a comprehensive review of pediatric psychopharmacology. Instead, it focuses primarily on the most commonly used agents and their adverse effects with an emphasis on illustrating those problems unique to the management of child and adolescent patients. Stimulants, heterocyclic antidepressants, and lithium are presented in more detail, given their widespread use and status as empirically defensible and symptom-specific treatments for certain disorders. Sedative hypnotics and alternatives to stimulants in the management of children with attention deficit-hyperactivity disorder (e.g., clonidine) are often misused and thus warrant specific mention. Side effects of antipsychotic drugs, mood stabilizers such as carbamazepine, and a variety of less frequently utilized agents including beta-blockers, anticholinergics, hypnotics, antihistamines, and opiate antagonists are either mentioned in passing or not addressed as their use and side effects differ very little from those encountered in adult practice.

Each drug class discussed in this chapter is presented in the context of relevant historical information and clinical indications and nonindications. A premium is placed on describing indications and nonindications, since the recognition and management of adverse drug effects in the pediatric population are inevitably complicated by: (1) errors resulting from the nonspecific use of medication or use in conditions where efficacy has not been demonstrated, (2) misdiagnosis, (3) failure to appreciate the importance of age dependent differences between adults and children in symptom expression and pharmacokinetics, and (d) decisions based on incorrect assumptions about potentially drug-responsive target symptoms.

BACKGROUND INFORMATION

As in adult psychiatry, the history of drug treatment in child and adolescent psychiatry reflects a growing reliance on research to guide clinical practice. Pharmacotherapy has become increasingly specific over time. The theoretical debates over the diagnostic validity of most major disorders and hypotheses that discount symptoms as epiphenomena referable to underlying conflict have given way to more precise descriptions of syndromes and their differential response to specific interventions.

Conditions such as major depression, bipolar disorder, panic disorder, obsessive-compulsive disorder, and others, formerly thought to arise during adulthood, are now recognized as disorders that often first become evident before puberty. Recent findings about natural history, comorbidity, the relationship between family aggregation and age of onset, as well as studies demonstrating significant functional impairment and long-term morbidity in affected individuals, often justify aggressive pharmacological intervention. In addition, the advantages of specific combinations of drug and nondrug treatments for certain disorders are now being identified.

Whether acknowledged explicitly or not, certain durable myths continue to influence clinical decisionmaking about pediatric psychopharmacology:

1. *Drug treatment as a nonspecific intervention of last resort.* Psychosocial treatments for children have historically enjoyed a favored status. They are sometimes viewed as more desirable, humane, and/or comprehensive because they address the causes of symptoms rather than the symptoms themselves. Consequently, pharmacotherapy may become a second class intervention used as a nonspecific last resort for those who either do not improve with psychotherapy or cannot be treated with it. Diagnostic imprecision and lack of information about potentially drug-responsive syndromes compound this problem.

2. *Convenience.* When viewed as a manifestation of social control or as a function of faulty caretaking (i.e., disinterested, poorly motivated teachers; incompetent, noncompassionate patients), objections to drug treatment as a form of chemical restraint and/or punishment are sometimes raised. Failure to appreciate the impact of psychiatrically impaired children on their caretakers and lack of information about the interaction between drug and nondrug treatments compound this problem.

3. *Favored theories of etiology.* Theories that view symptoms as a manifestation of conflict or a response to external, environmental variables alone commonly result in underdiagnosis of potentially drug-responsive disorders. At best, medication may be viewed as a temporary intervention and, at worst, as antithetical to genuinely corrective treatment because it addresses symptoms rather than their hypothesized causes.

4. *One drug-one disorder myth.* Inevitably, whenever a medication appears to be beneficial in a particular psychiatric disorder, the risk of indiscriminate overuse rises. Lack of accurate information about alternative nondrug treatments, the interaction between specific drug and psychosocial interventions, and overzealous diagnosing to justify use of a particular medication may result in widespread exposure of children to unnecessary risk with only marginal hope for benefit. Temporal fads and the "pendulum effect" often influence clinical practice more profoundly than

the dissemination of scientific knowledge, particularly in settings where resources necessary to deliver comprehensive treatment are limited.

DIFFERENCES BETWEEN ADULT PATIENTS AND CHILD/ADOLESCENT PATIENTS

Cognitive, social, psychological, and biological differences between adults and children and adolescents appear so obvious that elaboration is unnecessary. However, the theory and practice of pediatric psychopharmacology are predicated on an explicit understanding of these differences.

Developmental Pharmacokinetics

In practice, child patients are sometimes treated as small adults who require lower doses of medication on the basis of stature and body weight. In reality, they exhibit developmentally mediated differences in drug distribution, metabolism, and excretion distinct from neonates and adults that enable them to tolerate higher weight adjusted doses of pharmacological agents than adults. Pubertal status is often highly relevant.

Because of a reduced capacity for albumin binding and smaller absolute adipose compartment, children often have higher circulating levels of free, unbound drug than adults. Hepatic biotransformation into active metabolites occurs more promptly in children given their greater liver mass to total body mass ratio, resulting in shorter drug half-life, sharper plasma level peaks, and greater exposure to potentially toxic metabolites than is the case for adults. Finally, childhood renal function results in more rapid clearance of drugs excreted by the kidney.

Central Nervous System Development

Neurotransmitter system development affects the phenomenology and age of onset of major psychiatric disorders in ways that are only beginning to be understood. Affect regulation, control of appetite and other neurovegetative functions, sleep, and cognitive indices such as concentration and attention span are examples of developmentally mediated functions central to the assessment and pharmacological management of children and adolescents. For example, stimulants, which generally exert a dose-dependent effect on affective expression resulting in euphoria in adults, only rarely affect prepubertal children the same way. Dysphoria and irritability are more commonly reported when children are treated with high doses of stimulants.

Dependent Status of Children

Children are, by definition, dependent on parents, families, and other adult caretakers. Their status as dependents with limited capacity to judge the risk and benefits of treatment is compounded by the fact that they rarely seek or have primary responsibility for their own treatment. Caretakers must be carefully assessed and thoroughly educated about safety, risk/benefit, starting and stopping medication, and what to do about missed doses.

Unsupervised use of psychotropics and failure to sufficiently educate parents about the hazards of drugs such as heterocyclic antidepressants and lithium are responsible for common but avoidable tragedies such as accidental ingestion and poisoning. Underdosing, resulting in inaccurate assessment of medication effectiveness, and overdosing (with dangerous consequences) can occur when several caretakers share responsibility for supervising administration of medication, expect children to take responsibility themselves, or become confused about changes in dose schedule and/or the strength of each single dose. Medication that can only be monitored safely via ECG, plasma level, or other laboratory measures must never be prescribed if access to such tests cannot be guaranteed. Finally, the use of multiple informants to correctly identify target symptoms and track clinical response and adverse drug effects is mandatory to ensure safe, effective treatment.

STIMULANTS

Introduction

Representative agents

Methylphenidate, dextroamphetamine, and pemoline are generally regarded as the first line of pharmacological intervention for attention deficit-hyperactivity disorder (ADHD). They have also been utilized in the treatment of narcolepsy and in a very limited fashion for depression. These central nervous system (CNS) stimulants are also classified as sympathomimetics with the exception of pemoline, which has only mild sympathomimetic characteristics (Goodman & Gilman, 1985).

Indications

When utilized in the treatment of ADHD, it is recommended that stimulants be combined with other effective interventions such as behavioral therapy within the home and school setting (Barkley, 1981; Pelham & Murphy, 1986). Education of patients, families, and teachers about the disorder; social skills training; and, if necessary, changes in classroom placement represent other useful adjunctive interventions. Since learning disorders are seen in over 50% of children with ADHD, psychoeducational testing should be considered an integral part of the assessment.

Other stimulant compounds such as L-amphetamine, deanol, and caffeine have been tested in clinical trials but are rarely (if ever) prescribed because of a variety of drawbacks including limited efficacy and a broad side effect profile.

Monitoring Efficacy

Inattention, impulsivity, motor overactivity, and problems with rule-governed behavior are the hallmarks of ADHD. Treatment response should be determined by an improvement in these target symptoms. Parent and teacher checklists are invaluable aids in monitoring response. Stimulant medication should always be titrated to a maintenance dose that maximizes improvement in behavioral, academic, and social situations and results in the fewest side effects possible. Although guidelines concerning dose-response characteristics and weight adjusted doses for these drugs are available to help the practitioner, the most effective dose for any particular child must be determined on an individual basis.

Contraindications

One of the few absolute contraindications to the use of stimulant medication is the presence of a thought disorder or psychotic symptoms. Relative contraindications include the coexistence of a tic disorder, pathological anxiety, and any medical condition that may be exacerbated by the sympathomimetic effects of these drugs, especially methylphenidate and dexedrine (Donnelly & Rapaport, 1985). The presence of Tourette's syndrome (TS) or a family history of TS may best be described as conferring an intermediate level of risk between the absolute and relative contraindications mentioned previously. The failure of alternate pharmacological approaches in this situation (e.g., tricyclic antidepressants, clonidine) coupled with an incomplete response to behavioral and other adjunctive interventions at home and in school may justify a carefully monitored trial of stimulants.

Finally, stimulants reportedly interact with several other drug classes causing either changes in their relative concentration, therapeutic efficacy, or side effect profile. These include sedative hypnotics, tricyclic antidepressants, anticoagulants, anticonvulsants, antiinflammatory agents, antipsychotics, and monoamine oxidase inhibitors (MAOIs). The MAOIs are of greatest clinical concern because of the potential for this combination to precipitate hypertensive crises (Cantwell & Carlson, 1978; see also Chapters 3 and 4).

Side Effects

Common Side Effects

The most commonly reported side effects of this drug class are insomnia and anorexia. Weight loss, abdominal discomfort, nausea, and headache are also reported fairly frequently. These side effects tend to be self-limiting after several weeks of stimulant use. Otherwise, a reduction in dose or a change in dose schedule may be required. Changes in dose schedule are commonly made to improve a patient's appetite, reduce nausea and abdominal discomfort, or treat insomnia. This can be accomplished by giving the medication after meals (especially breakfast) or by giving the last dose earlier in the day to avoid insomnia. Other modifications such as sanctioning large (compensatory) bedtime snacks to guarantee adequate caloric intake or altering the child's bedtime schedule to facilitate falling asleep may also prove useful. Affective changes such as moodiness, tearfulness, oversensitivity, and isolation (wanting to be left alone, appearing subdued, losing their "spark") can be among the most distressing side effects to parents and teachers. This necessitates close observation of affect and social interaction during treatment (Klein, Gittelman, Quitkin, & Rifkin, 1980), especially since side effects such as social withdrawal, overfocusing, and blunting of affect may be confused with such desirable drug effects as diminished intrusiveness, a reduction of disruptive behavior, and diminished motor overactivity. Fortunately, such affective changes are generally dose-related and respond promptly either to a reduction of maintenance dose or a change from one stimulant to another. Treatment must be discontinued if depressive symptoms persist or worsen, and alternative pharmacological interventions should be considered.

Occasional Side Effects

Occasionally, other side effects such as drowsiness, dizziness, anxiety, euphoria, and mild elevation in pulse and blood pressure are reported. In general, these side effects are usually time-limited and respond well to a reduction in dose. Abnormal involuntary motor movements (repetitive jaw clenching, lip or cheek biting, picking at the skin around fingernails or on the palmar surfaces of the hands) are occasionally seen when high doses of amphetamine or pemoline are prescribed. Dose reduction or titration with a more gradual progression to most effective dose generally solve this problem.

Rare Side Effects

Rare but serious side effects such as toxic psychosis may occur, but at therapeutic dosages one should question the presence of an underlying thought disorder in the differential; this issue is discussed further in Chapter 17. Allergic and hypersensitivity phenomena occur infrequently and hematological abnormalities such as leukopenia and anemia have been reported. The role of stimulants in the latter is questionable (Dulcan, 1985). Unlike methylphenidate and dexedrine, pemoline has been associated with elevations in liver injury enzymes that require termination of drug treatment (Klein et al., 1980). Baseline measures of serum glutamic-oxaloacetic transaminase (SGOT) and serum glutamic-pyruvic transaminase (SGPT) before beginning pemoline are advisable.

Miscellaneous Side Effects

Tolerance to the stimulants does not appear to be a common difficulty though some decrement in efficacy may develop at higher doses (Winsberg, Matinsky, Kupietz, & Richardson, 1987). The risk of developing a secondary substance abuse disorder based on exposure to stimulants as a treatment for ADHD appears to be low, although it is frequently questioned by parents and teachers who confuse comorbid risk (e.g., ADHD and conduct disorder) with cause and effect. Stimulants, especially amphetamine, may affect rapid eye movement (REM) and stage IV sleep. The effect of stimulants on electroencephalogram (EEG) synchronization is less clear, resulting in conflicting findings (Cantwell & Carlson, 1978). However, there are some reports that stimulants, at doses used to treat ADHD, may have a stabilizing effect on EEG activity (Dulcan, 1985), whereas very high or toxic doses may be destabilizing and tend to lower seizure threshold. It has also been postulated that EEG abnormalities may predict a better response to stimulants (Satterfield, Cantwell, Saul, Lesser, & Podosin, 1973).

Information concerning behavioral rebound is limited. Nonetheless, a small percentage of children treated with stimulants at breakfast and lunch seem to exhibit a clear intensification of preexisting target symptoms in the evening as drug effects wear off (Johnston, Pelham, Hoza, & Sturges, 1988). Clinicians unfamiliar with this escape phenomenon may inadvertently exacerbate the problem by prescribing even larger daytime stimulant doses. Dose reduction or the addition of a late afternoon (or early evening) dose represent more effective corrective strategies.

Relatively few long-term side effects of stimulants have been identified. Probably the most controversial of these is the hypothesized relationship between chronic maintenance on stimulants and inhibited growth velocity. In general, the potential for small annual reductions in growth appears to exist while on stimulants, with dextroamphetamine being implicated more so than methylphenidate or pemoline. Risk appears to be compounded by chronicity of use and higher doses of medication. However, there is ample evidence that growth rebound or compensation occurs in most children exhibiting reduced growth velocity once treatment with stimulants is stopped (Gittelman-Klein & Mannuzza, 1988).

Potential mechanisms to explain reduced growth velocity in response to chronic treatment with stimulant drugs were reviewed by Greenhill (1981) and include the following: (1) stimulants may cause anorexia and weight loss, resulting in compromised nutritional status and growth retardation; (2) stimulants may directly interfere with human growth hormone secretion, resulting in reduction in the rate of growth; (3) stimulants may suppress somatomedin and thus interfere with cartilage synthesis; or (4) stimulants suppress the secretion of prolactin during sleep, ultimately compromising growth rate. Although further clarification is needed, the first two hypotheses appear unlikely based on current information while the latter two appear much more plausible. Close monitoring of height and weight, calculations of change in growth velocity rather than absolute stature alone, the introduction of drug holidays over weekends and during the summer (when appropriate), and the use of the smallest effective dose are generally sufficient. It is always advisable to address this concern directly with parents before initiating treatment with stimulants.

Alternative Drug Treatments

Clonidine, a centrally acting alpha-2 adrenergic agonist, is most noted for its antihypertensive effects. In children, it is most commonly used in the treatment of Tourette's syndrome. In addition, it may be effective in reducing symptoms of ADHD in a subgroup of children. The greatest improvement appears to occur with target symptoms such as motor overactivity and conduct problems (Hunt, Minderaa, & Cohen, 1985). The dose of clonidine used to treat ADHD is 4–5 μg/kg/day on a q.i.d. schedule as reported by Hunt et al. It is also available in a transdermal patch, which may be preferable for some children (Hunt, 1987).

The major side effect of clonidine is sedation with dry mouth, nausea, lightheadedness, sensitivity to bright lights and, at higher doses, hypotension and PR interval prolongation that do not appear significant (Young, Leven, Knott, Leckman, & Cohen, 1985). When withdrawing a patient from clonidine, the potential for rebound hypertension is significant. Therefore, as when initiating therapy, withdrawal of medication should proceed slowly in increments of .05 mg of medication. The use of the transdermal patch formulation has been associated with local skin irritation.

ANTIANXIETY AGENTS

Anxiety

Although many adults consider childhood and adolescence to be carefree periods of life, anxiety during these times is common to the point of ubiquity. As with adults, this creates diagnostic dilemmas. In addition to being a normal emotion during stressful times or events, anxiety also appears as a symptom of a wide variety of disorders. The decision of whether (and how) to treat anxiety in a child or adolescent is complicated not only by the differential diagnosis of anxiety, but also by theoretical questions regarding the appropriateness of anxiety to particular developmental tasks and the possible utility of the experience of anxiety in the accomplishment of those tasks. Nonetheless, most child psychiatrists would agree that prolonged and/or intense anxiety is more likely to impede than to enhance normal development. This, coupled with the significant discomfort associated with chronic or severe anxiety, makes it a worthy target of treatment.

Indications

The specific conditions that would prompt a physician to consider the use of anxiolytic medication in a child or adolescent include overanxious disorder (essentially the child and adolescent equivalent of generalized anxiety disorder, a chronic condition in which anxiety is prominent and bothersome), acute or severe situational anxiety or insomnia, night terrors, separation anxiety disorder (generally with school avoidance or other significant phobic behavior), and panic disorder. Although nonpharmacological approaches to the management of these problems exist and are often effective either independently or as adjuncts to drug therapy, a discussion of them is beyond the scope of this chapter. Also, as discussed elsewhere in this chapter, antidepressant medication may be the pharmacotherapy of choice for some anxiety disorders in this age group.

Evidence for Efficacy

Although the advent of the benzodiazepine anxiolytics has revolutionized the treatment of anxiety in adults, specific information regarding the uses and drawbacks of this class of drugs in children and adolescents is scant. Coffey, Shader, & Greenblatt (1983) have studied the pharmacokinetics of these agents in children, finding that, after 5 months of age, children metabolize diazepam more rapidly than adults. As with some other types of drugs, this may imply that children require larger weight-adjusted doses than adults to achieve comparable effects, although this has not been delineated. The paucity of controlled clinical studies of these compounds in children and adolescents makes statements regarding indications for this use, as well as side effects and toxicities, necessarily tentative.

Side Effects

Based on extensive experience with the use of benzodiazepines for the treatment of anxiety in adults, one might expect the most common side effects encountered in young people to be sedation and motor incoordination, particularly at higher doses. In addition, the possibility that disinhibition of undesirable behaviors may occur with the use of these agents should be kept in mind, despite the fact that no rigorous data are available to determine the risk of this specifically in children and adolescents. Nonetheless, particular caution is necessary when contemplating the use of benzodiazepines in the context of mental retardation, autism, and other evidence of gross brain dysfunction. Whether "paradoxical" behavioral effects are dose-related or are more likely with particular drugs in this class than with others remains to be shown. There is some evidence that high doses and sustained treatment may intensify risk (Gittelman-Klein, 1978).

Theoretical Concerns

Another parameter that deserves particular concern in this age group is cognition. Despite the fact that Simeon and Ferguson (1987) found no significant changes in attention or memory tasks in the patients they treated with alprazolam, the possibility that important adverse effects on learning may occur with these (or any CNS-depressing) agents certainly remains and needs careful study. The practice of prescribing potentially addictive drugs is a topic with political and social overtones that cannot be ignored in our current regulatory atmosphere, particularly when children and adolescents are involved.

HETEROCYCLIC ANTIDEPRESSANTS

Recognition of the existence (and relative frequency) of depressive illnesses in the child and adolescent age group has made information concerning the safe use and potential drawbacks of antidepressant agents in children and adolescents a topic of importance for psychiatrists. Recent advances in the standardization of diagnostic criteria strongly support the validity of depression as a syndrome in childhood carrying a significant enough morbidity to warrant treatment with medication (Puig-Antich, 1981; Puig-Antich & Gittleman, 1982). Although results to date regarding pharmacotherapy of adolescent depression have been discouraging, the existence of an apparent relationship between tricyclic plasma levels and response to treatment in childhood depression suggests a place for this treatment in depressed children.

Indications

Although depression is probably the most common indication for the administration of antidepressant drugs to youngsters, other reported uses include separation anxiety disorder, panic disorder, obsessive-compulsive disorder, eating disorders, and attention-deficit hyperactivity disorder. Another common condition for which antidepressants have enjoyed widespread use is enuresis. The generally self-limited nature of this disorder and the success of nonpharmacological treatments may make this the least reasonable indication among those mentioned for these agents (Rancurello, 1985).

As with all drugs, to understand the literature on antidepressant pharmacotherapy in the pediatric age group, basic principles of pediatric pharmacology must be kept in mind. Children tend to exhibit developmentally dependent differences in how they distribute, metabolize, and excrete drugs. These pharmacokinetic differences may influence dosing schedules, and total daily doses. For instance, the prototypical heterocyclic antidepressant imipramine (IMI) has a halflife that ranges from only 6 to 15 hours in children. On the other hand, because of the reduced capacity for albumin binding and the smaller absolute adipose compartment in children compared to adults, higher circulating levels of free, unbound drug can be expected. When combined with the fact that hepatic biotransformation into active metabolites occurs more promptly in children because of their greater liver mass to total body ratio, there is reason to believe that, with IMI, the risk of exposure to cardiotoxic metabolites such as 2-OH-imipramine may be greater in children than adults (Pollock & Perel, 1989).

Side Effects

The broad categories of side effects encountered with these agents in children and adolescents are the same as for adults, and include anticholinergic effects, cardiovascular effects, and dose-related phenomena encountered in poisoning, among others.

Anticholinergic

In general, central and peripheral anticholinergic side effects are more annoying than serious. They include sedation, blurred vision, dry mouth, drying of bronchial secretions, constipation, and urinary retention. The precipitation of narrow-angle glaucoma, although rare, is serious and requires prompt attention.

Cardiovascular

Cardiovascular side effects are clearly the most serious and potentially treatment-limiting pharmacological actions encountered. Recently, sudden, unexplained cardiac death has been reported in three pubertal children treated with desipramine (Abramowicz, 1990; Geller, 1991; Popper & Elliott, 1990; Riddle et al., 1991). Thus, it is imperative that physicians be thoroughly familiar with the indications, risks, limitations, and safety criteria for the use of cyclic antidepressants in children and adolescents. Virtually all agents marketed in the United States exert a quinidine-like effect that slows conduction time and repolarization, thus prolonging ECG indices such as PR, QRS, QTc, and HV intervals (also see Chapter 23). The overwhelming majority of children maintained on doses greater than or equal to the equivalent of 3.5 mg/kg/day of IMI exhibit a significant prolongation of the PR interval. Those children with the shortest pretreatment PR intervals tend to exhibit the greatest magnitude of change, although it is uncommon to exceed the 0.1 to 0.2 second normal range seen in 5–16 year olds unless unexpected complications such as unusually slow metabolism or hydroxylation defects are encountered. QRS complex widening, although relatively uncommon at doses under 5 mg/kg/day, is likely to be encountered at higher doses. Except in the case of acute toxicity, arrhythmias tend to be suppressed rather than accentuated by these drugs. Riddle et al. (1991) recommend that "an ECG with a rhythm strip obtained at baseline and during medication loading and steady state, with specific emphasis on measurement of the QTc, may be helpful in identifying potentially vulnerable children. It may be contraindicated to administer tricyclic antidepressants to children who have prolonged QTcs at baseline, and it may not be wise to continue medication in any patient whose QTc exceeds 0.425 to 0.450 seconds while on medication."

Similarly, anticholinergic effects on atrioventricular (AV) node firing and refractory time are seen in most children, resulting in a mean increase in resting heart rate of 10 to 20 beats per minute. Although blood pressure commonly drops in a dose-dependent manner in adults, children may exhibit a paradoxical increase in blood pressure. They are also subject to the same idiosyncratic dose-independent orthostatic hypotensive effects seen occasionally in adults.

Initial safety standards proposed by Puig-Antich (1981) have recently been modified based on clinical experience and normative pediatric cardiovascular data (Birmaher, Zuberbuhler, and Beerman, 1991; Ryan, 1990). At this time it appears prudent to observe different safety standards for children younger and older than

10 years of age (Birmaher et al., 1991). In all children and adolescents, the QRS interval should not be permitted to exceed 0.12 seconds or widen more than 50% over baseline, and QTc should be maintained at or below 0.48 seconds. It is important that the manometer used to measure blood pressure be well calibrated, and that the cuff completely encircle the arm while covering approximately 75% of the upper arm between the shoulder and the olecranon. Recommended safety criteria are summarized in Table 1.

Overdose

Toxicity associated with overdose represents a serious danger that is not limited to intentional or accidental drug ingestion (also see Chapter 4). Children with unusually short antidepressant drug half-lives (less than 7 hours) may fail to respond to doses many practitioners consider to be "standard" because their plasma levels are inadequate. In the absence of careful plasma-level monitoring, higher doses may be prescribed and thus expose the child to greater risk. Similarly, those with unusually lengthy halflives (greater than 12 hours) or those with genetically mediated defects in their ability to metabolize these drugs through hydroxylation are at risk and may unintentionally be made toxic on even low or modest doses. Fatalities after the accidental ingestion of IMI, nortriptyline, and amitriptyline have been described (Abramowicz, 1990; Goel & Shanks, 1974; Popper & Elliott, 1990; Saraf, Klein, & Gittleman-Klein, 1974), with most deaths attributed to heart block and/or tachyarrhythmias. Mild symptoms may include drowsiness, restlessness, vomiting, mydriasis, hallucinations, and tachycardia, whereas more serious symptoms range from ataxia, convulsions, and systolic hypertension to coma, hypotension, tachyarrhythmias, and cardiorespiratory arrest. Severe symptoms may be seen in children who have ingested up to 10 mg/kg of amitriptyline and are almost always present when higher doses have been ingested (Steel, O'Duffy, & Brown, 1967).

Miscellaneous

In addition to the untoward effects just noted, several others bear mention. Rapid withdrawal from maintenance doses greater than or equal to 3.5 mg/kg/d of the prototypical agent IMI is likely to be accompanied by uncomfortable flu-like symptoms such as nausea, vomiting, abdominal pain, drowsiness, diminished appetite, tearfulness, apathy, and headache. Cholinergic rebound has been implicated as the most likely cause for this syndrome in children (Law, Petti, & Kazdin, 1981) and has received support in the adult literature. Because these symptoms are rarely encountered when medication is discontinued slowly, it is recommended that

Table 1 Recommended cardiovascular safety criteria for children and adolescents

Cardiovascular indices	Under 10 years old	Over 10 years old
PR interval	≤ 0.18 seconds	≤ 0.20 seconds
QRS interval	≤ 0.12 seconds (≤ 50% over baseline)	Same
Corrected QT (QTc)	≤ 0.48 seconds	Same
Heart rate (resting)	≤ 110 bpm	≤ 100 bpm
Blood pressure (resting)	≤ 140/90 (or 130/85 50% of time over 3 weeks)	150/95 (or 140/85 50% of time over 3 weeks)

children be withdrawn gradually over a 1–2-week period. Finally, there is evidence, although controversial, that tricyclics may precipitate mania in vulnerable or predisposed adults. The applicability of these findings to children is unclear. However, in a group of rigorously diagnosed depressed adolescents, the most statistically significant predictor of early onset bipolar illness was the precipitation of mania by tricyclics (Strober & Carlson, 1982).

MONOAMINE OXIDASE INHIBITORS

Although the monoamine oxidase inhibitors (MAOIs) were the first drugs with specific antidepressant effects to be marketed and formally tested in treatment trials with adults, they have been much less studied than the heterocyclic antidepressants in the pediatric age group. Given the poor response to heterocyclic antidepressants shown by adolescent depressives (in contrast to childhood depressives) studied to date, future research may well point the way toward greater use of MAOIs in adolescence. Reasoning from the finding that young adult depressives more frequently than older adult depressives exhibit the "atypical" features of depression that predict greater efficacy of an MAOI (phenelzine) than (Casper et al., 1985; Liebowitz et al., 1984), Ryan and associates (1988b) have hypothesized that depressed adolescents may respond better to an MAOI than to imipramine. They reported a series of 23 adolescents openly treated with MAOIs alone or in combination with heterocyclic antidepressants for depression. All but two of them had undergone adequate but unsuccessful treatment trials with heterocyclic antidepressants before initiation of MAOI therapy. Seventy percent of these patients had "good" or "fair" responses to this treatment.

Side Effects

Side effects of MAOIs often include orthostatic hypotension, weight gain, and insomnia, although the series of adolescents reported by Ryan et al. (1988b) experienced side effects with approximately the same frequency and intensity as with heterocyclic antidepressants. It is, however, the need to follow a low-tyramine diet to avoid potentially serious hypertensive episodes that causes concern among physicians contemplating the use of MAOIs for their depressed patients (see Chapters 4 and 24). Patients and their families must understand both the diet they must follow and the possible consequences of noncompliance. In addition to accidental or deliberate dietary noncompliance, adolescents who abuse cocaine or amphetamines are at risk for serious reactions if these are taken while on an MAOI. Ryan et al. conclude that, despite the potential relief MAOI treatment may bring, the risks with MAOIs outweigh possible benefits in adolescents who use drugs, are impulsive, or are unreliable or have unreliable families (1988b).

LITHIUM

As previously noted, the recent history of child and adolescent psychiatry has witnessed a growing recognition of depressive disorders in this age group. Similarly, the early onset of bipolar disorder also has received greater attention, although the considerable proportion of bipolar adults who experience their first episode of illness during adolescence (or before) has been known for some time (Carlson, Davenport, & Jamison, 1977; Kraepelin, 1921; Loranger & Levine, 1978).

Indications

Mania (or hypomania) in childhood and adolescence is often treated with lithium salts, in spite of the relative lack of empirical support for this practice, as compared to treatment of the adult form of the condition. As with adults, lithium is also used for prophylaxis against manic or depressive recurrence in youngsters with bipolar disorder.

Although lithium is probably not useful alone as a treatment for acute depressive episodes, it may have an augmenting effect when added to cyclic antidepressants when those agents have provided unsatisfactory results in depressed patients. Paralleling studies with depressed adults, Ryan et al. (1988a) have reported on the use of lithium in augmenting antidepressant response in 14 depressed adolescents whose responses to antidepressant therapy alone were inadequate. In this retrospective chart review, six of the patients showed a good response to this combination treatment. Another clinical use of lithium has been as an "antiaggressive" agent, an indication that apparently may not require on the presence of affective illness to be effective (Jefferson, 1982).

The fact that lithium treatment may benefit a variety of mood and behavioral syndromes in the pediatric age group makes the question of predictability of benefit an important one. Factors that seem to militate in favor of lithium responsiveness include a history of classic manic and depressive episodes, episodic and remitting courses of nonclassic illness marked by affective or aggressive components (Jefferson, 1982), and family history of bipolar disorder or lithium responsiveness (Youngerman & Canino, 1978).

Side Effects

Common/Expected

Mild symptoms, often likely to occur in association with peaks in serum lithium concentration, are common and include tremor, diarrhea, drowsiness, and blurred vision. Polyuria and polydipsia are commonly seen, and nausea following the ingestion of lithium on an empty stomach can be eradicated by taking the drug with meals. Probably because of lithium's effect on intracellular electrolyte balance, cell membrane permeability, and action potential threshold in the heart, sinus node depression can occur, resulting in bradycardia that is reversible after discontinuing the drug. Flattening of T waves may be common but is of little concern, and at toxic blood levels the QT interval can be prolonged.

Metabolic and Endocrine

Metabolic and endocrine side effects of lithium pose more serious problems for use with children. A reduction in circulating thyroid hormone with compensatory hypersecretion of thyroid-stimulating hormone as well as clinical hypothyroidism are commonly observed but tend to be reversible once the drug is withdrawn. Adverse effects on carbohydrate metabolism and a transient increase in cortisol levels have been reported to occur in adults but have not been evaluated in children. Perhaps of even more concern in children who are still growing are reports of hypercalcemia and bone demineralization said to occur in some adults maintained on lithium for long periods of time. This effect on calcium metabolism has been hypothesized to be mediated at the renal level by elevated levels of circulating parathyroid hormone.

Toxicity

Neurotoxicity can be seen in overdoses or accidental poisoning with large doses of lithium. Initial symptoms are exaggerations of the more commonly encounterd mild side effects and include lethargy, nausea, vomiting, diarrhea, and polydipsia. Progression to confusion, ataxia, muscle fasciculation, marked hypoactivity, and diffuse EEG slowing can lead to coma and sometimes death. Severe toxicity may be difficult to manage clinically. Because lithium excretion is regulated by sodium exchange rates in the proximal kidney tubules, any factors that result in sodium wasting (concurrent use of diuretics, low salt diets, fluid loss through perspiration during vigorous exercise) tend to simultaneously increase serum lithium concentration and predispose the individual to potentially toxic side effects. Fatalities have been reported.

Miscellaneous

Miscellaneous side effects include leukocytosis, skin rashes, acne, hair loss, and reversible nephrogenic diabetes insipidus. Another controversy beyond the scope of this chapter is the potentially damaging effect of long-term lithium maintenance on the microanatomy of the kidney, although this worry seems to have been exaggerated in the past (Schou, 1989).

ANTIPSYCHOTICS

Both high- and low-potency antipsychotic medications have been used in the treatment of child and adolescent psychiatric disorders since chlorpromazine was first widely marketed. Low-potency agents such as chlorpromazine and thioridizine were, for many years, overutilized for management of disruptive behavior in children, and mentally retarded children, adolescents, and adults. Although the side effect profile of this drug class is virtually the same when used in the treatment of children, adolescents, and adults, a few critical distinctions are worth making. In addition, more specific agents are now available for the treatment of several disorders and symptom clusters formerly treated with antipsychotic medication, altering the risk/benefit assessment of this drug class in a negative way. Teicher and Glod (1990) have addressed the indications and rational guidelines for the use of the antipsychotic drugs in children and adolescents in an excellent review article.

Accepted indications for the use of antipsychotic medications in child and adolescent patients include acute psychotic symptoms (associated with bipolar disorder, delusional major depression, schizoaffective disorder, schizophreniform and/or schizophrenic disorders, and drug-induced psychotic disorders), Tourette's syndrome, and hyperaggressive behavior disorders refractory to other interventions. Episodic dyscontrol syndromes, borderline personality disorder, and the temporary control of dangerous agitation represent other defensible indications, particularly when other treatments have proved ineffective. Despite the widespread use of low-potency agents (e.g., thioridazine) in the past for the management of anxiety, school refusal, and attention-deficit hyperactivity disorder, more specific pharmacological and nonpharmacological treatments with far fewer side effects are now available. The possible exception to this generalization is the adjunctive use of high-potency antipsychotic medication in hyperaggressive children with attention-deficit hyperactivity disorder who only respond partially to treatment with stimulants (Weizman, Weitz, Szeckly, Tyaho, & Belmaker, 1984). The "reflex" practice of prescribing antipsychotic medication to even moderately disruptive children and adolescents (including those who are mentally retarded and/or autistic) cannot be condoned given the risk of tardive dyskinesia and the adverse effect this drug class has on cognition and learning.

Side Effects

Common Side Effects

As with adults, the most common side effects encountered when children and adolescents are treated with antipsychotic drugs include sedation, fatigue, anticholinergic symptoms, hypotension, weight gain, akathisia, and parkinsonism. Impaired cognition (cognitive blunting and interference with learning) may not be seen more frequently in children than in adults, but obviously represents a more serious threat to "occupational functioning" when one considers the importance of school and social learning during childhood.

Occasional Side Effects

Acute dystonia, tardive dyskinesia, and withdrawal-emergent dyskinesia are also problematic in this age group. Clinical experience prompts most clinicians to consider the risk of acute dystonia, particularly in adolescent patients. However, the risk of tardive dyskinesia is often underestimated given the fact that children are frequently treated with small doses of low-potency antipsychotics. Campbell, Grega, Green, and Bennett (1983) report that 8–51% of juveniles treated with antipsychotic medication over a long period of time will develop dyskinetic movements during treatment, following dose reduction or once antipsychotic maintenance is discontinued. A 30% prevalence rate of dyskinesia was reported in a prospective study of autistic children treated with haloperidol (Campbell, Adams, Perry, Spencer, & Overall, 1988). Although 80% of the affected children had withdrawal-emergent dyskinesia, none developed permanent (irreversible) movement disorders.

Rare Side Effects

All rarely encountered antipsychotic drug side effects reported in adults are also theoretically possible in children and adolescents. Neuroleptic malignant syndrome, agranulocytosis, pigmentary retinopathy, endocrine dysfunction (amenorrhea, galactorrhea, gynecomastia, inhibited orgasm, impotence), photosensitivity, and alteration of the seizure threshold must be considered in this population. Cardiac conduction defects are of most concern with drugs like pimozide, where up to one quarter of adults and children treated for Tourette's syndrome exhibit ECG changes (Young, Leven, Knott, Leckman, & Cohen 1985).

REFERENCES

Abramowicz M, 1990: Sudden death in children treated with a tricyclic antidepressant. *The Medical Letter on Drugs and Therapeutics, 32*(53).

Barkley R, 1981: *Hyperactive children: A handbook for diagnosis and treatment.* New York: Guilford Press.

Beaudry P, Fontaine R, Chouinard G, Annable L, 1986: Clonazepam in the treatment of patients with recurrent panic attacks. *Journal of Clinical Psychiatry, 47*, 83–85.

Biederman J, 1987: Clonazepam in the treatment of pubertal children with panic-like symptoms. *Journal of Clinical Psychiatry, 48*(10, suppl), 38–41.

Birmaher B, Zuberbuhler J, Beerman L, 1991: Revised EKG and blood pressure guidelines for the use of tricyclic antidepressants in children and adolescents. Personal communication and internal document concerning standards of practice, Western Psychiatric Institute and Clinic.

Campbell M, Adams P, Perry R, Spencer EK, Overall JE, 1988. Tardive and withdrawal dyskinesia in autistic children: A prospective study. *Psychopharmacology Bulletin, 24*, 251–255.

Campbell M, Grega DM, Green WH, Bennett WG, 1983. Neuroleptic-induced dyskinesias in children. *Clinical Neuropharmacology, 6*, 207–222.

Campbell M, Spencer EK, 1988: Psychopharmacology in child and adolescent psychiatry: A review of the past five years. *Journal of American Academy of Child and Adolescent Psychiatry, 27*(3), 209–279.

Cantwell D, Carlson G, 1978: Stimulants. In: *Pediatric psychopharmacology: The use of behavior modifying drugs in children,* edited by J Werry. New York: Brunner/Mazel.

Carlson GA, Davenport YB, Jamison K, 1977: A comparison of outcome in adolescent- and late-onset bipolar manic-depressive illness. *American Journal of Psychiatry, 134*, 919–922.

Casper RC, Redmond DE, Katz MM, Schaffer CB, Davis JM, Koslow SH, 1985: Somatic symptoms in primary affective disorder: Presence and relationship to the classification of depression. *Archives of General Psychiatry, 42*, 1098–1104.

Coffey B, Shader RI, Greenblatt DJ, 1983: Pharmacokinetics of benzodiazepines and psychostimulants in children. *Journal of Clinical Psychopharmacology, 3*, 217–225.

Donnelly M, Rapoport J, 1985: Attention deficit disorder. In: *Diagnosis and psychopharmacology of childhood and adolescent disorders,* edited by JM Weiner. New York: Wiley Interscience.

Dulcan M, 1985: The psychopharmacologic treatment of children and adolescents with attention deficit disorder. *Psychiatric Annals, 15*(2), 69–86.

Garfinkle BD, Carlson GA, Weller EB (Eds.), 1990: *Psychiatric disorders in children and adolescents.* Philadelphia: W. B. Sanders.

Geller B, 1991: Clinical comment: Commentary on unexplained deaths of children on Norpramin. *Journal of the American Academy of Child and Adolescent Psychiatry, 30*(4), 682–684.

Gittelman-Klein R, 1978: Psychopharmacological treatment of anxiety disorders, mood disorders, and Tourette's disorder in children. In: *Psychopharmacology: A generation of progress,* edited by MA Lipton, A DiMascio and KF Killam. New York: Raven Press.

Gittelman-Klein R, Mannuzza S, 1988: Hyperactive boys grown up. *Archives of General Psychiatry, 45*(12), 1131–1134.

Goel KM, Shanks RA, 1974: Amitriptyline and imipramine poisoning in children. *British Medical Journal, 1*, 265–275.

Goodman L, Gillman A (Eds.), 1985: *The pharmacologic basis of therapeutics,* 7th edition. New York: MacMillan.

Greenhill L, 1981: Stimulant-related growth inhibition in children: A review. In: *Strategic interventions for hyperactive children,* edited by M Gittelman. New York: M. E. Sharpe.

Hunt R, 1987: Treatment effects of oral and transdermal clonidine in relation to methylphenidate: An open pilot study in ADD-H. *Psychopharmacology Bulletin, 23*(10), 111–114.

Hunt R, Minderaa R, Cohen D, 1985: Clonidine benefits with attention deficit disorders and hyperactivity: Report of a double-blind placebo-crossover therapeutic trial. *Journal of the American Academy of Child and Adolescent Psychiatry, 24*(5), 617–629.

Jefferson JW, 1982: The use of lithium in childhood and adolescence: An overview. *Journal of Clinical Psychiatry, 43*, 174–176.

Johnston C, Pelham W, Hoza J, Sturges J, 1988: Psychostimulant rebound in attention deficit disordered boys. *Journal of the American Academy of Child and Adolescent Psychiatry, 27*(6), 806–810.

Klein D, Gittelman R, Quitkin F, Rifkin A, 1980: Diagnostic and drug treatment of childhood disorders. In: *Diagnosis and drug treatment of psychiatric disorders: Adults and children*, 2nd edition, edited by D. F. Klein. Baltimore: Williams and Wilkins.

Kraepelin E, 1921: *Manic Depressive Insanity and Paranoia*. Edinburgh: E&S Livingstone.

Last CG, Hersen M, 1990: *Handbook of child psychiatric diagnosis*. New York: John Wiley & Sons.

Law W, Petti TA, Kazdin AE, 1981: Withdrawal symptoms after graduated cessation of imipramine in children. *American Journal of Psychiatry, 138*(5), 647–650.

Liebowitz MR, Quitkin FM, Steward JW, McGrath PJ, Harrison W, Rabkin J, Tricamo E, Markowitz JS, Klein DF, 1984: Phenelzine vs. imipramine in atypical depression. A preliminary report. *Archives of General Psychiatry, 41*, 669–677.

Loranger AW, Levine PM, 1978: Age at onset of bipolar affective illness. *Archives of General Psychiatry, 35*, 1345–1348.

Pelham W, Murphy HA, 1986: Attention deficit and conduct disorders. In: Pharmacological and behavioral treatment: *An integrative approach*, edited by M Hersen. New York: Wiley.

Pollock BG, Perel JM, 1989: Hydroxy metabolites of tricyclic antidepressants: Evaluation of relative cardiotoxicity. In: *Clinical Psychopharmacology in Psychiatry*, edited by SG Dahl and LF Gram (pp. 232–236). Springer-Verlag.

Popper CW, Elliott GR, 1990: Sudden death and tricyclic antidepressants: Clinical considerations for children. *Journal of Child and Adolescent Psychopharmacology, 1*(2), 125–132.

Puig-Antich J: Antidepressant treatment in children: Current state of the evidence. In: *Depression and antidepressants: Implications for cause and treatment*, edited by E Friedman, S Gershon, and J Mann. New York: Guilford.

Puig-Antich J, Gittelman R, 1982: Depression in childhood and adolescence. In: *Handbook of affective disorders*, edited by ES Paykel. New York: Guilford.

Puig-Antich J, Perel JM, Lupatkin W, Chambers WJ, Tabrizi MA, King J, Goetz R, Davies M, Stiller RL, 1987: Imipramine in prepubertal major depressive disorders. *Archives of General Psychiatry, 44*, 81–89.

Rancurello MD, 1985: Clinical applications of antidepressant drugs in childhood behavioral and emotional disorders. *Psychiatric Annals, 15*(2), 88–100.

Riddle MA, Nelson CJ, Kleinman CS, Rasmussen A, Leckman JF, King RA, Cohen DJ, 1991: Sudden death in children receiving Norpramin: A review of three reported cases and commentary. *Journal of the American Academy of Child and Adolescent Psychiatry, 30*(1), 104–108.

Ryan ND, 1990: Heterocyclic antidepressants in children and adolescents. *Journal of Child and Adolescent Psychopharmacology, 1*(1), 21–31.

Ryan ND, Meyer V, Dachille S, Mazzie D, Puig-Antich J, 1988a: Lithium antidepressant augmentation in TCA-refractory depression in adolescents. *Journal of the American Academy of Child and Adolescent Psychiatry, 27*, 371–376.

Ryan ND, Puig-Antich J, Rabinovich H, Fried J, Ambrosinia P, Meyer V, Torres D, Dachille S, Mazzie D, 1988b: MAOI treatment of adolescent major depression unresponsive to tricyclic antidepessants: A pilot clinical report. *Journal of the American Academy of Child and Adolescent Psychiatry, 27*, 755–758.

Saraf K, Klein D, Gittelman-Klein R, Groff S, 1974: Imipramine and side effects in children. *Psychopharmacologia, 37*, 265–275.

Satterfield J, Cantwell D, Saul R, Lesser L, Podosin R, 1973: Response to stimulant drug treatment in hyperactive children: Prediction from EEG and neurological findings. *Journal of Autism and Childhood Schizophrenia, 3*(1), 36–48.

Schou M, 1989: Lithium prophylaxis: Myths and realities. *American Journal of Psychiatry, 146*, 573–576.

Simeon JG, Ferguson HB, 1987: Alprazolam effects in children with anxiety disorders. *Canadian Journal of Psychiatry, 32*, 570–574.

Spier SA, Tesar GE, Rosenbaum JF, Woods SD, 1986: Treatment of panic disorder and agoraphobia with clonazepam. *Journal of Clinical Psychiatry, 47*, 238–242.

Steel CM, O'Duffy J, Brown SS, 1967: Clinical effects and treatment of imipramine and amitriptyline in children. *British Medical Journal, 3*, 663–667.

Strober M, Carlson G, 1982: Bipolar illness in adolescents with major depression. *Archives of General Psychiatry, 39*, 549–555.

Teicher MH, Glod CA, 1990: Neuroleptic drugs: Indications and guidelines for their rational use in children and adolescents. *Journal of Child and Adolescent Psychopharmacology, 1*(1), 33–56.

Weizman A, Weitz R, Szeckly GA, Tyano S, Belmaker RH, 1984: Combination of neuroleptic and stimulant treatment in attention deficit disorder with hyperactivity. *Journal of the American Academy of Child Psychiatry, 23*(3), 295–298.

Winsberg B, Matinsky S, Kupietz S, Richardson E, 1987: Is there dose dependent tolerance associated with chronic methylphenidate therapy in hyperactive children: Oral dose and plasma considerations. *Psychopharmacology Bulletin, 23*(1), 107–110.

Young JD, Leven L, Knott P, Leckman J, Cohen D, 1985: Tourette's syndrome and tic disorders. In: *Diagnosis and psychopharmacology of childhood and adolescent disorders,* edited by J Weiner. New York: Wiley Interscience.

Youngerman J, Canino IA, 1978: Lithium carbonate use in children and adolescents: A survey of the literature. *Archives of General Psychiatry, 35,* 216–224.

7

Adverse Drug Effects in the Older Adult

John S. Kennedy

The older adult population, spanning age 55 and greater, often presents a challenge to the physician seeking to treat the patient's psychiatric disorder. Frequent features of the older population that complicate therapy include the accumulating burden of chronic illnesses, which may require multiple medicines. As discussed in Chapter 3, this results in the potential for interactions between medical problems and psychotropic medicines (e.g., hypotension associated with diabetes mellitus and tricyclic antidepressants) and presentation of unexpected drug-drug interactions (e.g., possible interaction between nortriptyline and chlorpropamide producing hypoglycemia) (True, Perry, & Burns, 1987). Other factors that complicate therapy include changes in physiological factors (Table 1), which are often reflected in pharmacokinetic changes (Greenblatt, Abernathy, & Shader, 1986), as well as pharmacodynamic differences (Casteden, George, Marcer, & Hallet, 1977; Meyer et al., 1984; Vestac, Wood, & Shand, 1979; Lawlor et al., 1989; Sunderland et al., 1987). Particularly in the old-old group (often defined as age 80 and above), increasing physical frailty as well as the increased prevalence of cognitive impairments are of special concern. This volume outlines in each of its chapters potential adverse problems that can arise in patients of any age; where appropriate, the risk that aging brings has been emphasized (Table 2). The physician treating the younger patient has the opportunity to prevent many adverse sequelae, such as movement disorders; this is often not the case for the physician attending the older patient who was managed in a less than optimal fashion at a younger age. This chapter focuses on pragmatic issues in the pharmacotherapy of the older population and discusses approaches to reduce the risk of adverse events in the management of the patient seen at maturity.

ASSESSMENT

The older adult patient requires a comprehensive physical assessment before therapy. Detailed review of systems, together with a physical examination, evaluation of the patient's cardiac conduction, and biochemical status, provides a background against which treatment options can be rationally considered (Alessi & Cassel, 1991; Shader & Kennedy, 1989). Psychological assessment is conducted not only to establish the patient's diagnosis and target symptoms but also to ascertain if cognitive impairment is present and to provide an understanding of the patient's attitudes toward medication use. The two former inquiries establish the need for medicines and outcome features to be followed. The two latter inquiries are necessary to estimate and allow anticipation of the likelihood of proper compliance with therapy. Social assessment—including inquiry concerning the availabil-

Table 1 Effects of aging on pharmacokinetic factors

Factor	Effects
Absorption	Decreased number of absorptive cells
	Decrease in some of the active transport processes
	Decrease in gastric acidity and greatly increased prevalence of achlorhydria
	Decrease in intestinal fluid volume, gastric emptying rate, gastrointestinal motility, and blood flow
Distribution	Decreased total body water
	Decreased lean body mass with increased fat to muscle ratio
	Decreased perfusion of tissues from increased cardiac output and decreased hepatic and renal blood flow
	Decreased plasma albumin ratio
Metabolism	Reduced oxidation enzyme activity of some P450 systems
	Reduced hepatic blood flow affecting medicines with high hepatic extraction ratios such as propranolol
Renal excretion	Decreased kidney weight and parenchymal cells
	Decreased renal blood flow and active tubular secretion

ity of regular observers of the patient, transportation, and other resources—assists in determining what therapies can be safely given. Collectively, the assessment of each of these patient domains provides the physician with the necessary under-standing of the likely limits to potential therapy, what therapy should be provided, and how the patients will be monitored after therapy is initiated.

MEDICATION SELECTION

Little available controlled data generally support the indications of safety and efficacy of psychotropic medicines often used specifically for the older adult popu-lation. Few controlled studies have evaluated chronic dosage regimens optimal for treatment of older patients with schizophrenia (Salzman, 1987), anxiety disorders (Shader, Kennedy, & Greenblatt, 1987), and well-characterized subforms of the organic mental disorders (Salzman, 1987; Risse & Barnes, 1986). Relatively few studies have evaluated the relevant antidepressants (Plotkin, Gershon, & Jarvik, 1987). The physician must be cautious when extending information from younger

Table 2 Conditions in which age may be a risk factor for adverse drug effects

Condition	Chapter
Drug-induced parkinsonism	9
Tardive dyskinesia	10
Neuroleptic malignant syndrome (possibly)	11
Akathisia	12
Anticholinergic effects	14
Iatrogenic delirium/psychosis	17
Adverse cognitive and psychomotor effects	18
Benzodiazepine withdrawal	19
Orthostatic hypotension	23
Hyponatremia	27
Psychotropic-induced agranulocytosis	28

patients to older patients. For example, fluoxetine may not be a good first-line treatment for many older patients because of its ability to promote weight loss, inhibition of metabolism of other medicines, apparent increased risk of causing profound hyponatremia in the elderly, and relatively long half-life; the minimum recommended daily adult dosage is 20 mg/day, which is four times greater than is required by many elderly patients. Many of these factors (i.e., weight loss, long half-life, inhibition of concurrent medicines) are often less of a concern in younger patients. Thus, limited available data sets and consequent uncertainty surrounding attempts to predict risk of adverse side effects support the need to be disciplined in following the recommendations discussed in the next five sections.

INITIATING THERAPY

Several benefits support the use of low initial dosages in older patients. These include the reality that many side effects are not dose related and may appear at low dosages. Low initial-dosing regimens also allow more rapid total clearance of the medicine if a problem has emerged early in therapy and reduces the time required to introduce an alternative. Slow and modest increments in dosage provide time to observe the effects of the dose change. This offers the greatest likelihood that if dose-related toxicity emerges and the medicine is discontinued, adverse effects will quickly diminish.

INDIVIDUALIZING REGIMENS

The older adult population is quite heterogeneous in oral-dosing regimens needed for effective therapy. Because of this reality, therapeutic drug-level monitoring of medicines with known therapeutic blood level ranges is often helpful in ascertaining the optimal oral dose. For example, nortriptyline should be monitored by blood levels during dose titration to characterize the adequacy of therapy. This strategy will reveal that some older patients may achieve an adequate level of 50–150 ng/ml with 10 mg given every second day, whereas another seemingly similar patient will tolerate and require more than 100 mg orally, every day. Although sources of such evident variation in pharmacokinetics are not fully understood, some contributing factors are discussed in Chapter 3, and common changes observed in the older adult are outlined in Table 2. For older patients, dosages of most medications that are more than one half the recommended younger adult maximum are not well supported in the literature (Shader & Kennedy, 1989).

IDENTIFYING AND MANAGING SIDE EFFECTS

As is noted throughout this text, many adverse side effects are common to several different classes of psychotropic drugs and many of these are most commonly observed in the older adult. Early identification and management is essential to avoid tragedy. To illustrate the importance of this principle, it is helpful to focus on early identification and management of hypotension.

Hypotension is a very common side effect of psychotropic therapy in the older patient. The management of this problem is discussed in Chapter 23. Hypotension may arise in association with normal changes in the older adult's cardiovascular system and may present as a consequence of drug-drug interactions (Table 3). Nonmanagement of hypotension is a common reason for discontinuing an otherwise good treatment. Failure to identify this problem early on and failure to attempt to manage or discontinue the medicine prolong unnecessary risks for potential sequelae of hypotension. Potential sequelae include falls with hip fracture, myocardial infarction, and ischemic brain injury among other potentially preventable problems.

SUPERVISING PATIENT COMPLIANCE

Inadequate compliance limits the success of therapy in patients of all ages (Sackett & Snow, 1979). Compliance problems may be more frequently a problem of the older adult in association with the expense and potential for confusion associated with requiring multiple medications for multiple medical problems. Four populations of older adults require particularly careful monitoring: (1) the patient who seeks medications from many physicians; (2) the patient who shares medicines with his or her spouse; (3) the patient who lives alone with even very mild cognitive impairment; and (4) the nursing home patient. The needs of the first two groups are often addressed by the assessment process, initiating the appropriate medications and psychological therapy, and having the patient's home cleaned out of all old and unnecessary prescriptions. This may be accomplished by family members, but the physician may have to visit the home to assist in this. Occasionally, this results in the jettisoning of one or two large garbage bags worth of pharmaceuticals. Follow-up of this procedure includes a letter or phone call to the patient's physicians and advice to the involved pharmacies of the discontinuation of the prescriptions. The physician's observance of the patient's response to the medication; frequent visits to the outpatient setting during the initial weeks of therapy; and frank discussion with the patients, spouse, and children about the attendant risk of medication-seeking and sharing of medicines are also important. This is a time-consuming process, not fully reimbursed by most insurers, but necessary to reduce the risk of adverse events.

The third problem patient—the cognitively impaired patient living in the community—requires careful integration of family, friends, and/or available community-based resources into the patient-monitoring process. Under some circumstances, community-based monitoring by paramedical professionals is supported by some insurers. Such attention is essential to ensure patient safety. With this process in place, a simple, consistently structured treatment regimen (such as taking medicines at meal and/or bedtimes, use of a commercial medication-organizing box, and phone calls from members of the patient's support network at predetermined times) is also essential. For many patients with nonprogressive cognitive impairment, a short period of intense monitoring results in training that is sufficient. For other patients, adequate monitoring will reveal if the time has arrived for them to live in a different environment such as an assisted living apartment or even more dependant care.

The final problem patient is found in the nursing home. Misuse of medications in the nursing home setting is a very serious problem (Roberts, 1988). It is not restricted to psychotropic medications; one survey that reviewed over 3,000 patients found that 90% of patients receiving cimetidine were doing so for unjustified

Table 3 Significant potential drug-drug interactions in psychogeriatrics

Interaction	Consequence
Salicylates	
Beta-adrenergic blockers	Decreased antihypertensive action
Hypoglycemics (chlorpropamide)	Large ASA doses may cause hypoglycemia
Lithium	Possible lithium toxicity
Valproate	Possible valproate toxicity
Nonsteroidal antiinflammatory medicines	
Beta blockers	Decreased antihypertensive action
Captopril	Indomethacin-decreased antihypertensive action
Furosemide	Decreased diuretic action and antihypertensive effect
Haloperidol	Possible severe sedation with indomethacin
Potassium	Indomethacin-induced hyperkalemia
Thiazide diuretics	Hyponatremia
Antidepressants: tricyclics	
Clonidine	Decreased antihypertensive effect
Disulfiram	Organic mental disorder
Guanethidine	Decreased antihypertensive effect
Hypoglycemics (chlorpropamide)	Doxepin-induced hypoglycemia
Nitroglycerin (sublingual;	
tolazamide)	Nortriptyline-induced hypoglycemia
Trimethoprim: sulfamethoxazole	Nitroglycerine may not dissolve; loss of antidepressant effect
Antidepressants: nontricyclic	
Tricyclics	Fluoxetine and maprotiline may inhibit metabolism of some tricyclics
Digoxin	Trazodone may increase risk of digoxin toxicity
Phenothiazines	Trazodone combined may produce severe hypotension
Carbamazepine (CBZ)	
Anticoagulants	Prothrombin time decreased
Cimetidine	CBZ levels increased
Desipramine (DMI)	CBZ and DMI levels increased
Diltiazem	Neurotoxicity
Metoclopramide	Neurotoxicity
Theophylline	Theophylline concentration decreased
Thiazide diuretics	Hyponatremia
Verapamil	CBZ levels increased
Beta-adrenergic blockers	
Alcohol	May block signs of delirium tremens
Cimetidine	Decreased beta-adrenergic blocker metabolism
Clonidine	Paradoxical hypertension
Diltiazem	Heart failure
Haloperidol	Profound hypotension
Sulfonylureas	Prolonged hypoglycemia with hypoglycemic overdose
Insulin	Prolonged hypoglycemia with hypoglycemic overdose
Maprotiline	Decreased maprotiline metabolism
Methyldopa	Hypertensive reaction
Nifedipine	Heart failure
Chlorpromazine	Levels increased of both medications
Thioridazine	Thioridazine levels increased
Sympathomimetic bronchlodilators	Decreased bronchodilatation
Theophyllines	Theophylline toxicity
Thiazide diuretics	Cardiac arrhthmias
Verapamil	Heart failure
Lithium	
Methyldopa	Lithium toxicity
Phenytoin	Lithium toxicity
Verapamil	Neurotoxicity, bradycardia

For further details, see Rizack & Martin, 1989; Ciraulo et al., 1989; Griffin & D'arcy, 1984.

reasons (Sherman, Avorn, & Campion, 1987). The simplest approach to resolving this problem is for physicians to follow the patient sent to the nursing home. This is not always practical. Physician contact with the nursing home physician can provide an effective alternative. Physicians send patients to nursing homes with a prescription order for *use as needed,* 50% of the time (Roberts, 1988). In the context of long-term care, relationships emerge between patient and institutional care personnel that reflect the breadth of complexity of all human relationships. Although exceptions exist, most nurses aids receive limited, if any, mental health education and know less about the issues in long-term care relationships than about medicines. It is not difficult to understand that the physician who consistently makes treatment decisions by relying on information primarily derived from such well-meaning but undereducated caregivers is unlikely to be able to make the most informed treatment decisions.

In an initial attempt to address the misuse of and excess use of psychotropic medicines in the long-term care setting, the U.S. Health Care Financing Administration (HCFA) has published rules for surveyors to use. These are paraphrased in Tables 4–7. The exact rules may be obtained from your local community department of health and are described in *State Operations Manual,* HCFA publication

Table 4   Guide to identifying potential drug therapy problems in the elderly (HCFA)

Type	Potential problem
General	Multiple orders of the same drug (by different brand names) for the same patient by the same route of administration.
	Medications administered regardless of established stop-order policies.
	PRN medication orders administered as directed everyday for more than 30 days.
Hypnotic anxiolytic therapy	Continuous use of hypnotics in Table 7 for more than 30 days.
	Use of two or more hypnotics in Table 7 at the same time or in excess of the listed maximum dose.
	Use of anxiolytic drugs in dosages over maximum in Table 7.
Antidepressant therapy	More than two changes of an antidepressant within a 7-day period.
	Use of an antidepressant for less than 3 days.
	Use in excess of daily maximum dosage of antidepressant drugs listed in Table 7.
Antipsychotic therapy	Use of antipsychotic medications for more than 3 days (exception: compazine used as an antinauseant).
	Use of two or more of the antipsychotics listed in Table 7 at the same time.
	Use of antipsychotic medications in excess of the listed maximum daily dosage.
	Use of the antipsychotic drugs in the absence of gradual dose reduction attempts every 6 months after therapy is started, unless the dose has already been reduced to the lowest possible dose to control symptoms.
	Use of PRN antipsychotic drugs more than five times in any 7-day period without a physician review of the patient.
	Use of an antipsychotic drug in the absence of documentation in the medical record of one of the specific conditions outlined in Table 5.
	Use of an antipsychotic when one or more of the behaviors listed in Table 6 is the only indication for its use.

Table 5 Specific conditions approved for antipsychotic usage (HCFA)

Type of disorder	
Schizophrenia	Atypical psychoses
Schizophreniform disorder	Delusional disorder
Schizoaffective disorder	Psychotic mood disorder
Acute psychotic episode	Tourette's syndrome
Brief reactive psychosis	Huntington's disease

Organic mental disorders

With psychoses and/or agitated features as defined by:

Documentation on the medical chart of specific behaviors that have been quantified as to number of episodes and that cause the patient to present as a danger to themselves or others (including staff) or interferes with staff's ability to provide care.

Continuous crying out, screaming, yelling or pacing—if these specific behaviors cause an impairment in functional capacity and if their length of time has been documented.

Psychotic symptoms (hallucinations, paranoia, delusions) not exhibited as specific behaviors (see above), if these behaviors cause an impairment in functional capacity.

no. 7 (through rev. 179). In reviewing Table 7, it should be apparent that the dosage guides are not a guide establishing an optimal standard of practice in the older adult population. For example, the effects of giving 800 mg of chlorpromazine per day to a psychotic Alzheimer's patient invites the patient's rapid demise although this dosage may, on occasion, be required to effectively treat a severely disturbed older patient with schizophrenia.

NEW TREATMENTS

Trials of new treatment should be avoided in an older patient, unless they have been established in younger patients or a second opinion has confirmed their appropriateness. This requirement is probably the most difficult to follow and is a usual result of a patient not responding well to attempted therapeutic regimens. The academic literature is filled with single case letters and reports of patients who "respond" to novel therapeutic approaches. Such approaches are often later tried by other physicians and found wanting—either because of lack of efficacy or untoward effects. Burdened by an illness appearing to require novel therapy, and a higher average risk of adverse effects of medications, most such older patients require hospitalization, careful observation, and diagnoses. This is then usually

Table 6 Behaviors that in isolation are not an indication for antipsychotic medication (HCFA)

Type of behavior	
Wandering	Insomnia
Poor self-care	Unsociability
Restlessness	Indifference to surroundings
Impaired memory	Fidgeting
Anxiety	Nervousness
Depression	Uncooperativeness
Unspecified agitation	

Table 7 Recommended maximum dosages of psychotropic medications used in
long-term care in the United States: patients age 65 and older (HCFA)

Drug	Max. dosage	
Hypnotics (usual maximum *single* dosages)		
Amobarbital	165	mg
Butabarbital	100	mg
Pentobarbital	100	mg
Secobarbital	100	mg
Ethchlorvynol	500	mg
Glutethimide	500	mg
Methyprylon	200	mg
Flurazepam	15	mg
Temazepam	15	mg
Triazolam	0.25	mg
Chloral hydrate	750	mg
Anxiolytics (usual maximum *daily* dosages)		
Alprazolam	2	mg
Chlordiazepoxide	40	mg
Clorazepate	30	mg
Diazepam	20	mg
Halazepam	80	mg
Lorazepam	3	mg
Oxazepam	60	mg
Prazepam	30	mg
Meprobamate	600	mg
Antidepressants (usual maximum *daily* dosage)		
Amitriptyline	150	mg
Amoxapine	200	mg
Desipramine	150	mg
Doxepin	150	mg
Maprotiline	150	mg
Nortriptyline	75	mg
Protriptyline	30	mg
Trazodone	300	mg
Trimipramine	150	mg
Antipsychotics (usual maximum *daily* dosage)		
Acetophenazine	150	mg
Butaperazine	80	mg
Chlorpromazine	800	mg
Chlorprothixene	800	mg
Fluphenazine	20	mg
Haloperidol	50	mg
Loxapine	125	mg
Mesoridazine	250	mg
Moloxidone	112	mg
Perphenazine	32	mg
Piperacetazine	80	mg
Thiothixene	30	mg
Trifluoperazine	40	mg
Triflupromazine	100	mg

followed later with well-considered conventional treatment. In the circumstance that a patient is not improved, a phone call to the author of the report of the novel intervention will often reveal its current value and the appropriateness of the patient for such an approach.

REFERENCES

Alessi CA, Cassel CK, 1991: Medical evaluation and common medical problems. In: *Comprehensive review of geriatric psychiatry,* edited by J Sadavoy, LW Lazarus, LF Jarvik. Washington, DC: American Psychiatric Press, Washington DC.

Casteden CM, George CF, Marcer D, Hallett C, 1977: Increased sensitivity to nitrazepam in old age. *British Medical Journal, 1,* 10–12.

Ciraulo DA, Shader RI, Greenblatt DJ, Greelman W, 1989: *Drug interactions in psychiatry.* Baltimore: Williams and Wilkins.

Greenblatt DJ, Abernathy DR, Shader RI, 1986: Pharmacokinetic aspects of drug therapy in the elderly. *Therapeutic Drug Monitoring, 8,* 249.

Griffin JP, D'arcy PF, 1984: *A manual of adverse drug interactions.* 3rd edition. Bristol: John Wright & Sons.

Lawlor BA, Sunderland T, Hill J, Mellow AM, Molchan SE, Mueller EA, Jacobsen FM, Murphy DL, 1989: Evidence for a decline with age in behavioral responsivity and the serotonin agonist m-chlorophenylpiperazine in healthy human subjects. *Psychiatry Research, 29,* 1–10.

Meyer BR, Lewin M, Dreyer DE, Pasmantier M, Lonski L, Reidenberg MM, 1984: Optimizing metoclopramide control of cisplatin induced emesis. *Annals of Internal Medicine, 100,* 393–395.

Plotkin DA, Gershon SC, Jarvik LF, 1987: Antidepressant drug treatment in the elderly. In: *Psychopharmacology,* edited by HY Meltzer. New York: Raven Press.

Risse SC, Barnes R, 1986: Pharmacologic treatment of agitation associated with dementia. *Journal of the American Geriatric Society, 34,* 368–376.

Rizack MA, Hillman CDM, 1989: *Handbook of adverse drug interactions.* New Rochelle, New York: The Medical Letter.

Roberts PA, 1988: Extent of medication use in long term care facilities. *American Journal of Hospitals and Pharmacies, 45,* 93–100.

Sackett KL, Snow JC, 1979: The magnitude of compliance and noncompliance. In: *Compliance in health care,* edited by RB Haynes, DW Taylor, DG Sackett. Baltimore: John Hopkins University Press.

Salzman C, 1987: Treatment of agitation in the elderly. In: *Psychopharmacology, generation of progress,* edited by HY Meltzer. New York: Raven Press.

Shader RI, Kennedy JS, 1989: Geriatric psychiatry: biological treatments. In: *Comprehensive textbook of psychiatry,* 5th edition, edited by HI Kaplan, BJ Sadock. Baltimore: Williams and Wilkins.

Shader RI, Kennedy JS, Grennblatt DJ, 1987: Treatment of anxiety in the elderly. In: *Psychopharmacology, the third generation of progress,* edited by HY Meltzer. New York: Raven Press.

Sherman DS, Avorn J, Campion EW, 1987: Cimetidine use in nursing homes: Prolonged therapy and excessive doses. *Journal of the American Geriatric Society, 35,* 1023–1027.

Sunderland T, Tariot PN, Cohen RM, Weingartner H, Mueller EA, Murphy DL, 1987: Anticholinergic sensitivity in patients with dementia of the alzheimer type and age-matched controls: a dose response study. *Archives of General Psychiatry, 44,* 418–426.

True Bl, Perry PJ, Burns EA, 1987: Profound hypoglycemia with the addition of a tricyclic antidepressant to maintenance sulfonylurea therapy. *American Journal of Psychiatry, 144,* 1220.

Vestal RE, Wood AJJ, Shand DG, 1979: Reduced beta adrenoreceptor sensitivity in the elderly. *Journal of Clinical Pharmacology and Therapeutics, 26,* 181–186.

Concluding Remarks

Adverse drug reactions are quite common in psychiatric practice and may be predictable or idiosyncratic and unpredictable. In many cases, it is possible to minimize or avoid significant adverse drug reactions by adhering to principles of wise prescribing: (1) ensure that the patient is comprehensively understood before treatment initiation; (2) offer an individualized treatment approach that is tailored to the patient's overall needs and conducted therapy in the setting of a good therapeutic alliance; (3) educate the patient (and, where appropriate, significant others) regarding the proposed treatment and the alternatives, as well as their risk and benefits; (4) choose the optimal treatment to be given for the indications; (5) monitor therapy to ensure compliance and to detect adverse occurrences early; (6) avoid unnecessary polypharmacy; (7) familiarize yourself with pharmacology of the drug being prescribed; (8) be alert to the potential for new drug reactions; and (9) be attentive to the patient's input into his or her treatment's both beneficial and adverse effects.

Legal Issues

Adverse effects of psychotropic agents and electroconvulsive therapy are a frequent cause for malpractice liability. The criteria for liability include the existence of a duty, deviance from standard practice, and direct damage as a result of the deviant practice. In psychopharmacology, liability could ensue from wrongful diagnosis, wrongful treatment indications, failure to diagnose and/or monitor adverse drug reactions, and failure to provide adequate informed consent. Treatment refusal is another problematic issue and needs skillful therapeutic management.

Drug Interactions

Improved and more rational pharmacotherapy is sometimes possible by concurrent administration of more than one drug. Such practice, unless used judiciously, may lead to adverse interactions; these may arise by either pharmacokinetic or pharmacodynamic mechanisms or both. Determining the nature and associated clinical significance of known drug-drug interactions is important in choosing how the patient is to be optimally managed.

Psychotropic Drug Overdose

Psychotropic drugs are among the most frequent drugs used in overdose attempts. Lithium and tricyclic agents are among the more lethal agents. Prompt, early recognition and intensive management of the overdose based on sound pharmacological principles can help in minimizing fatalities and residual morbidity in the majority of cases. Prompt diagnosis requires a careful history, knowledge of toxic syndromes, and examination for telltale signs of specific overdose effects. Simple blood tests (e.g., serum lithium) may be confirmatory. Treatment of drug poisoning requires immediate symptomatic therapy and life supports, termination of exposure and removal of poison from the body, and, in select cases, administration of antidotes.

Teratogenicity

Reliable data on possible effects of psychotropic drugs on fetal development are still limited. However, there is evidence that lithium causes adverse effects on fetal development and should be avoided in the first trimester. Carbamazepine, which could have possible effects on intrauterine growth as well, should also be avoided. In deciding to treat a pregnant woman pharmacologically, all data about her case should be assessed and a risk benefit analysis be done, leading to an appropriate choice of treatment.

Adverse Drug Effects in Children and the Elderly

The practice of pediatric psychopharmacology requires a good understanding of cognitive, social, developmental, and biological differences between children and adults. These differences have pharmacokinetic and pharmacodynamic implications and therefore affect the prescribing practices of psychotherapeutic drugs, as well as the side effects profile. The recognition and management of adverse drug effects in children are complicated by erroneous prescribing practices, misdiagnosis, failure to appreciate developmental differences in symptom patterns and drug responses, and decisions based on false assumptions about pediatric psychopharmacotherapy.

Similar issues are involved in psychopharmacological practice with the other extreme of age (i.e., the older adult). Features of this heterogeneous population that complicate therapy include coexistence of multiple medical illnesses; coadministration of multiple medications; age-related physiological changes affecting pharmacokinetics and pharmacodynamics. Comprehensive medical and psychosocial assessment, use of smaller dosages, appropriate choice of therapeutic agents, individualization of treatment regimen, and close monitoring of patient compliance are all necessary for rational pharmacotherapy in the elderly.

II

DRUG-INDUCED
NEUROPSYCHIATRIC
SYNDROMES

This section aims to review the potential adverse neuropsychiatric effects of psychotherapeutic drugs. Prominent among neurological complications are the extrapyramidal effects of antipsychotic drugs. The acute extrapyramidal syndromes (i.e., dystonia and parkinsonism) are initially reviewed; this is followed by reviews of longer term and serious extrapyramidal complications (i.e., tardive dyskinesia and neuroleptic malignant syndrome). Akathisia and a phenomenologically similar syndrome—jitteriness induced by tricyclic antidepressants—are reviewed next.

Psychotherapeutic drugs may also cause psychiatric dysfunction encompassing affective, psychotic, and adverse cognitive reactions. These are reviewed with emphasis on principles of their diagnosis, prevention, and management. Anticholinergic antiparkinsonism drugs are associated with cognitive, affective, and psychotic disturbances. Because of this wide range and unique constellation of adverse effects, the authors have chosen to discuss this as a separate chapter. Likewise, the diverse cognitive, affective, and systemic complications of electroconvulsive treatment are also discussed separately.

8

Drug-Induced Dystonias

Sandra Steingard

Extrapyramidal symptoms are well-known side effects of antipsychotic medications. Until recently, the occurrence of movement disorders, such as cataplexy, in rats exposed to these medications was used as a marker for potential antipsychotic efficacy. Drug-induced extrapyramidal syndromes are commonly divided into acute, persistent, and tardive types (Table 1). Dystonia refers to the sustained spasm or twisting of one or more muscle groups. This chapter will discuss acute and tardive forms of dystonia.

EPIDEMIOLOGY

In one study that evaluated 352 chronically hospitalized psychiatric patients, 1.5% were found to have dystonia (Friedman, Kucharski, & Wagner, 1987). This is in contrast to an estimated overall prevalence of dystonia in the U.S. population of 0.3 per 100,000. Of the cases they identified, 4 were male and 1 was female; 3 had subnormal intellects and 2 had received electroconvulsive therapy. Yassa, Nair, and Dimitry (1986) evaluated 351 chronic antipsychotic-treated psychiatric patients for the presence of dystonic movements. Patients were more carefully screened to rule out other causes of dystonia than in the former study. Yassa et al. found a 2% prevalence of dystonia, without any significant difference between sexes. In these 7 patients, 5 had other signs of tardive dyskinesia.

In a series of articles, Burke and colleagues have reported on a total of 93 patients who they had evaluated and treated (Burke et al., 1982; Burke and Kang, 1988; Kang, Burke, & Fahn, 1986). They also reviewed 15 other cases of tardive dystonia reported in the literature before 1982. This collection forms the most comprehensive clinical review of this class of patients. The age range of the patients was 5 to 89 years. In contrast to traditional tardive dyskinesia, in which the elderly and women are at greatest risk, young *and* older patients tended to be equally at risk for development of tardive dystonia. Although there was no statistically significant difference between the sexes, more men than women were affected and the males had an earlier age of onset (34 years versus 44 years). Cranial and neck regions were the most frequently affected body parts (83% of patients had involvement of these regions). Retrocollis was the single most common dystonia (49%). At onset, 61% of patients had focal dystonia, 38% segmental, and 1.6% generalized. In contrast to idiopathic torsion dystonia (Chapter 10), the legs or trunk were never affected in the absence of neck or cranial involvement. Generalized dystonia tended to be seen in younger patients. The time period for which patients were exposed to antipsychotics before developing dystonia ranged from 3 days to 37.5 years. All classes of antipsychotic medication were implicated. It was uncommon for patients to have had acute dystonic reactions during the earlier course of treatment. In the study by Kang, Burke, and Fahn (1988) of 67 patients, over half had evidence of oral-lingual-buccal tardive dyskinesia. Multiple psychiatric syndromes, including schizophrenia, depression, hyperemesis gravidarum, anxiety, and "aggressive disorder," were represented. Singh and Jankovic (1988) have reported two patients with Tourette's disorder who developed sustained dystonic movements after being treated with antipsychotic medications.

PATHOPHYSIOLOGY

Acute Dystonia

The etiology of dystonia is not clearly established. However, several hypotheses have been proposed. Most theories are concerned with dopamine (DA) and acetylcholine (ACh) imbalances in the basal ganglia. A relative decrease in DA as compared to ACh is believed to cause hypokinetic movement disorders. The most classic example of this is idiopathic Parkinson's disease in which there is a degeneration of the DA-containing neurons in the substantia nigra. On the other hand, the hyperkinetic movement disorders are thought to result from a relative excess of DA in comparison to ACh.

Marsden and Jenner (1980) and Rupnick et al. (1986) in thorough reviews of their own and others' work, have discussed alternative theories. They suggest that, paradoxically, acute dystonia may occur as a result of a relative increase in dopamine. Their argument is based on the fact that shortly after receiving antipsychotics, there is an increase in dopamine turnover. In studies on rats who have received a single dose of butaperazine, a phenothiazine antipsychotic, they followed the course of apomorphine-induced stereotypy and striatal concentrations of dopamine, homovanillic acid (HVA), and dihydroxyphenylacetic acid (DOPAC). This allowed them to compare dopamine receptor sensitivity and dopamine turnover. Initially there was a complete absence of apomorphine-induced stereotypy. At 24 hours, however, stereotypy was normally observed, whereas HVA and DOPAC levels were still elevated. They interpreted this to mean that there is a point at which postsynaptic receptor blockade has diminished but dopamine turnover is still increased. The time course for these events parallels the time course in which acute dystonic movements are typically seen. They also point out that the effectiveness of anticholinergics, along with other preclinical data, suggests that excessive cholinergic activity is also involved. Dystonia appears shortly after beginning antipsychotic medications that are well known to be potent DA receptor antagonists. These symptoms respond promptly to treatment with anticholinergics agents. The most common explanation for these symptoms is that they are caused by a relative deficiency of dopamine and a relative excess of acetylcholine (Stahl & Berger, 1982). Garver et al. (1976a, b) studied the relationship between the pharmacokinetics of butaperazine and the occurrence of acute dystonia. They found that although red blood cell and plasma levels peaked 2 to 8 hours after a single 40-mg oral dose, dystonic reactions did not occur for at least 23 hours when levels were about 20% of their peak values. They suggest that the dystonia occurs when the concentration of drug has fallen below the level necessary to block ACh receptors but is still high enough to block DA receptors.

Tardive Dystonia

There is no consensus on whether the pathophysiology of tardive dystonia is related to acute dystonia, tardive dyskinesia, or alternatively is distinct from both of these movement disorders. The dominant theory of the pathophysiology of tardive dyskinesia suggests that the movement disorder is caused by supersensitivity of postsynaptic dopamine receptors that develops after prolonged exposure to antipsychotic drugs (Tarsy & Baldessarini, 1970). If supersensitivity does occur, then drugs that deplete presynaptic DA stores should lead to improvement of symptoms. On the other hand, anticholinergic agents should exacerbate symptoms. If tardive dystonia has the same pathophysiology as acute dystonia, then anticholinergic drugs would be expected to improve the condition. Both of these strategies have been used in treatment and pharmacological probe studies. The response of tardive dystonia to various pharmacological strategies is not completely consistent with any theory. For instance, in one study (Lieberman, Pollack, Lesser, & Kane, 1988) 15 patients with tardive movement disorders were treated with single doses of each of the following types of drug: a DA agonist (bromocriptine), a DA antagonist (haloperiodol), an ACh agonist (physostigmine), and an ACh antagonist (benztropine). According to the DA supersensitivity theory, one would predict that the DA agonist and ACh antagonist would worsen tardive dystonia and the DA antagonist and ACh agonist would improve it. They did not find any consistent effects of the medications when they analyzed the results of all 15 patients.

When they analyzed the results of the patients according to whether they had predominantly choreoathetoid versus dystonic movements in the neck and trunk regions, the nondystonic groups ($N = 10$), consistent with the DA supersensitivity theory, worsened with the DA agonist and improved with the DA antagonist. However, the movements also worsened with the cholinergic agonist, in contradiction to the theory. The dystonic group ($N = 5$) tended to improve with both the cholinergic agonist and antagonist, but these changes were not significant. They had minimal response to the DA agonist and antagonist. The marked heterogeneity of response was seen not only among patients but also within individuals. A given patient might have different patterns of response in different body regions. Although there was a suggestion that choreoathetoid tardive dyskinesia may be pathophysiologically distinct from tardive dystonia, the difference did not consistently support either the DA supersensitivity theory or its opposite for either of these disorders.

Dystonia/Dyskinesia and Mood Disorders

Another interesting aspect of tardive dystonia refers to the observations of this movement disorder occurring in cyclical pattern in patients with affective disorders. Praveena, Saxena, & Mohan (1988) report the case of a 44-year-old man in whom manic episodes alternated with periods of dystonic movements. Kwentus, Schultz, and Hart (1984) describe a 52-year-old woman whose dystonic movement disorder first occurred when she was depressed. Treatment with electroconvulsive therapy improved both the mood and movement disorders. Previously, Cutler, Post, Rey, & Bunney (1981) had described 2 patients in whom choreoathetoid tardive dyskinesia became significantly worse during periods of depression and improved during periods of mania. Keshavan and Goswamy (1983) described a patient in whom the opposite phenomenon occurred. These cases suggest that there is some relationship between the pathophysiology of mood disorders and both tardive dystonic and dyskinetic movement disorders. However, the nature of this relationship remains unclear.

CLINICAL DESCRIPTION

The areas of the body that can be involved in dystonia include the ocular muscles (oculogyric crisis), neck (torticollis), facial and laryngeal muscles, and muscles in the extremities and about the spine. Dystonia can be painful and frightening to the patient. When persistent, dystonia can be associated with hypertrophy of the involved muscles.

Acute Form

The acute forms of antipsychotic-induced dystonias are well recognized. They typically begin 24 to 72 hours after the medications are begun (Gardos, 1981). They have been estimated to occur in anywhere from 10–94% of patients exposed to these medications, and they are more typically associated with high-potency antipsychotics (Swett, 1975; Arana, 1988). When the acute forms involve the laryngeal muscles, their spasms can lead to respiratory obstruction and potentially death (Flaherty & Lahmeyer, 1978; Menuck, 1981). Fortunately, as will be discussed later, acute dystonias rapidly respond to treatment.

Acute dystonias occur more commonly in younger, male patients (Swett, 1975; Keepers et al., 1983). Although most commonly seen early in treatment, they may occur later. Patients who have other tardive movement disorders are not immune from developing acute dystonia (Gardos, 1981; Nasrallah, Pappas, & Crowe, 1980; Munetz, 1980). Late-onset "acute" dystonia differs from tardive dystonia in its rapid onset and response to treatment in the manner that earlier occurring acute dystonias do.

Table 1 Acute and tardive dystonias: Clinical characteristics

	Acute dystonia	Tardive dystonia
Description	Sustained spasm or twisting of or more muscles in groups; frequently painful	Slow twisting movements; frequently associated with choreoathetoid movements
Areas involved	Ocular, neck, facial, laryngeal muscles, extremities, spine	Limbs, trunk, neck, or face
Prevalence	10–94% of patients exposed to antipsychotics	1.5–2.0% of patients exposed to antipsychotics
Onset	24 to 72 hours after exposure to antipsychotics	Days to years after exposure to antipsychotics
Risk factors	Young males	Males > females; all ages
Treatment	Dramatic response to benztropine or diphenhydramine	Generally unsatisfactory response (Table 3)

Tardive Forms

Less well recognized are the late occurring forms of dystonic movement disorders that occur in patients who have been chronically exposed to antipsychotic medications. Several recent reviews have clearly documented their occurrence (Burke et al., 1982; Burke & Kang, 1988; Kang et al., 1988; Yassa et al., 1986; Friedman, Kuchersky, & Wagner, 1987). Dystonic movements occur less commonly than the well-recognized choreoathetoid tardive disorders. It has therefore been difficult to collect rigorous epidemiological data that would clarify the relationship between tardive dystonia and antipsychotic exposure (Kang et al., 1988). Nevertheless, many clinicians who work with these patients have come to recognize dystonia as an important form of tardive dyskinesia (Kang et al., 1988). Unlike acute dystonias, the tardive form is more likely to be persistently disabling.

Tardive dystonic movements are typically slow, twisting movements that involve the limbs, trunk, neck, or face (Burke et al., 1982). The sustained nature of these movements renders them more disabling than other forms of tardive dyskinesia.

Dystonia Variants

There are two syndromes that have received particular attention in the literature and are worth mentioning here. In the Pisa syndrome, there is a tonic flexion and rotation of the trunk, resulting in a posture resembling the Pisa Tower. This has been described as occurring as both an acute (Ekbom, 1972) and tardive (Guy, Raps, & Assad, 1986; Saxena, 1986; Yassa, 1985) syndrome. This is most likely a subtype of acute and chronic dystonia.

Meige's syndrome was originally described as an idiopathic disorder manifested by blepharospasm and oromandibular dystonia. There have been several reports of this syndrome occurring in patients who have been exposed to antipsychotics, raising the question of whether this is a drug-induced tardive dystonia variant (Ananth, Edelmuth, & Dargan, 1988; Glazer, Moore, & Hansen, 1983; Weiner, Nauseida, & Glantz, 1981). Because of the small numbers of patients involved, it remains impossible to establish whether this is a coincidental occurrence, a variant of tardive dystonia, or a distinct entity that is, nevertheless, related to antipsychotic exposure. This condition is further discussed in Chapter 10.

DIAGNOSIS

The diagnosis of acute dystonia is straightforward. The occurrence of the characteristic spasms after exposure to an antipsychotic agent and the rapid response to anticholinergic medication are adequate to confirm the diagnosis.

When the movements occur after prolonged exposure to antipsychotic medications and they do not improve with anticholinergic medication, then alternative diagnoses must be considered. There are numerous disorders that can produce dystonic movements (Table 2). Many of these can be ruled out with a careful history and physical examination. These include Huntington's chorea, Wilson's disease, Hallervorden-Spatz disease, intracranial mass lesions, cerebral lipido-

Table 2 Differential diagnosis of dystonias

Hereditary	Sporadic	Toxins
Idiopathic torsion dystonia (dystonia musculorum deformans)	Intracranial mass lesions	Manganese
	Postencephalitic parkinsonism	Carbon disulfide
Wilson's disease	Spasmodic torticollis	Carbon monoxide
Hallervorden-Spatz disease	Retrocollis	
Huntington's chorea	Writer's cramp	
Cerebral lipidoses	Meige's syndrome	
Fahr's syndrome	Perinatal injury	
	Hysterical movement disorders	

sis, and idiopathic torsion dystonia (also see Chapter 10). Because several of these disorders are familial, it is important to obtain a careful family history.

Phenomenologically, tardive dystonic movements do not distinguish these patients from those with idiopathic torsion dystonia (dystonia musculorum deformans). However, in the latter disorder, movements often begin in the limbs, and the legs and trunk can be involved without involvement of the face. As noted earlier, the face and neck are most commonly involved in tardive dystonia. In addition, the movements tend to be more disabling (Burke et al., 1982) in idiopathic torsion dystonia.

Additional studies should include serum ceruloplasmin, tests of liver function, and slit-lamp ophthalmological examination to look for Kayser Fleischer rings, all of which are associated with Wilson's disease. Patients may also require a computed tomography or magnetic resonance imaging scan, particularly if there are other neurological findings.

TREATMENT

Acute Dystonia

The treatment of acute dystonia is also straightforward (Baldessarini, 1977; Schatzberg & Cole, 1986). It responds quickly to anticholinergic agents such as diphenhydramine 25 or 50 mg, benztropine 2 mg, biperiden 2 mg, trihexyphenidyl 5 mg, and procyclidine 5 mg. Diphenhydramine and biperiden are available for intravenous and intramuscular administration. Benztropine is available for intramuscular administration. When the acute dystonia is severe, the drugs should be administered intravenously or intramuscularly. The onset of action is within minutes when it is given via these routes. Diazepam has also been reported to be effective in the treatment of acute dystonia (Director & Muniz, 1982; Gagrat, Hamilton, & Belmaker, 1978).

What remains as a somewhat controversial point is whether patients should be started on an anticholinergic agent when they are started on antipsychotic drugs (Lake et al., 1986; McEvoy, 1983). Some psychiatrists recommend this since the onset of these side effects can be distressing and may lead a patient to discontinue the antipsychotic. There is some indication that prophylactic treatment may decrease the incidence of dystonia and other extrapyramidal side effects (EPSE) (Arana, Goff, Baldessarini, & Keepers, 1988; Boyer, Honeycutt-Bakalar, & Lake, 1987; Keepers, Clappison, & Casey, 1983; Manos, Lavrentiadis, &

Gkiouzepas, 1986; Sramek et al., 1986; Winslow et al., 1986). On the other hand, the majority of patients will not develop dystonia and they would needlessly be exposed to the autonomic and adverse cognitive effects of the anticholinergic agents. An alternative strategy would be to treat patients with minimal doses of antipsychotic agents (McEvoy, 1983). There is recent evidence that doses of antipsychotics that produce only minimal extrapyramidal side effects may be the optimal effective dose for the treatment of schizophrenic psychoses (Lake et al., 1986; McEvoy, in press). In general, there is increasing evidence that patients may respond to doses of antipsychotic drugs that might cause fewer EPSE (Balderssarini, Cohen, & Teicher, 1988). This preliminary evidence supports the view that one should avoid routine prophylactic treatment of EPSE (also see Chapters 3 and 9 for a further discussion). Acute dystonia can require urgent attention if it occurs as a severe problem producing pain or occlusion of larynx, or if it presents as an oculogyric crisis. To address this possibility patients should receive and carry a filled prescription for an anticholinergic. They should be instructed to use the medicine only if problems emerge. This, of course, applies to patients who are deemed capable of carrying out these requirements. Patients who are unlikely to adhere to this requirement should be hospitalized throughout the period of greatest risk or started on prophylactic therapy.

Once anticholinergic agents are given, they should be prescribed once or twice a day for several months if the antipsychotics are also continued. After that time, the dose can be decreased to establish whether the patient continues to have the side effect for which the medication was started. Frequently, patients will be less likely to require these medications over time, particularly when the symptom being treated is acute dystonia (McEvoy, 1983).

The treatment of acute dystonia is well established. Issues that need to be considered are the risk that a given patient will develop EPSE from a particular antipsychotic drug, the likelihood that a given patient might discontinue the antipsychotic if a side effect were to occur, and the risks and impact of the autonomic and adverse cognitive effects of the anticholinergic drugs. Once an anticholinergic agent has been started, the dose can often be reduced or discontinued after several months (see also Chapter 9).

Tardive Dystonia

Since the prevailing notions of movement disorders suggest abnormalities in the dopamine-acetylcholine balance in the basal ganglia, most treatment strategies have involved medications that affect these neurotransmitters. There are a few controlled clinical treatment studies of tardive dystonia. There is, however, a larger literature of open-label studies and single case reports. What generally stands out from these studies is that, overall, tardive dystonia is poorly responsive to treatment (Table 3).

Drug Discontinuation

Kang et al. (1988) were able to discontinue antipsychotic medications in 42 of the 67 patients they followed. Only 5 patients had complete remissions, which occurred over 2.8 ± 2 years. The patients who remitted were, on the average, younger than the nonremitted patients. They had shorter lengths of exposure to

Table 3 Treatment of tardive dystonia

Drug class	Design	Results	Dose
Dopamine depleters			
Reserpine			
Kang et al. (1988)	Open label	4/8 improved; 6/8 improved on reserpine in combination with other drugs	2–9 mg/day
Tetrabenzine			
Asher & Aminoff (1981)	Open label, blind rating of videotapes	6/12 with tardive dyskinesia improved; 2/8 with dystonia improved, not clear if any patients had tardive dystonia	Up to 200 mg/day
Jankovic & Orman (1982)	Double blind, 1 patient with tardive dystonia	Patient improved	200 mg/day
Jankovic & Orman (1988)	Open label in treatment refractory patients	14/15 patients with tardive dystonia had moderate/fair improvement	Up to 100 mg/day
Kang et al. (1988)	Open label	3/7 improved; 10/16 improved on tetrabenazine in combination with other drugs	12.5–250 mg/day
Anticholinergics			
Trihexyphenidyl			
Kang et al. (1988)	Open label	3/8 improved; 4/9 improved in combination with other drugs	10–32 mg/day
Wolf & Koller (1985)	Open label, blind rating of videotapes	2/3 patients improved, in one of these choreic movements worsened	15 mg/day
Ethopropazine			
Kang et al. (1988)	Open label	3/11 improved; 5/12 improved in combination with other drugs	100–450 mg/day
Other drugs			
Bromocriptine			
Luchins & Goldman (1985)	Open label; single case	Patient improved	20 mg b.i.d.
Lisuride			
Quinn et al. (1985)	Open label	2/3 patients improved by 40%	Up to 5 mg/day
Ethyl alcohol			
Biary & Koller (1985)	Double blind, IV infusion	No improvement	
Diltiazem			
Falk et al. (1988)	Open label, single case	Transient improvement	Up to 60 mg q.i.d.
Baclofen			
Rosse et al. (1986)	Open label, single case	Improved	60 mg/day
Naloxone			
Sandyk & Snider (1985)	Open label, single case	Improvement in movements and psychosis	0.8 mg IM/b.i.d.
Antipsychotic discontinuation			
Kang et al. (1988)	Open label	5/42 patients had complete remissions over 2.8 ± 2 years	

antipsychotics, and they were treated for the dystonia sooner than the other patients. None of these comparisons reached statistical significance, possibly because of the small number of remitted patients.

Dopamine-Depleting Drugs

Tetrabenazine and reserpine are the best studied and probably the most effective drugs used in the treatment of tardive dystonia. In their large, clinical study of 67 patients with tardive dystonia, Kang et al., (1988) found that 50% (4/8) of patients responded to reserpine alone and 55% (6/11) responded to this medication in combination with other drugs. Their data were collected from a retrospective chart review of patients who had been evaluated and treated in their movement disorders clinic. They do not give information on their criteria for response or duration of effect. They used daily doses ranging from 2 to 9 mg. Forty-three percent (3/7) responded to tetrabenazine alone and 63% (10/16) responded to it in combination with other drugs. Their daily dosage range was 12.5 to 250 mg. Jankovic (1982) performed a double-blind study of tetrabenazine in patients with movement disorders, one of whom had tardive dystonia. This patient did improve on this medication. In a later open study, Jankovic evaluated the effects of this drug on 217 patients with movements disorders. Of the 15 patients with tardive dystonia, 14 had fair or moderate improvement. Lang and Marsden (1982) openly studied the effects of tetrabenazine in 48 patients, 3 of whom had tardive dystonia. One of these patients had an 89% improvement in the involuntary movement score; however, this was complicated by severe parkinsonism. Asher and Aminoff (1981) also studied the effects of tetrabenazine in patients with a variety of movement disorders. One half of the patients with tardive dyskinesia improved as compared to 25% of the patients with dystonia. However, it is not clear from the paper whether any of these patients had antipsychotic-induced tardive dystonia.

Anticholinergic Agents

In their study, Kang et al. (1988) found that 38% (3/8) responded to trihexyphenidyl alone and 44% (4/9) responded to it in combination with other drugs. They used daily dosages of 10–32 mg. They had similar results with ethopropazine in dosages ranging from 100–400 mg. Wolf and Koller (1985) treated 3 patients with the anticholinergic, trihexyphenidyl, in an open-label study that used blind videotape ratings. Two of these patients responded to 15 mg of trihexyphenidyl; however, in one patient the choreoathetoid movements were exacerbated by this medication. Both patients had less response to 20 mg of the drug.

Clozapine

Lieberman, Saltz, Johns, Pollack, & Kane (1989) reported on their experience with clozapine in patients with tardive dyskinesia and dystonia. This novel antipsychotic is only a weak DA antagonist (Ljungberg & Ungenstedt, 1978) and does not cause receptor supersensitivity. Since these effects of antipsychotics are thought to be involved in the pathophysiology of tardive dystonia, clozapine holds promise as an antipsychotic that might not cause tardive movement disorders. In their open study of the course of antipsychotic-induced movement disorders in patients treated with clozapine, they found that the patients with dystonia were more likely to improve than those without it. It was not clear whether the improvement was a result of the discontinuation of the offending antipsychotic or to an ameliorative effect of clozapine. In either case, this medication may hold therapeutic promise for patients with tardive dystonia who require ongoing treatment with an antipsychotic.

Other Drugs

Drugs reported to be occasionally effective include bromocriptine (Luchins, 1985), lisuride (Quinn, Lang, Sheeh, & Marsden 1985), baclofen (Kang et al., 1988; Rosse, Allen & Lux, 1986), naloxone (Sandyk & Snider, 1985), and benzodiazepines (Kang et al., 1988). On the other hand, the following drugs have been used without success: ethyl alcohol (Biary & Koller, 1985), diltiazem (Falk, Wojick, & Gelenberg, 1988), propranolol (Cooper, Doherty, & King, 1989), levodopa, amantadine, carbamazepine, valproate, and deanol acetaminobenzoate (Kang et al., 1988).

CONCLUSION

First-line treatment of dystonia would include early identification followed by discontinuation of antipsychotic medication when possible. Kang et al. (1986, 1988), the group that probably has the largest reported clinical experience with this disorder, recommend trying pharmacological agents only if the movements are disabling. Unfortunately, the results of treatment are not generally robust and are difficult to predict. In general, dopamine depleting drugs or anticholinergics are the first-line agents. If these are not effective either alone or in combination, then sequential trials of some of the other agents that have been reported to be occasionally effective would be warranted. Clozapine may hold promise as a antipsychotic that is not likely to exacerbate and may even benefit the movement disorder.

REFERENCES

Ananth J, Edelmuth C, Dargan B, 1988: Meige's syndrome associated with neuroleptic treatment. *American Journal of Psychiatry, 145*(4), 513–515.

Arana GW, Goff DC, Baldessarini RJ, Keepers GA, 1988: Efficacy of anticholinergic prophylaxis for neuroleptic-induced acute dystonia. *American Journal of Psychiatry, 145*(8), 993–996.

Asher SW, Aminoff MJ, 1981: Tetrabenazine and movement disorders. *Neurology, 31,* 1051–1054.

Baldessarini RJ, 1977: *Chemotherapy in psychiatry.* Cambridge, MA: Harvard University Press.

Baldessarini RJ, Cohen BM, Teicher MH, 1988: Significance of neuroleptic dose and plasma level in the pharmacological treatment of psychoses. *Archives of General Psychiatry, 45,* 79–91.

Biary N, Koller W, 1985: Effect of alcohol on dystonia. *Neurology, 35,* 239–240.

Boyer WF, Honeycutt-Bakalar N; Lake CR, 1987: Anticholinergic prophylaxis of acute haloperiodl-induced acute dystonic reactions. *Journal of Clinical Psychopharmacology, 7*(3), 164–166.

Burke RE, Fahn S, Jankovic J, Marsden CD, Lang AE, Golomp S, Ilson J, 1982: Tardive dystonia: Late-onset and persistent dystonia caused by antipsychotic drugs. *Neurology, 32,* 1335–1346.

Burke RE, Kang UJ, 1988: Tardive dystonia: Clinical aspects and treatment. In: *Advances in neurology, vol. 49: Facial dyskinesias,* edited by J Jankovic and E Tolosa. New York: Raven Press.

Cooper SJ, Doherty MM, Kig DJ, 1989: Tardive dystonia: The benefits of time. *British Journal of Psychiatry, 155,* 113–115.

Cutler NR, Post RM, Rey AC, Bunney WE, 1981: Depression-dependent dyskinesias in two cases of manic-depressive illness. *New England Journal of Medicine, 304*(18), 1088–1089.

Director KL, Muniz CE, 1982: Diazepam in the treatment of extrapyramidal symptoms: A case report. *Journal of Clinical Psychiatry, 43*(4), 160–161.

Ekbom K, Lindholm H, Lundberg L, 1972: New dystonic syndrome associated with butyrophenone therapy. *Neurology, 202,* 94–103.

Falk WE, Wojick JD, Gelenberg AJ, 1988: Diltiazem for tardive dyskinesia and tardive dystonia. *Lancet, 1,* (8589), April 9, 824–825.

Flaherty JA, Lahmeyer HW, 1978: Laryngeal-pharyngeal dystonia as a possible cause of asphyxia with haloperidol treatment. *American Journal of Psychiatry, 135,* 1414–1415.

Friedman JH, Kucharski LT, Wagner RL, 1987: Tardive dystonia in a psychiatric hospital. *Journal of Neurology, Neurosurgery and Psychiatry, 50,* 801–803.

Gagrat D, Hamilton J, Belmaker R, 1978: Intramuscular diazepam in the treatment of neuroleptic induced acute dystonia and akathisia. *American Journal of Psychiatry, 135,* 1232–1233.

Gardos G, 1981: Dystonic reaction during maintenance antipsychotic therapy. *American Journal of Psychiatry, 138*(1), 114–115.

Garver DL, Davis JM, Dekirmenjian H, Ericksen S, Gosenfeld L, Haraszti J, 1976a: Dystonic reactions following neuroleptics: Time course and proposed mechanisms. *Psychopharmacology, 47,* 199–201.

Garver DL, Davis JM, Dekirmenjian H, Jones FD, Casper R, Haraszti J, 1976b: Pharmacokinetics of red blood cell phenothiazine and clinical effects: Acute dystonic reactions. *Archives of General Psychiatry, 33,* 862–886.

Glazer WM, Moore DC, Hansen TC, Brenner LM, 1983: Meige syndrome and tardive dyskinesia. *American Journal of Psychiatry, 140*(6), 798–799.

Guy N, Raps A, Assael M, 1986: The Pisa syndrome during maintenance antipsychotic therapy. *American Journal of Psychiatry, 143*(11), 1492.

Jankovic J, 1982: Treatment of hyperkinetic movement disorder with tetrabenazine: A double blind crossover study. *Annals of Neurology, 11,* 41–47.

Jankovic J, Orman J, 1988: Tetrabenazine therapy of dystonia, chorea, tics, and other dyskinesias. *Neurology, 38,* 391–394.

Kang UJ, Burke RE, Fahn S, 1986: Natural history and treatment of tardive dyskinesia. *Movement Disorders, 1*(3), 193–208.

Kang UJ, Burke RE, Fahn S, 1988: Tardive dystonia. In *Advances in neurology, vol. 50: Dystonia 2,* edited by S Fahn, CD Marsden, and DB Calne. New York: Raven Press.

Keepers GA, Clappison VJ, Casey DE, 1983: Initial anticholinergic prophylaxis for neuroleptic-induced extrapyramidal syndromes. *Archives of General Psychiatry, 40,* 1113–1117.

Keshavan MS, Goswamy U, 1983: Tardive dyskinesia less severe in depression. *British Journal of Psychiatry, 142,* 207–208.

Kwentus JA, Schulz SC, Hart RP, 1984: Tardive dystonia, catatonia, and electroconvulsive therapy. *Journal of Nervous and Mental Diseases, 172*(3), 171–173.

Lake CR, Casey DE, McEvoy JP, Siris SG, Boyer WF, Simpson G, 1986: The "pros" and "cons" of anticholinergic prophylaxis. *Psychopharmacology Bulletin, 22,*(3), 981–984.

Lal KP, Saxena S, Mohan D, 1988: Tardive dystonia alternating with mania. *Biological Psychiatry, 23,* 312–316.

Lang AE, Marsden CD, 1982: Alphamethylparatyrosine and tetrabenazine in movement disorders. *Clinical Neuropharmacology, 5*(4), 375–387.

Lieberman J, Pollack S, Lesser M, Kane J, 1988: Pharmacologic characterization of tardive dyskinesia. *Journal of Clinical Psychopharmacology, 8,* 254–260.

Lieberman JA, Saltz BL, Johns CA, Pollack S, Kane JM, 1989: Clozapine effects on tardive dyskinesia. *Psychopharmacology Bulletin, 25*(1), 57–62.

Ljungberg T, Ungerstedt U, 1978: Classification of neuroleptic drugs according to their ability to inhibit apomorphine induced locomotion and gnawing: Evidence for two different mechansims of action. *Psychopharmacology* (Berlin), *56,* 239–247.

Luchins DJ, Goldman M, 1985: High-dose bromocriptine in a case of tardive dystonia. *Biological Psychiatry, 20,* 179–181.

Manos N, Lavrentiadis G, Gkiouzepas J, 1986: Evaluation of the need for prophylactic antiparkinsonian medication in psychotic patients treated with neuroleptics. *Journal of Clinical Psychiatry, 47*(3), 114–116.

Marsden CD, Jenner P, 1980: The pathophysiology of extrapyramidal side-effects of neuroleptic drugs. *Psychological Medicine, 10,* 55–72.

McEvoy JP, 1983: The clinical use of anticholinergic drugs as treatment for extrapyramidal side effects of neuroleptic drugs. *Psychopharmacology, 3,* 288–302.

McEvoy JP, Hogarty GE, Steingard S (in press): Optimal dose of neuroleptic in acute schizophrenia: A controlled study of the neuroleptic threshold. *Archives of General Psychiatry.*

Menuck M, 1981: Laryngeal-pharyngeal dystonia and haloperidol. *American Journal of Psychiatry, 138*(3), 394–395.

Munetz MR, 1980: Oculogyric crises and tardive dyskinesia. *American Journal of Psychiatry, 137*(12), 1628.

Nasrallah HA, Pappas NJ, Crowe RR, 1980: Oculogyric dystonia in tardive dyskinesia. *American Journal of Psychiatry, 137*(7), 850–851.

Quinn NP, Lang AE, Sheehy MP, Marsden CD, 1985: Lisuride in dystonia. *Neurology, 35,* 766–769.

Rosse RB, Allen A, Lux WE, 1986: Baclofen treatment in a patient with tardive dystonia. *Journal of Clinical Psychiatry, 47*(9), 474–475.

Rupniak MJ, Jenner P, Marsden CD, 1986: Acute dystonia induced by neuroleptic drugs. *Psychopharmacology, 88,* 403–419.

Sandyk R, Snider SR, 1985: Naloxene and tardive dyskinesia. *Biological Psychiatry, 20,* 1335–1336.

Saxena S, 1986: Tardive dystonia and Pisa syndrome. *British Journal of Psychiatry, 149,* 524.

Sayers AC, Burki HR, Ruch W, Asper H, 1975: Neuroleptic induced hypersensitivity of striatal dopamine receptors in the rat as a model of tardive dyskinesia: Effects of clozapine, haloperidol, loxapine and chlorpromazine. *Psychopharmacology* (Berlin), *41,* 97–104.

Schatzberg AF, Cole JO, 1986: *Manual of clinical psychopharmacology.* Washington, DC: American Psychiatric Press.

Singh SK, Jankovic J, 1988: Tardive dystonia in patients with tourette's syndrome. *Movement Disorders, 3*(3), 274–280.

Sramek JJ, Simpson GM, Morrison RL, Heiser JF, 1986: Anticholinergic agents for prophylaxis of neuroleptic induced dystonic reactions: A prospective study. *Journal of Clinical Psychiatry, 47,* 305–309.

Stahl SM, Berger PA, 1982: Bromocriptine, physostigmine, and neurotransmitter in the dystonias. *Neurology, 32,* 889–892.

Swett C, 1975: Drug-induced dystonia. *American Journal of Psychiatry, 132,* 523–534.

Tarsy D, Baldessarini RJ, 1970: The pathophysiologic basis of tardive dyskinesia. *Biological Psychiatry, 12,* 431–450.

Weiner WJ, Nausieda PA, Glantz RH, 1981: Meige syndrome (blepharospasm-oromandibular dystonia) after long-term neuroleptic therapy. *Neurology, 31,* 1555–1556.

Winslow RS, Stillner V, Coons DJ, Robinson MW, 1986: Prevention of acute dystonic reactions in patients beginning high potency neuroleptics. *American Journal of Psychiatry, 143,* 706–710.

Wolf ME, Koller WE, 1985: Tardive dystonia: Treatment with trihexyphenidyl. *Journal of Clinical Psychopharmacology, 5*(4), 247–248.

Yassa R, 1985: The Pisa syndrome: A report of two cases. *British Journal of Psychiatry, 146,* 93–95.

Yassa R, Nair V, Dimitry R, 1986: Prevalence of tardive dystonia. *Acta Psychiatrica Scandinavica, 73,* 629–633.

9

Drug-Induced Parkinsonism

Kashinath G. Yadalam

In the year 1817, James Parkinson wrote "An Essay on the Shaking Palsy," wherein he described an ailment characterized by "involuntary tremulous motion with lessened muscular power, in parts not in action and even when supported; with a propensity to bend the trunk forward, and to pass from a walking to a running pace: the senses and intellects being uninjured" (Parkinson, 1817). He referred to this condition as "shaking palsy" or its Latin equivalent paralysis agitans. It is now clear that tremor need not be a part of this syndrome; also, true paralysis is not common. Hence, the term shaking palsy is somewhat inaccurate (Klawans, 1973). Parkinsonism is a syndrome, not a disease; a descriptive term should precede to indicate the type. Postencephalitic parkinsonism implies etiology, and drug-induced parkinsonism (DIP) implies a specific pathogeneis. The term Parkinson's disease is used to refer to the idiopathic form as described by Parkinson. DIP is reversible as opposed to idiopathic and postencephalitic types. Clinically, the different forms of this syndrome are identical.

Exposure to a variety of neurotoxic compounds such as carbon monoxide, carbon disulfide, manganese, and MPTP (1-methyl-4-phenyl-1,2,3,6-tetrahydropyridine) also cause parkinsonism; their course and neuropathology are varied and are not discussed here.

Similarities between DIP and Parkinson's disease in areas other than the extra-pyramidal system continue to be reported; examples are the high prevalence of seborrheic dermatitis (Binder & Jonelis, 1983) and visual contrast sensitivity loss, which may reflect generalized dopaminergic deficiency (Bulens, Meerwaldt, Van Der Wildt, & Keeminck, 1989).

RISK FACTORS

Age

DIP affects all age groups, including children and neonates. In two retrospective chart reviews (Keepers, Clappison, & Casey, 1983; Moleman et al., 1986), the incidence of DIP was greater in patients 40 years and younger. Some state the opposite (Ayd, 1961; Crane, 1974). In the Moleman et al. (1986) report, the dose, sex, and duration of treatment were examined in a logistic regression model. Examining the data published in the aforementioned works and other studies, it appears that the risk of DIP peaks in two age groups. It is high in teens and declines gradually to about the fourth decade and increases gradually again from the fifth decade onward. The increased incidence in older subjects is consistent with the fact that concentrations of dopamine, tyrosine hydroxylase, and nigral cell counts all decline with advancing age (McGeer & McGeer, 1977).

Gender

Gender difference in the incidence of DIP (females > males) has been reported, but when the dose of the antipsychotic is converted to mg/kg, there appears to be no difference (Levinson, 1990). In one report (Gratton, 1960), a higher incidence of DIP was found in premenopausal women as compared with postmenopausal women; DIP was precipitated within 24–48 hours after estrogen administration in women taking phenothiazines. The dopamine-blocking properties of estrogen may be relevant in this regard (Gordon, Borison, & Diamond, 1980).

Discontinuation of antipsychotics results in the alleviation of DIP within a few weeks. Occasionally, in the elderly, these symptoms may persist for several months or even as long as one year (Klawans, Bergen, & Bruyn, 1973). Cases of permanent parkinsonism sometimes occur following drug withdrawal in elderly individuals; these are probably patients with latent Parkinson's disease uncovered by dopamine blockers (Tarsy, 1983). Sometimes severe parkinsonian reactions occur after abrupt discontinuation of anticholinergic drugs, even if antipsychotics have been discontinued at the same time. The most likely cause is cholinergic rebound and the continued dopamine blockade of the slowly excreted antipsychotic (Simpson & Kunz-Bartholini, 1968).

Drug Factors

All the antipsychotic drugs now marketed cause akinesia, including clozapine. The route of administration appears to affect the speed of onset and the incidence of these side effects. Depot fluphenazine has been reported to induce akinesia more quickly than oral fluphenazine (Ayd, 1974). On the other hand, in a small study with raters blind to the route of administration, 4 patients receiving intravenous haloperidol had less extrapyramidal symptoms (EPS) than 6 patients receiving an equal amount of oral haloperidol (Menza, Murray, Holmes, & Rafuls, 1987). The explanation for these differences could, among others, include pharmacodynamics, the first pass effect, the role of metabolites, and the ratio of the metabolite(s) to the parent compound.

Attempts to correlate the total drug dose with DIP have not shown a clear relationship, suggesting a role for individual vulnerability. One study (Simpson & Kunz-Bartholini, 1968), which examined the risk of individual vulnerability, found that the dose of trifluperazine required to produce a similar degree of parkinsonism ranged from 20 to 480 mg. Individual variability may also explain why some patients are more prone to develop one of the DIP side effects than another; in 12 patients receiving more than 800 mg of trifluperazine per day, none exhibited rigidity but all had tremor (Simpson, 1983).

Plasma Levels

There is often a several-hundred-fold variation in plasma levels between individuals treated with the same antipsychotic drug (Simpson & Yadalam, 1985,

1990) and an anticholinergic drug (Tune & Coyle, 1981). The oral dosage generally does not correlate with the severity of these symptoms. Two other approaches have yielded meaningful results. In a 4-week, fixed-dose, oral fluphenazine study, higher mg/kg dosage (greater than 0.3 mg/kg/day) was associated with more severe DIP (Levinson et al., 1990). There are many studies examining the relationship of plasma level of various antipsychotic drugs to clinical response and side effects. Plasma level of haloperidol higher than 10.7 ng/ml (Itoh, Fujii, & Ichikawa, 1984) and 9 ng/ml (Morselli, Bianchetti, & Dugas, 1982) and plasma level of perphenazine greater than 2–3 nmol/L have been demonstrated to possibly correlate with increased incidence of DIP (Bolvig-Hansen & Larsen, 1985). These findings are only preliminary and require further evaluation in well-designed studies before being recommended for routine clinical care. Few well-designed studies have examined the relationship between plasma level of anticholinergic drugs and DIP response. In one study (Bamrah, Krska, & Soni, 1988), 68 schizophrenic patients with DIP maintained on a single antipsychotic drug and an anticholinergic were assessed using an extrapyramidal rating scale. The dosages of antipsychotic drugs were converted to chlorpromazine equivalents (CPZ Eq; Davis, 1974) and the doses of anticholinergic drugs were converted to orphenadrine equivalents (Orph Eq; Klett & Caffey, 1972); the serum anticholinergic levels were measured using a radioreceptor assay. The severity of EPS score was unrelated to plasma level of antipsychotic drug, CPZ Eq, and Orph Eq. The radioreceptor assay employed measured the total muscarinic receptor blockade, which takes into account the combined effects of antipsychotic drugs and anticholinergic drugs. When a serum level of 4.5 pmol/ml atropine equivalents was used as a cut-off point, 25 of the 44 patients exhibited EPS, whereas only 2 of 23 above this level demonstrated this side effect.

Individual susceptibility seems to play a major role, and it may be more important than age, sex, dose, type, and duration of antipsychotic treatment in causing DIP. The evidence for this comes from several areas including pharmacokinetics and brain biochemistry, brain morphology, and the influence of genetics.

Dopamine

A group of investigators (Chase, Schur, & Gordon, 1970) reported that patients with DIP had lower levels of homovanillic acid (HVA) in the cerebrospinal fluid (CSF), suggesting that these subjects were less able to mount a compensatory increase in dopamine turnover. Another group (Van Praag & Korf, 1976) examined CSF HVA responses to probenecid (believed to be a measure of dopamine turnover) before and after administration of dopamine-blocking agents in acutely ill psychotic patients. Patients who developed more DIP had a greater increase in HVA response after drug treatment than patients without such side effects. This group also reported a lower pretreatment HVA response in probenecid-treated patients who developed DIP than those who did not. Both these studies indicate that the development of DIP is dependent on an individual sensitivity that is more closely tied to pretreatment dopamine turnover than posttreatment HVA response to antipsychotic treatment.

Calcium

The role of calcium ion in causing DIP has been controversial. In a recent prospective study (Kuny & Binswanger, 1989), 11 patients who developed EPS had significantly lower ionized calcium levels and a significantly lower ionized/total calcium ratio in the predrug period than the 13 patients without these side effects.

Organic Factors

Schizophrenic patients with a history of lobotomy are more prone to develop DIP (Holden, Itil, & Keskiner, 1969). Two groups of investigators examined the relationship of DIP and brain morphology as observed on CT scans. Twenty young patients, most having schizophrenia, were treated with a fixed dose of chlorpromazine for 5 weeks. Eight patients developed DIP. The lateral ventricular brain ratio (VBR) in this group was larger than the 12 patients who did not require antiparkinsonian drug treatment (Luchins, Jackman, & Meltzer, 1983). In a second study of 21 patients over the age of 55 years diagnosed with schizophrenia and receiving various antipsychotics, 16 patients had DIP. The severity of parkinsonism was significantly associated with larger VBR (Hoffman, Labs, & Casey, 1987).

Genetic Factors

It is well known that genetic factors play an important role in some movement disorders. Based on this, a group of investigators (Meltzer et al., 1989) examined the prevalence of human leukocyte antigen (HLA) in DIP. Of the 52 white male chronic schizophrenic patients, 29 developed DIP and 23 did not. There were no differences between the two groups with respect to age or duration of antipsychotic treatment. One HLA antigen, B44, was significantly more prevalent in the DIP group. The authors postulate that HLA-B44 may play a role in genetic or immunologic susceptibility to develop DIP in white schizophrenic individuals. Another group (Galdi, Reider, Silber, & Bonato, 1981) found that schizophrenia patients with relatives having a history of depression experienced more severe DIP.

PATHOPHYSIOLOGY

The striatum contains the highest concentrations of acetylcholine and dopamine in the brain (Bertler, 1961; Feldberg & Vogt, 1948). The syndrome of parkinsonism appears whenever there is a decreased activity of dopamine in the striatum leading to an imbalance between these two neurotransmitters. In Parkinson's disease, there is a decreased quantity of dopamine in the striatum because the cells projecting to it from the substantia nigra degenerate. In DIP, sometimes referred to as "pseudoparkinsonism," dopamine is decreased in the striatum. The dopamine decrease in the striatum is produced by various drugs with diverse mechanisms of action (Table 1). Despite the fact that parkinsonism results from a primary disturbance in the striatal dopaminergic system, changes in the cholinergic function can influence parkinsonian features. Two groups of investigators have reported an exacerbation of phenothiazine-induced parkinsonism in patients simultaneously ex-

Table 1   Drugs causing parkinsonism

Name	Mechanism
Antipsychotic agents	Block postsynaptic striatal dopamine receptors
Reserpine and tetrabenazine	Deplete synaptic stores of dopamine
Alpha methyl dopa	Acts as a false neurotransmitter
MPTP	Selectively destroys dopaminergic neurons in the substantia nigra (A8 and A9 cells)

posed to physostigmine (Ambani, Van Woert, & Bowert, 1973; Gerlach, Reisby, & Randrup, 1974).

CLINICAL FEATURES

The cardinal features of parkinsonism are akinesia, tremor, rigidity, and abnormalities of posture and gait. The individual components of the full syndrome are described in Table 2. Akinesia, sometimes referred to, in its milder form, as bradykinesia or hypokinesia, is often the earliest, the most common, and at times the only manifestation of DIP. Akinesia (and rigidity) in its severe form results in a marked reduction of all spontaneous movements, masked facies, absent arm swing, soft and monotonous speech, and slowness in the initiation and execution of all voluntary movements. A subtle reduction in facial expressions usually heralds the onset of akinesia. Unlike early Parkinson's disease, the akinesia in DIP is symmetrical in distribution (Tarsy, 1983). The behavioral dimension of akinesia includes diminished spontaneity characterized by limited gestures, unspontaneous

Table 2   Clinical features of DIP

Features	Specific effects
Akinesia	Muscle fatigue and weakness Reduction in physical activity Joint and muscle pain in advanced stage
Rigidity	Absent arm swing Stiffness and slowness of all voluntary movements Gait and posture disturbance Masked facies Cogwheel-type rigidity Shuffling gait Slow monotonous speech Stooped posture Dysarthria
Tremor	Rhythmic 4–6 oscillations per second Resting tremor that disappears on volition May involve head, perioral area ("rabbit syndrome"), trunk or lower extremities
Autonomic nervous system	Drooling Hyperhidrosis and heat intolerance Sialorrhea and seborrhea

This table was adapted from Donlon, PT, Stenson, RL, 1976:

speech, apathy, and difficulty with initiating usual activities (Rifkin, Quitkin, & Klein, 1975).

The tremor, when present, is more prominent in the distal part of the upper extremities. This tremor is present at rest and disappears on movement and may reappear if the volitional act is continued. The tremor may, at times, be masked by the patient assuming purposeful activity such as holding a cigarette, grasping his knees, or clutching the arms of his chair. The frequency of the tremor is similar to the kind observed in Parkinson's disease, which is about 4–6 oscillations per second. On the other hand, the typical pill-rolling tremor of Parkinson's disease is uncommon in DIP.

Rigidity or increased muscle tone, which appears from days to weeks after the onset of akinesia, is present in the larger joints of the extremities, neck, or trunk. The rigidity can be either cogwheel or lead-pipe type or both. The variable or constant resistance of the agonist and antagonist muscle groups lead to the former and latter types of rigidity. An early sign of muscle rigidity may be slowness in the speed of arm drop (Simpson & Angus, 1970).

Micrographia is often present, and this can be elicited by asking the patient to copy a paragraph of text. The amount of time taken and the area of the copied paragraph are both useful; repeating this procedure periodically provides an objective measure of change in the course of the syndrome (Simpson & Angus, 1970). Difficulties in postural fixation, righting reflexes, and gait abnormalities appear later.

Accurate and elaborate techniques involving several instruments have been developed to quantitatively measure the various aspects of DIP; these methods are useful when comparing the effects of several drugs and in research settings to eliminate observer bias (May, Lee, & Bacon, 1983).

In a large survey (Ayd, 1974), 90% of DIP cases developed within the first 72 days after taking oral antipsychotic drugs, and these side effects appeared within 2–5 days following parenteral fluphenazine preparations. Akinesia was the first symptom to appear that was not relieved by methylphenidate but was responsive to anticholinergic drugs. In this survey, almost every patient receiving a clinically effective dose of an antipsychotic drug developed mild akinesia (Ayd, 1974). The reported incidence of akinesia varies widely. This wide discrepancy (in patients receiving conventional dosages of antipsychotics) suggests that physicians differ greatly in their ability to detect these symptoms, particularly akinesia (Van Putten, 1978). An examination of patients with schizophrenia residing in a community board and care facility revealed that 59% of the patients maintained on an average daily dose of 760 mg chlorpromazine equivalents were at least mildly akinetic (Van Putten & Spar, 1979).

DIAGNOSIS

Much of the DIP literature in psychiatry has focused on akinesia because it has been notoriously confused with or misdiagnosed as depression (Van Putten, 1978), somatic delusions (Quitkin, Rifkin, & Klein, 1975), catatonic psychoses (Gelenberg & Mandel, 1977), demoralization (Rifkin, Quitkin, & Klein, 1975), and negative symptoms associated with schizophrenia.

Many patients, family members, or others visiting a psychiatric ward can attest to the fact that these side effects are common. Unfortunately, they are often ignored, misdiagnosed, or improperly treated by the staff. Patients may not report these symptoms because of the assumption that it is the nature of the illness they are suffering from and give the benefit of doubt to their doctors.

The proper diagnosis of DIP requires training and not all institutions have psychiatrists who are skillful in assessment of this problem. All the signs and symptoms described previously as clinical features should be assessed systematically. The examination can be divided into different areas. Akinesia, tremor, absence of spontaneous movements, and gait disturbances are observable phenomena. Rigidity of the various muscle groups (shoulders, elbows, wrists, neck, and knees) and the swiftness of the shoulder drop can be quickly and easily detected by performing a simple physical examination (Simpson & Angus, 1970). Because DIP does not affect all the muscle groups in a symmetric fashion, each part of the body must be examined. These examinations must be repeated often in the acute inpatient ward, following initiation and dosage changes of the antipsychotic drugs and anticholinergic drugs. Specific questions pertaining to the behavioral aspects of the syndrome, such as apathy and nonspontaneity, should be asked.

The most difficult problem with diagnosis is in differentiating DIP from the syndrome of depression and the so-called negative syndrome of schizophrenia. Symptoms such as flat affect, apathy, psychomotor retardation, nonspontaneity, and emotional withdrawal are common in all three syndromes, although different terms are used to describe the "same" sign or symptom. A group of investigators (Prosser et al., 1987) attempting to delineate these syndromes report preliminary evidence that in patients with low anticholinergic activity, negative symptoms may be associated with higher plasma antipsychotic activity. If replicated, this observation supports the notion that at least in some cases, the "negative symptoms" are actually DIP. This phenomenological overlap is often responsible for the dilemma, confusion, and controversy. Some have postulated that a decreased dopaminergic transmission can result in a defect state (Chouinard & Jones, 1978). Speculative extension of this view suggests that there may even be a common biochemical substrate for DIP and negative symptoms. Several approaches may help to delineate these syndromes but none meet with success all the time. A careful history pertaining to the chronology and severity of these symptoms and their relation to the initiation of antipsychotic treatment should be obtained.

The initial treatment approach is to reduce the dosage of the antipsychotic drug if the psychotic symptoms permit. If the dosage of the antipsychotic drug can be reduced, this will often decrease the intensity of DIP. Improvement in movement or the lack of change in the other symptoms may provide some clues. Because antipsychotics have long half-lives, an immediate change in DIP cannot be expected. This dose reduction approach is of most relevance while reducing the dosage of depot preparations (Simpson & Yadalam, 1990). An intramuscular injection of benztropine sometimes decreases akinesia but almost always relieves rigidity and drug-induced retardation. Prescribing antidepressants does not help in differential diagnosis and may worsen the patient's illness particularly if it is schizophrenia. If benefit is obtained, this does not necessarily indicate a depression is present; improvement is expected if the antidepressant used possesses significant anticholinergic properties.

TREATMENT

Some of the common reasons for DIP in susceptible individuals are high dosages of antipsychotics, inadequately low dosages of anticholinergic drugs, and frequently both, at the same time. These can be corrected as an initial step. Although plasma levels and receptor assays of these drugs may ultimately prove useful, clinicians today must use their clinical skills before resorting to these methods, if available. Freyhan (1958) noted that even when DIP is diagnosed correctly, patients may not receive adequate treatment because some clinicians believe that akinesia is " . . . a regular effect of antipsychotic drugs, part and parcel of their therapeutic action, which in many instances makes it seem arbitrary to define borderlines between therapeutic quanta of hypomotility and early signs of parkinsonism." This remains true today.

Patients and family members may be helpful in identifying DIP early on in its presentation, and as part of the informed consent they should be educated and fore-warned about the various side effects that may occur with treatment. They should also be encouraged to report them early and be reassured that side effects are common in the course of treatment and that they can be alleviated by changing the dose or adding other medications. If patients and family members are treated as active participants in treatment, the compliance and the benefits of therapy are enhanced.

There are several antiparkinsonian drugs available, and there are important differences among them. These drugs differ in their propensity to bind to plasma proteins, which may in part explain the differences in potency. Only 70% of benztropine is protein-bound compared to 93% for benzhexol and 99% for procyclidine (Bamrah et al., 1988). The various antiparkinsonian drugs and their special characteristics are described in Table 3 (adapted from Friend, 1963; Hoffman, 1981; Richardson, 1965).

It is often the practice to treat patients receiving high-potency dopamine blockers with antiparkinsonian agents from the start of treatment. However, this remains controversial (Davis, Barter, & Kane, 1989). A further discussion of this issue may be found in Chapter 12. Anticholinergic drugs prevent the occurrence of certain dramatic side effects such as acute dystonia, thereby improving compliance to drug treatment. The dose of the antiparkinsonian agent is titrated depending on the intensity of side effects; the dose range of the various agents is described in Table 3. Because these drugs have short half-lives, they should be prescribed in divided doses.

Unlike the other antiparkinsonian agents, amantadine alleviates DIP by releasing dopamine from the neuronal storage sites (Grelak, Clark, Stump, & Vernier, 1970). In a double-blind, placebo-controlled crossover study of 39 inpatients, amantadine and trihexyphenidyl were equally effective in treating DIP, and amantadine produced fever and less severe side effects (Fann & Lake, 1976). Some (Gelenberg, 1978; Gelenberg & Mandel, 1977) have found amantadine useful when other antiparkinsonian agents failed and in severe forms of parkinsonism. Amantadine is also useful for patients receiving antipsychotic agents who have urinary retention, glaucoma, or constipation, or who are elderly. Because 90% of this drug is excreted in the urine, toxicity may occur if used in patients with renal disease (Ing et al., 1979). Also, livedo reticularis of the lower extremities may occur with long-term use (Hamlin, 1975).

There is disagreement about the chronic use of these agents. A group of investi-

Table 3 Antiparkinsonian drugs

Type	Drug	Dose range (mg)	Actions
Antihistamine	Orphenadrine	150–250	A mild stimulant; main effect on rigidity and akinesia. Less useful in tremor.
Antihistamine and anticholinergic	Diphenhydramine	25–200	Highly sedating.
	Benztropine	0.5–8	Sedating; a muscle relaxant; has a relatively long half-life. Relieves rigidity, sialorrhea, and tremor. Can be used intravenously. Drug of choice for tremors.
	Ethopropazine	50–400	
Anticholinergic	Procyclidine	7.5–20	Less effective than others; fewer side effects.
	Trihexyphenidyl	1–15	Less sedating; shorter half-life; very potent. Relieves rigidity, weak for tremor.
Dopamine agonist	Amantadine	100–300	Useful in patients who are prone to anticholinergic side effects, especially the elderly.

gators (Manos, Gkiouzepas, & Logothetis 1981) abruptly discontinued trihexyphenidyl in a blind study in a group of chronic patients receiving antipsychotic drug treatment. This procedure resulted in worsening of EPS in 68% (58/75) of the subjects sufficient to necessitate withdrawal from the study, and another 28% showed less severe worsening. These investigators (Manos, Gkiouzepas, Tzotzoras, & Tzanetoglou, 1981) repeated the study but withdrew the antiparkinsonian agents gradually and the results were the same. As a principle of therapy, the need for these medications should be periodically reevaluated in patients receiving them on a chronic basis. One approach is to periodically review the presence of DIP and the dose of antipsychotic drug every 3 to 6 months and to reduce the antipsychotic dose if indicated. The comparison of side effects before and after the dose reduction determines the need for further reduction, stabilization at the new dose, or a return to the previous level. Although time consuming, when this procedure is followed it results in the lowest, effective dose of the antipsychotic agent and assists in clarifying the need for continued anticholinergic drug therapy.

REFERENCES

Ambani LH, Van Woert MH, Bowers MB, 1973. Physostigmine effects on phenothiazine-induced parkinsonism. *Archives of Neurology, 29,* 444–446.

Ayd FJ, 1961: A survey of drug-induced extrapyramidal reactions. *Journal of the American Medical Association, 175,* 102–108.

Ayd FJ, 1974: Side effects of depot fluphenazines. In: *The phenothiazines and structurally related drugs,* edited by IS Forrest, CJ Carr, and E Usdine. New York: Raven Press.

Ayd FJ, 1983: Early-onset neuroleptic-induced extrapyramidal reactions: A second survey, 1961–1981. In: *Neuroleptics, behavioral and clinical perspectives,* edited by JT Coyle and SJ Enna. New York: Raven Press.

Bamrah JS, Krska J, Soni SD, 1988: Relationship between extrapyramidal symptoms and serum anticholinergic levels in treated chronic schizophrenics. *Journal of Psychopharmacology, 2*(1), 39–46.

Bertler A, 1961: Occurrence and localization of catecholamines in the human brain. *Acta Physiologica Scandinavica, 51,* 97–107.

Binder RL, Jonelis FJ, 1983: Seborrheic dermatitis in neuroleptic-induced parkinsonism. *Archives of Dermatology, 119,* 473–475.

Bolvig-Hansen L, Larsen NE, 1985: Therapeutic advantages of monitoring plasma concentrations of perphenazine in clinical practice. *Psychopharmacology, 87,* 16–19.

Bulens C, Meerwaldt JD, Van Der Wildt GJ, Keemink CJ, 1989: Visual contrast sensitivity in drug-induced parkinsonism. *Journal of Neurology, Neurosurgery and Psychiatry, 52,* 341–345.

Chase TN, Schur JA, Gordon EK, 1970: Cerebrospinal fluid monamine catabolites in drug-induced extrapyramidal disorders. *Neuropharmacology, 9,* 265–275.

Crane GE, 1974: Factors predisposing to drug-induced neurological effects. In: *The phenothiazines and structurally related drugs,* edited by IS Forrest, CJ Carr, and E Usdin. New York: Raven Press.

Chouinard G, Jones BD, 1978: Schizophrenia as dopamine deficiency disease. *Lancet, 2,* 99–100.

Davis JM, 1974: Dose equivalents of the antipsychotic drugs. *Psychiatry Research, 11,* 65–69.

Davis JM, Barter JT, Kane JM, 1989: Antipsychotic drugs. In: *Comprehensive textbook of psychiatry,* 5th edition (vol. 2), edited by HI Kaplan and BJ Sadock. Baltimore: Williams and Wilkins.

Donlon PT, Stenson RL, 1976: Neuroleptic-induced extrapyramidal symptoms. *Diseases of the Nervous System, 37,* 629–635.

Fann WE, Lake CR, 1976: Amantadine and trihexyphenidyl in the treatment of neuroleptic-induced parkinsonism. *American Journal of Psychiatry, 133,* 940–943.

Feldberg W, Vogt M, 1948: Acetylcholine synthesis in different regions of the central nervous system. *Journal of Physiology, 107,* 372–381.

Freyhan FA, 1958: Psychomotility and parkinsonism in treatment with neuroleptic drugs. *Archives of Neurology and Psychiatry, 78* 465–471.

Friend DG, 1963: Antiparkinsonism drug therapy. *Journal of Clinical Pharmacology and Therapeutics, 1963,* 815–822.

Galdi J, Reider Ro, Silber D, Bonato RR, 1981: Genetic factors in the response to neuroleptics in schizophrenia. *Psychological Medicine, 11,* 713–728.

Gelenberg AJ, 1978: Amantadine in treatment of benztropine refractory extrapyramidal disorders induced by antipsychotic drugs. *Current Therapeutic Research 23,* 375–380.

Gelenberg A, Mandel MR, 1977: Catatonic reactions to high-potency neuroleptic drugs. *Archives of General Psychiatry, 34,* 947–950.

Gerlach J, Reisby N, Randrup A, 1974: Dopaminergic hypersensitivity and cholinergic hypofunction in the pathophysiology of tardive dyskinesia. *Psychopharmacology, 34,* 21–35.

Gordon TH, Borison RL, Diamond BI, 1980: Estrogen in experiemental tardive dyskinesia. *Neurology, 30,* 551–554.

Gratton L, 1960: Neuroleptiques, parkinsonnisme, et schizophrenie. *Union Medicale du Canada, 89,* 679–684.

Grelack RP, Clark R, Stump JM, Vernier VG, 1970. Amantadine-dopamine interaction: Possible mode of action in parkinsonism. *Science, 169,* 203–204.

Hamlin T, 1975: Current concepts in therapy: Agents for treatment of Parkinson's disease. *New England Journal of Medicine 256,* 699–701.

Holden JMC, Itil TM, Keskiner A, 1969: The treatment of lobotomized schizophrenic patients with butaperazine. *Current Therapeutic Research, 11,* 418–428.

Hoffman BF, 1981: The diagnosis and treatment of neuroleptic-induced parkinsonism. *Hospital and Community Psychiatry, 32,* 110–114.

Hoffman WF, Labs SM, Casey, 1978: Neuroleptic-induced parkinsonism in older schizophrenics. *Biological Psychiatry, 22,* 427–439.

Ing TS, Daugirdas JT, Soung LS, Klawans HL, Mahurkar SD, Hayashi JA, Geis WP, Hano JE, 1979: Toxic effects of amantadine in patients with renal failure. *Canadian Medical Association Journal, 120,* 695–698.

Itoh H, Fujii Y, Ichikawa K, 1984: Blood level studies of haloperidol. In: *Advances of human psychopharmacology,* edited by GD Burrows and JS Werry. Greenwich: Jai Press.

Keepers GA, Clappison VJ, Casey DE, 1983: Initial anticholinergic prophylaxis for neuroleptic-induced extrapyramidal syndromes. *Archives of General Psychiatry, 40,* 1113–1117.

Klawans HL, 1973: The pharmacology of extrapyramidal movement disorders. Basel, Switzerland: S. Karger.

Klawans HL, Bergen D, Bruyn GW, 1973: Prolonged drug-induced parkinsonism. *Confin Neurologica, 35,* 368–377.

Klett CJ, Caffey E, 1972: Evaluating the long term need for antiparkinsonian drugs by chronic schizophrenics. *Archives of General Psychiatry, 25,* 374–379.

Kuny S, Binswanger U, 1989: Neuroleptic-induced extrapyramidal symptoms and serum calcium levels. *Neuropsychobiology, 21,* 67–70.

Levinson DF, 1990: Personal communication.

Levinson DF, Simpson GM, Singh H, Yadalam KG, Jain A, Stephanos MJ, Silver P, 1990: Fluphenazine dose, clinical response and extrapyramidal symptoms during acute treatment. *Archives of General Psychiatry, 47,* 761–768.

Luchins DJ, Jackman H, Meltzer HY, 1983: Lateral ventricular size and drug-induced parkinsonism. *Psychiatry Research 9,* 9–16.

Manos N, Gkiouzepas J, Logothetis J, 1981: The need for continuous use of antiparkinsonian medications with chronic schizophrenic patients receiving long-term neuroleptic therapy. *American Journal of Psychiatry, 138,* 184–188.

Manos N, Gkiouzepas J, Tzotzoras T, Tzanetoglou A, 1981: Gradual withdrawal of antiparkinson medication in chronic schizophrenics. Any better than the abrupt? *Journal of Nervous and Mental Diseases, 169,* 659–661.

May PRA, Lee MA, Bacon RC, 1983: Quantitative assessment of neuroleptic-induced extrapyramidal symptoms: Clinical and nonclinical approaches. *Clinical Neuropharmacology, 6*(s1), S35–51.

McGeer PL, McGeer EG, 1977: Aging and extrapyramidal function. *Archives of Neurology, 34,* 33–35.

Menza MA, Murray GB, Holmes VF, Rafuls WA, 1987: Decreased extrapyramidal symptoms with intravenous haloperidol. *Journal of Clinical Psychiatry, 48,* 278–280.

Metzer WS, Newton JE, Steele RW, Claybrook M, Paige SR, McMillan DE, Hays S, 1989: HLA antigens in drug-induced parkinsonism. *Movement Disorders, 4*(2), 121–128.

Moleman P, Janzen G, von Bargen BA, Kappers EJ, Pepplinkhuizen L, Schmitz PIM, 1986: Relationship between age and incidence of parkinsonism in psychiatric patients treated with haloperidol. *American Journal of Psychiatry, 143,* 232–234.

Morselli PL, Bianchetti G, Dugas M, 1982: Haloperidol plasma level monitoring in neuropsychiatric patients. *Drug Monitoring, 4,* 51–58.

Parkinson J, 1817: *An essay on the shaking palsy.* London: Sherwood/Neely P & Jones.

Prosser ES, Csernansky JG, Kaplan J, Thiemann S, Becker TJ, Hollister LE, 1987: Depression, parkinsonian symptoms, and negative symptoms in schizophrenics treated with neuroleptics. *Journal of Nervous and Mental Diseases, 175,* 100–105.

Quitkin F, Rifkin A, Klein DF, 1975: Very high dosage vs. standard dosage fluphenazine in schizophrenia. *Archives of General Psychiatry, 32,* 1276–1281.

Richardson JC, 1965: Drugs for parkinsonism. *Canadian Medical Association Journal, 92,* 928–929.

Rifkin A, Quitkin F, Klein DF, 1975: Akinesia—a poorly recognized drug-induced extrapyramidal behavioral disorder. *Archives of General Psychiatry, 32,* 672–674.

Simpson GM, 1983: Editorial. *Clinical Neuropharmacology, 6*(s1), s1–s2.

Simpson GM, Angus JWS, 1970: A rating scale for extrapyramidal side effects. *Acta Psychiatrica Scandinavica, 212* (suppl), 11–19.

Simpson GM, Kunz-Bartholini, 1968: Relationship of individual tolerance, behavior, and phenothiazine produced extrapyramidal system disturbance. *Diseases of the Nervous System, 29,* 269–274.

Simpson GM, Yadalam KG, 1985: Blood levels of neuroleptics: State of the art. *Journal of Clinical Psychiatry, 46*(5, sec. 2), 22–28.

Simpson GM, Yadalam KG, 1990: Single dose pharmacokinetics of fluphenazine after fluphenazine decanoate administration. *Journal of Clinical Psychopharmacology,* in press.

Tarsy D, 1983: Neuroleptic-induced extrapyramidal reactions: Classification, description, and diagnosis. *Clinical Neuropharmacology, 6*(s1), 9–26.

Tune L, Coyle JT, 1981: Acute extrapyramidal side effects: Serum levels of neuroleptics and anticholinergics. *Psychopharmacology, 75,* 9–15.

Van Praag HM, Korf J, 1976: Importance of dopamine metabolism for clinical effects and side effects of neuroleptics. *American Journal of Psychiatry, 133,* 1171–1176.

Van Putten T, 1983: Vulnerability to extrapyramidal side effects. *Clinical Neuropharmacology, 6*(sl), 27–34.

Van Putten T, May PRA, 1978: Akinetic depression in schizophrenia. *Archives of General Psychiatry, 35,* 1101–1107.

Van Putten T, Spar J, 1979: The board and care home. *Hospital and Community Psychiatry, 30,* 461–464.

10

Tardive Dyskinesia

James B. Lohr

The discovery of the antipsychotic effects of chlorpromazine in the early 1950s revolutionized the treatment of mental illness and was one of the primary factors ushering in the modern age of psychopharmacology. Yet in spite of the dramatic effects of these medications and their high therapeutic index, antipsychotics are associated with several unwanted side effects. Most of these are primarily a source of discomfort rather than a serious problem, although any unwanted side effect can adversely affect compliance. The side effect tardive dyskinesia (TD) has gained particular notice, since it may persist long after discontinuation of the antipsychotics.

About 5 years after the discovery of the antipsychotic effects of chlorpromazine, the first probable cases of TD were described (Schonecker, 1957). The tardive disorders, distinct from the acute extrapyramidal syndromes, most often occur late in the course of antipsychotic treatment and may persist after discontinuation of the antipsychotic. Another distinguishing characteristic is that an increase in the dose of antipsychotic may suppress the movements, at least temporarily. This leads to the paradoxical observation that the causative agent can also be palliative. Another commonly observed paradoxical feature is that, following decrease or discontinuation of the offending antipsychotic, the disorder may actually increase in severity. Although several different tardive disorders have been described, the prototype, and still by far the most common, is tardive dyskinesia. Here we run into confusion with terminology, since "dyskinesia" in principle refers to any movement disorder, usually of a hyperkinetic nature. Tardive dystonia, tardive tics, and so forth are also forms of a tardive "dyskinesia." Here the term *tardive dyskinesia* is used to refer to a specific disorder characterized by choreoathetoid movements.

TD occurs in approximately 20–25% of patients treated with antipsychotic medications for long periods (Jeste & Wyatt, 1982). Among younger patients on chronic antipsychotics, the yearly incidence is about 4% per year, at least during the initial 5 years or so of treatment. Also, in younger patients there is no clear period of maximum risk; rather the risk continues at an approximately linear yearly rate. However, in older patients the prevalence is much higher, probably greater than 50%. In this patient group, the yearly incidence is also probably much higher, perhaps more than 10%.

RISK FACTORS

Advanced age is the most consistently described risk factor for TD and is discussed in more detail in the next section. Female gender is another risk factor that is commonly accepted (Jeste & Wyatt, 1982b). Perhaps the one risk factor with the greatest clinical importance is the presence of a mood disorder, either unipolar of bipolar (Gardos & Casey, 1984). There is evidence that patients with a mood disorder who are treated with antipsychotics may develop TD more frequently and more severely than other patients (such as those with schizophrenia). It is suggested that antipsychotics be used sparingly in the elderly, especially elderly women, because of the risk of TD. To this should be added their sparing use in patients with mood disorders. Antipsychotics should be used for as short a time as possible in patients with psychotic depression or mania.

Other proposed risk factors are more controversial. These include mental retardation, brain damage (or dementia), length of antipsychotic exposure, use of anticholinergic drugs, history of acute extrapyramidal side effects, antidepressant drugs, depot antipsychotics, history of drug interruptions or holidays, elevated serum antipsychotic concentration (especially in the elderly), smoking, and late-onset psychosis. Even if anticholinergic medications are not a risk factor for TD, they do appear to increase the severity of TD when it is present and can unmask latent TD.

Aging and TD

It is now clear that elderly patients are at greater risk for the development of TD than younger patients (Baldessarini et al., 1980; Casey, 1985; Jeste & Wyatt, 1987). Not only is TD more common in the elderly, but also it appears to be more persistent. Why should this be so? Jeste and Wyatt (1987) in a recent review of TD in the elderly concluded that the increased incidence of TD in the elderly is not a result of differences in dosages or the use of other drugs, such as anticholinergics. However, there are several potential mechanisms by which age could predispose to the development of TD:

1. *Pharmacokinetic mechanisms:* Jeste, Linnolia, Wagner, and Wyatt, (1982) observed that older patients (over age 50) have a three-fold greater serum antipsychotic concentration than younger patients on similar doses. Thus, the pharmacokinetics of antipsychotics are probably altered with age, although it is still not clear if a greater antipsychotic concentration predisposes to more TD.

2. *Age-related brain changes:* A variety of age-related phenomena have been reported in the brain, including neuronal loss and alterations in neurochemical receptors, which could relate to the development of TD (Lohr & Bracha, 1988).

3. *Mood disorders:* TD may be more common in patients with mood disorders, compared to patients with schizophrenia (Gardos & Casey, 1984). Because mood disorders have a later age of onset than schizophrenia, older populations will have a greater proportion of patients with unipolar and bipolar disorders than younger populations, and, therefore, possibly a higher prevalence of TD.

4. *Medical illnesses:* It appears that a variety of medical disorders can be associated with the development of choreoathetoid movements. Elderly patients with medical illnesses are more likely to have orofacial dyskinesias than healthy elderly patients (Lieberman et al., 1984). The age-related increase in medical disease may thus be associated with an increase in TD, especially if TD, like

spontaneous orofacial movements, is more likely to occur in the presence of medical disease.

In some cases, specific medical conditions have been thought to place the elderly at increased risk for TD. For example, it has been suggested that diabetes mellitus, which increases with age, may be a risk factor for TD (Mukherjee, Wisniewski, Bilder, & Sackeim, 1985). Also, some investigators have proposed that a decrease in estrogen may be associated with the emergence of TD, because the risk of TD is especially high for elderly women. In other words, estrogen may exert a protective or masking effect on TD, but this idea so far lacks proof (Gordon, Borison, & Diamond, 1980; Villeneuve, Langlier, & Bedard, 1978). Finally, dental problems, including edentulousness, which are more prevalent in geriatric patients, have been shown to be associated with orofacial dyskinesias and may be associated with greater severity of TD. Perhaps some cases of supposed persistent TD following antipsychotic withdrawal actually are related to edentulous dyskinesias that may have escaped notice before the institution of antipsychotic treatment.

5. *Increased antipsychotic exposure:* If length of exposure or cumulative antipsychotic dose are true risk factors for TD, then this factor alone could account for a general delay in the appearance of TD, shifting it toward older populations of people who receive chronic antipsychotic treatment. Also, cases of persistent TD will be cumulative, additionally increasing the prevalence with age.

PATHOPHYSIOLOGY

The pathophysiology of TD is not known. There is evidence to suggest that neurotransmitter abnormalities are involved, but the exact importance of these remains unclear. One of the oldest theories is that TD involves supersensitivity of dopamine receptors (Lieberman, 1989). The basic hypothesis is that dopamine supersensitivity develops in response to prolonged dopamine blockade by the neuroleptic. Although dopamine is probably involved in some manner in many cases of TD, there is actually very little evidence that dopamine supersensitivity is the mechanism (Jeste, Lohr, Kaufmann, & Wyatt, 1986; Lieberman, 1989). Some investigators have suggested that there may be a balance between D_1 and D_2 receptors in the brain, which is disturbed in TD—an idea supported by the possible efficacy of SKF38393 (a D_1 agonist) in some TD patients (Davidson et al., 1990). This idea requires further research.

There is also evidence that there may be noradrenergic hyperactivity in the brains of some patients with TD (Glazer, 1989; Jeste, Linnoila, & Fordis, 1982), which is supported by studies of norepinephrine and dopamine beta hydroxylase, and by treatment studies using noradrenergic antagonists. Gamma aminobutyric acid (GABA) may also be involved in some patients with TD. For example, there are reports of reduced GABA in the cerebrospinal fluid of TD patients and studies demonstrating the efficacy of GABA agonists in the condition (Nguyen, Thaker, & Tammings, 1989; Thaker et al, 1987).

At present, it is not clear how these various reports of alterations in different neurotransmitter systems relate to one another. It is possible that there may be several, if not many, different neurochemical changes in patients with TD. Another possibility is that there are subgroups of TD patients, each with a different neurochemical abnormality.

The occurrence of persistent TD has led some investigators to suggest that, apart from neurochemical alterations in TD, neuropathological changes may also occur. Gross obvious neuropathology does not appear to occur in TD, so such changes, if present, are probably subtle (Lohr, Wisniewski, & Jeste, 1986). The mechanism by which persistent neuropathological changes could occur is also not clear, but one possibility is that long-term antipsychotic medication may damage neurons through oxidative mechanisms (Elkashef, Ruskin, Bacher, & Barret, 1990; Lohr et al., 1988).

CLINICAL FEATURES

Description

The abnormal movements of TD are usually termed choreoathetoid in appearance. This means there is a combination of athetoid movements, which are slow, writhing, sinuous movements of small amplitude, and choreiform movements, which are faster, more erratic, and of larger amplitude. In most cases the movements of TD appear athetoid, but severe TD can have a choreiform component. Although choreoathetoid movements are considered to be completely irregular, as seen in the movements of Huntington's disease, the movements of TD often show considerable rhythmicity and repetitiveness. This is especially true when the movements are mild, or involve a joint around which there are limited degrees of freedom of motion (e.g., the big toe). The rhythmic nature of some of the movements of TD can cause confusion with parkinsonism. In such cases it is important to observe the frequency of the movements, because those of TD are usually slow (3 second/or less), whereas the frequency of parkinsonian tremor is faster (4-7/ second range) (Caliguiri & Lohr, 1990; Wirshing, Freidenber, Cummings, & Bartzokis, 1989).

Tongue involvement is extremely common, and two types of movements are seen. The first is thrusting or writhing movements involving displacement of the tongue in space. The tongue may stick out of the mouth, sometimes very quickly, or may protrude into the cheek. The second type of movement consists of vermicular or wormlike movements of the tongue, so called because the random-appearing contraction of fascicles of the tongue resembles the motion of a bag of worms. It is important to observe the tongue at different times and under different conditions, because the movements can be exacerbated or suppressed in ways that differ from patient to patient. Therefore, the tongue should be observed with the mouth open and the tongue at rest on the floor of the mouth. Then the patient should protrude and hold the tongue out for at least 10-15 seconds. Also the tongue should be examined when the patient is engaged in some manual activity; many people have tongue movements when performing some act requiring manual dexterity, and this often brings out dyskinetic tongue movements in patients with TD. Some patients have a worsening of tongue movements on protrusion of the tongue, whereas other patients appear to stabilize the tongue with this maneuver and hence suppress the movements.

Lip and jaw movements, consisting of pursing or puckering the lips, and anteroposterior, lateral, or rotatory chewing movements of the jaw are also common in TD. It may be difficult to tell if there are separate lip and jaw movements in the presence of considerable tongue movement. Occasionally there are repetitive blinking and brow movements, but these are less common than movements of the lower face. TD involving the face should be distinguished from facial parkinsonian tremor involving the lips and jaw, sometimes called rabbit syndrome.

After the face, the hands are the most commonly affected part of the body. Usually there are writhing movements of the fingers, although in milder cases the only movements may be repetitive flexion and extension of the thumb on one or both sides. The feet may be involved, but again the movements may be quite mild, involving only the big toe or the ankle.

More severe TD involves the trunk and more proximal extremities. Very severe TD can involve the intercostal, pharyngeal, and diaphragmatic muscles. With mild TD, disability is usually also mild, although there is often some embarrassment and social withdrawal. With more severe TD, there may be problems with speaking and eating, and manual deficits can occur. Very severe TD can result in mouth excoriations, dental problems, and difficulty breathing and swallowing. It is interesting that regardless of the severity of the movements, they disappear during sleep. Stress makes the movements worse.

Although the movements of TD are involuntary, they are not totally outside of the patient's control. For short periods a patient may be able to decrease the movements consciously, sometimes to the point of total suppression. This is often observed during the interview with the patient. The best time to look for signs of subtle TD may be when the patient is not aware that he or she is being observed, such as while in the waiting room.

Research diagnostic criteria for TD have been developed by Schooler and Kane (1982). There are basically three criteria:

1. A history of at least 3 months of exposure to antipsychotics. The 3 months of exposure do not have to be in a single continuous episode, but may occur over a longer time.

2. Abnormal movements of at least a moderately severe nature (AIMS score of 3 or more) in one body area or of at least a mild nature (AIMS score of 2 or more) in two body regions. For example, a person with moderately severe abnormal movements only of the tongue would qualify—or of mild movements of the tongue and lips. Mild movements of the tongue alone would not qualify for a diagnosis of TD, although the clinician should be suspicious that this represents subclinical early TD.

3. The absence of any other disorders that could cause the abnormal movements. Therefore, all patients who develop what may be TD should have a complete movement disorder work-up, which is described later.

It is important to remember that TD may occur with all antipsychotic medications (except perhaps clozapine). These include medications such as metoclopramide (Reglan), if long-term administration is required.

SUBTYPES OF TD

A variety of different subtyping schemes have been proposed for TD. The most commonly used schemes divide TD according to course, severity, distribution, and type of movement.

Course

TD has been divided into two main forms, reversible (lasting less than 3–6 months) and persistent (lasting longer than 6 months). The term withdrawal dyskinesia is used to refer to abnormal movements that appear only after antipsychotic discontinuation (or reduction). If the movements disappear within 3–6 weeks, then it is considered to be a self-limited withdrawal dyskinesia. If withdrawal dyskinesia persists beyond 6 weeks or so, it has been termed withdrawal TD or unmasked TD.

Severity

TD is usually graded as mild, moderate, or severe (corresponding to global AIMS scores of 2, 3, and 4, respectively). In the majority of patients of TD, the dyskinesia is mild and does not constitute a serious physical disability. In a minority of cases TD develops after relatively brief treatment with antipsychotics, rapidly increases in severity, and does not improve on antipsychotic withdrawal. This type of TD has been called malignant TD. There is no published definition of malignant TD and its exact incidence is unknown. It probably accounts for about 5% of the cases of TD in younger patients and approximately 10% among patients over 50. Malignant TD is not the same as severe TD or persistent TD, although these categories do overlap.

Distribution

Some investigators have proposed dividing TD according to body regions involved (Barnes, Kidger, Trauer, & Taylor, 1980; Kidger, Barnes, Trauer, & Taylor, 1980). TD has been divided into a central or orofacial vs a peripheral or limb-truncal form. The orofacial form may be more common in the elderly and the limb-truncal more common in younger patients.

Type of Movement

In recent years a variety of tardive movement disorders have been described (Burke et al., 1982; Lohr & Jeste, 1988). They are, strictly speaking, all TDs, but the term *tardive dyskinesia* usually refers to the choreoathetoid disorder. The other conditions are termed tardive dystonia, tardive akathisia, and tardive tic or tardive Tourette's disorder. These conditions share with typical TD their occurrence late in the course of antipsychotic treatment and their suppression after an increase in antipsychotic dosage.

Of these other disorders, tardive dystonia is the most common (Chapter 8) and may coexist with more typical TD. Unlike typical TD, which usually worsens or shows no change following administration of anticholinergic medications, tardive dystonia often responds to these drugs. The dystonia can involve any body part, although the neck (torticollis, retrocollis), jaw, limbs, or back are most commonly involved. Just as with TD, many classes of antipsychotics have been implicated. The disorder can last for years after discontinuation of the antipsychotic. Other tardive syndromes may include tardive myoclonus and tardive parkinsonism, although little is known about these conditions.

COURSE

The course of TD has been difficult to investigate because of the long delay in developing the disorder, the inherent variability in the condition, the effects of different treatments and changes in antipsychotics, and the loss of patients to follow-up. Only in recent years has it been possible to put together an idea of what happens to the condition under different circumstances.

Unlike chronic progressive conditions like Huntington's disease, TD is a condition that usually increases in severity over a fairly brief period of time (usually months) and then stabilizes. After someone has had TD for a year or more, or after it has stabilized for 6 months or so, it appears unlikely to become much worse unless the dose of antipsychotic is significantly changed (Casey, 1985; Kane, Woerner, & Lieberman, 1985). Unfortunately, if a patient is seen early in the course of TD, it is impossible to say exactly how severe it may become. After the movements have appeared and become relatively stable, it is useful to distinguish the course of TD under two conditions: when antipsychotics are stopped and when they are continued.

Discontinuation of Antipsychotics

If antipsychotics are discontinued, there are several possible outcomes. First, the movements may improve quickly and may disappear. Second, there may be a temporary exacerbation of the movements followed by improvement. This latter occurrence may be a withdrawal dyskinesia superimposed on the TD. These two courses probably account for between one third and two thirds of cases in which antipsychotics are continued and comprise reversible (or partially reversible) TD. Antipsychotic withdrawal results in remission of dyskinesia after a 3-month period in about 40% of patients. After a year of antipsychotic withdrawal, probably between at least one half and two thirds of patient may have a significant reduction of dyskinesia (Glazer et al., 1984; Jeste & Wyatt, 1982).

The third possibility is that the dyskinesia continues to exist, termed persistent TD. Many cases of persistent TD improve over the years and some may even gradually disappear. There is, however, a group of patients who continue to have TD virtually unchanged for many years, and sometimes these cases have been termed irreversible TD. This term is not commonly used because there is always the possibility of improvement in the disorder with time. Rarely, some patients, after discontinuing antipsychotics, may have a worsening of TD that does not improve because of the masking effects of antipsychotics on TD.

Continuation of Antipsychotics

If antipsychotics are continued, again there is usually improvement in the TD, although it is more gradual. An increase in antipsychotic dosage may suppress the TD for a time, but it usually recurs. In some cases of very severe TD, however, an increase in the dose of antipsychotic may suppress the dyskinesia for many months, if not indefinitely. On the other hand, occasionally patients demonstrate a gradual worsening of TD over months to years with continued antipsychotics.

TD usually develops over a period of months and then stabilizes. If antipsychotics are discontinued, the majority of patients have a marked improvement in the condition, but a third or more can have persistent TD, which may or may not gradually improve over the years. If antipsychotics are continued, again most patients will have a gradual improvement in TD, but in a large number the TD will remain the same or gradually worsen. An increase in the dose of antipsychotic can suppress the movements, usually only temporarily, but occasionally for long periods. Although there are not enough data to support the idea, many clinicians believe that the earlier antipsychotics are decreased or discontinued after the first development of abnormal movements, the better the chances for improvement.

DIFFERENTIAL DIAGNOSIS

Other Antipsychotic-Induced Disorders

It is important to distinguish TD from antipsychotic-induced parkinsonism. One complicating factor, however, is the coexistence of TD with other antipsychotic-induced movement disorders (such as parkinsonism), which may occur in as many as 50% of patients with TD. When TD occurs with parkinsonism the diagnosis of both becomes difficult. Also, TD and parkinsonism need not occur in different body regions; they can coexist even in the same finger.

Rabbit syndrome is a parkinsonian tremor of the orofacial region marked by small rhythmic movements of lips at a frequency of about 5 per second. Sometimes there is a popping sound when the lips are opened (Todd, Lippman, Manshadi, & Chang, 1983). The tongue may or may not be involved; when it is, tongue movements are of a tremulous nature. Like other parkinsonian symptoms and unlike TD, rabbit syndrome may respond to anticholinergic agents.

Akathisia is another antipsychotic-induced movement disorder that usually appears within a few weeks of starting treatment. When mild, there is a feeling of anxiety or agitation often accompanied by a desire to move. With increasing severity, the patients demonstrate excessive movement, usually in the lower extremities. This consists of foot tapping, crossing and uncrossing the legs, and various postural changes. When standing, patients may shift weight repeatedly from one foot to the other, or walk around the room. Patients occasionally state that moving decreases the discomfort, but this is not true in every case. Unlike TD, the movements are fairly repetitive and are more pronounced in the legs and trunk. When severe, however, the condition can be difficult to distinguish from TD. There is probably a tardive form of akathisia also. Akathisia can be very difficult to treat, but may respond to anticholinergic medications, beta-blockers, or benzodiazepines.

Movement Disorders Involving Primarily the Orofacial Region

Bruxism is a common condition consisting of regular, repetitive jaw movements in which the teeth are brought into contact and grind against each other. This condition frequently occurs at night and can be easily suppressed volitionally, unlike TD.

Senile chorea or senile buccolinguomasticatory (BLM) dyskinetic disorder is very common in the elderly and often indistinguishable from orofacial TD. BLM dyskinesias in the elderly are common, but usually occur in patients with medical or psychiatric illness (Lieberman et al., 1984). Most senile choreoathetoid disorders are mild.

Edentulous dyskinesia also is a condition usually seen in the elderly (Koller, 1983; Sutcher, Underwood, Beatty, & Sugar, 1971), but may occur in younger patients with dental abnormalities. The incidence is not known. The movements are usually mild and may resemble oral TD. There is no involvement of other body regions. It is often improved by dentures.

Meige's syndrome, which has also been called blepharospasm-oromandibular dystonia syndrome, is a disorder that usually occurs later in life. It may present with either blepharospasm, oromandibular dystonia, or both (Marsden, 1976). Patients may later develop dystonias in other body parts, such as in the neck and upper extremity. Like TD, the condition appears to be more common in women than in men. It may be severely incapacitating and the blepharospasm can render patients virtually blind; the oral dystonia may significantly impair eating and speaking and, rarely, breathing. Depression occurs in approximately one third of patients. Meige's syndrome is more dystonic than typical TD, although it may occasionally occur as a form of tardive dystonia.

Generalized Movement Disorders

Parkinson's disease is a chronic progressive disorder usually beginning in late middle age years. It is characterized by the clinical tetrad of tremor, rigidity, bradykinesia, and postural abnormalities. Although occasionally parkinsonian tremor may be confused with TD, it is usually more rhythmical, regular, and faster, in the range of 4–7 cycles per second.

Huntington's disease is a hereditary degenerative disease with an autosomal dominant mode of inheritance, marked by progressive clumsiness and choreoathetoid movements. Variants have been described that are characterized more by progressive rigidity—especially of the trunk and proximal limb musculature—than by choreoathetoid movements. The majority (as many as 90%) of patients have some form of psychopathology, although there appears to be less psychopathology with later-onset cases. In approximately half of patients, psychiatric symptoms are the reason for first admission. In two thirds of cases the psychopathology appears before the abnormal movements. Many different psychiatric conditions can occur, including mood disorder (mainly depression), a schizophrenia-like psychosis, and personality disorders. Dementia is very common in chronic cases. The movements are generalized, affecting virtually all body regions, which is unlike all but the most severe cases of TD. Also, there is always a family history, although it may not always be available. CT scans show evidence of basal ganglia atrophy to a much greater extent than in cases of TD.

Sydenham's chorea is a delayed reaction to group A streptococcal infection. Although it typically occurs in children and adolescents, it is important to note that post-Sydenham's patients may show evidence of continuing abnormalities in extrapyramidal function. These include a predilection to redevelop chorea after stimulants or estrogens, or during pregnancy (chorea gravidarum). Psychopathology usually consists of neuroses and personality disorders, the latter having at times been called "post-choreic personality." There may be fidgetiness, dizziness, irritability, and excitability that can last long after the chorea has disappeared (Schwartzmann, 1950). The onset is more acute than TD and the movements are more choreiform and asymmetrical. There is usually a history of rheumatic fever, and some patients demonstrate elevated antistreptolysin O (ASO) titers.

Wilson's disease is a degenerative disorder caused by an abnormality in copper metabolism, although the exact defect is not known. There is a decrease in the bound product of copper and apoceruloplasmin (ceruloplasmin), and an elevation of free copper concentration in the blood. Urinary copper excretion is increased, and there is deposition of copper in the tissues, most notably the brain (predominantly the basal ganglia) and the liver. The disease has an autosomal recessive mode of inheritance. It commonly manifests with hepatic cirrhosis and jaundice, renal tubular damage, and neuronal damage in a variety of brain areas, especially in the basal ganglia. Kayser-Fleischer rings are a hallmark of the condition. These are observed initially on slit-lamp evaluation as brownish-red or green crescents in the superior and inferior aspects of the corneoscleral junction. The movement disorder may consist of any combination of rigidity, coarse proximal tremor ("wing-beating"), choreoathetosis, and dystonia. There may be dysarthria and dysphagia also. In as many as one fifth of patients, psychiatric symptoms precede the onset of other abnormalities. Such symptoms include impulsivity, irritability, restlessness, and personality and mood changes. Psychosis, usually paranoid in nature, is uncommon. Rarely, severe psychiatric symptoms may be the presenting feature. The abnormal movements are more dystonic and rhythmical than TD, and the copper abnormalities and Kayser-Fleischer rings are diagnostic.

Hallervorden-Spatz disease is a very rare hereditary disorder that usually begins in late childhood or early adolescence. It is marked by the accumulation of a brown iron-containing pigment in the basal ganglia, particularly the globus pallidus and substantia nigra pars reticulata. The condition is slowly progressive and the abnormal movements consist of choreoathetosis, dystonia, and rigidity. Occasionally there may also be spasticity, hyperreflexia, and dysarthria. Psychiatric symptoms usually consist of either mental retardation or dementia, although depression can occur.

Dystonia musculorum deformans (torsion dystonia) is the name for a group of disorders that typically begin in late childhood or early adolescence and are marked by the progressive development of slow irregular contorting movements. Primary psychiatric problems are rare. The movements are usually more severe, progressive, and dystonic in nature than those of TD.

Tourette's disorder is a condition that usually begins in childhood and is characterized by tics of the face and extremities. Other common features include vocal tics, echolalia, echopraxia, coprolalia, compulsive and avoidant behavior, and attentional problems. Tics may range from simple to complex and are more highly repetitive than the movements of TD (although tardive tic disorders may be indistinguishable from Tourette's disorder).

Other Movement Disorders

Some investigators have noted the presence of movement disorder in patients with schizophrenia and other psychiatric and catatonic disorders (sometimes called spontaneous dyskinesias). This literature has been summarized by Casey and Hansen (1984). It appears that the overall prevalence of spontaneous dyskinesias in schizophrenia is probably about 5%. Just as is the case with TD, women, the elderly, and patients with organic mental disorders appear to be at greatest risk for developing spontaneous dyskinesias. Although it is possible that in some cases the movements may be similar in appearance to those of TD, this is not completely clear. Schizophrenic and manic patients with catatonia may of course have stereotypical movements, but these are usually more complex and repetitive than TD. They often resemble routine actions or fragments of actions. For further discussion on the distinction between stereotypical movements and TD, see Lohr and Wisniewski (1987).

There are many other conditions in which abnormal movements may be observed, which should be distinguished from TD. These include other drug-induced or toxin-induced disorders (such as stimulant-induced or heavy metal-induced dyskinesias), familial paroxysmal choreoathetosis, chorea-acanthocytosis, hyperthyroidism, polycythemia, and systemic lupus erythematosus.

ASSESSMENT

The work-up of TD begins with a complete history—with special attention devoted to exposure to antipsychotics (including metoclopramide) and to L-dopa, lithium, estrogens, stimulants (including street drugs and diet pills), and toxins (including carbon monoxide, manganese, other transition metals). Inquiries should be made regarding a history of rheumatic fever or Sydenham's chorea early in life or a history of chorea gravidarum (which may be a recurrence of Sydenham's chorea appearing during pregnancy). Questions should be asked about thyroid disease, polycythemia, and systemic lupus erythematosus. A family history of movement disorder is very helpful in identifying Huntington's disease. A complete physical exam should be performed, including detailed neurological and mental status examinations. Finally, laboratory investigations should include bloodwork (including electrolytes, glucose, complete blood count, thyroid function tests) a urine drug screen for stimulants, phencyclidine and transition metals, an electroencephalogram, and a CT scan.

PREVENTION AND TREATMENT

There are two approaches to reducing TD: preventing it and treating it after it has developed. The primary preventive measure is, of course, not to prescribe antipsychotics, since it is mainly agents with antipsychotic-like properties that are known to cause TD. Although this sounds simple and easy to carry out, many clinicians, when confronted with psychosis, almost reflexively think "antipsychotic treatment." It is at this stage, before antipsychotics are prescribed, that the situation should be carefully considered, because patients may be continued on antipsychotics beyond the point necessary. For example, patients may be transferred from one physician to another, and other physicians may feel uncomfortable discontinuing the drugs for fear of a recurrence of psychosis and subsequent destabilization of the patient. For this and other reasons, starting antipsychotics should be considered very carefully. The physician should ask, "Will this psychosis resolve spontaneously without antipsychotics?" "Will this psychotic mania resolve with carbamazepine or lithium alone, or this psychotic depression with antidepressants alone?" and "Can I use a benzodiazepine or propranolol to control the psychotic agitation instead of an antipsychotic?" Once antipsychotics are initiated, consideration should be given to discontinuing them as soon as possible.

On the other hand, for those patients who require chronic antipsychotic treatment, such treatment should not be withheld simply because of the risk of TD. The patient should be counseled about TD, but it should be noted that most of the time TD is mild and frequently reversible. The patient and the family should be taught about the signs of TD and instructed to notify the caregiver as soon as any of these are seen. Also, all of this should be documented in the chart. It is important to discuss with the patient which symptoms are most distressing. Many patients can tolerate abnormal movements much better than hallucinations. Other patients are not bothered much by hallucinations, but find abnormal movements very distressing. Although anticholinergic drugs can exacerbate TD, patients frequently complain more about parkinsonism than about TD, and this must be taken into account when making a clinical decision. It is essential to work with the patient to achieve the best result possible. It is often very useful to explain the nature of the dilemma to the patient. Even those patients with fairly severe psychopathology can often understand what is happening and make informed decisions.

After TD has developed, the primary treatment is reduction and, if possible, discontinuation of antipsychotics. When antipsychotics are being used appropriately, the patient should already be on the minimum effective dose. At this point, anticholinergic medication and any stimulant medication (including diet pills and many over-the-counter cough and cold medications) should be reduced to a minimum, as these can exacerbate the movements. Switching to a different antipsychotic is occasionally beneficial, especially if the patient is switched to clozapine.

Clozapine is an atypical antipsychotic that was released in the United States in February 1990. Although it does not appear to cause TD, it is associated with a high incidence (around 1%) of agranulocytosis, which is potentially fatal. For this reason all patients receiving the drug must be enrolled in a monitoring system requiring a weekly blood analysis. The initial monitoring system "Clozaril Patient Management System (CPMS)" is expensive and cumbersome, limiting the availability of the drug, but is available for selected patients with moderate to severe TD who continue to require antipsychotics. Fortunately, there are a number of new antipsychotics currently under development that may offer the advantage of therapeutic efficacy without TD and that hopefully will not have such a common serious side effect as clozapine. These other "atypical" antipsychotics may become available within the next decade.

Sometimes a medication can be added to the antipsychotic, which will allow for a reduction in the antipsychotic dosage. For example, if the patient has considerable agitation as a component of the psychosis, a benzodiazepine may be added to allow reduction in the antipsychotic. The addition of lithium or carbamazepine may occasionally reduce the amount of antipsychotic drug needed.

Apart from these approaches, the treatment of TD is largely empirical. There is no single generally effective treatment, so a variety of approaches may be tried. A trial of a GABA-ergic agonist such as the benzodiazepine clonazepam (Thaker et al., 1990) or a noradrenergic antagonist such as propranolol (if medically feasible) may be helpful. For further discussion of the pharmacological treatment of TD, see Jeste and Wyatt (1982a) and Jeste, Lohr, Clark, and Wyatt, (1988).

Finally, in cases of severe incapacitating dyskinesias that are unresponsive to other pharmacological manipulations, it may be necessary to attempt to suppress the dyskinesia by giving higher doses of antipsychotic. This is far from optimal, however, because of the possibility that the dyskinesia may further worsen and reerupt at the higher dose.

REFERENCES

Baldessarini RJ, Cole JO, Davis JM, Gardos G, Preskorn SH, Simpson GM, Tarsy D, 1980: *Tardive dyskinesia: A task force report of the American Psychiatric Association.* Wasington, DC: American Psychiatric Association.

Barnes TRE, Kidger T, Trauer T, Taylor P, 1980: Reclassification of the tardive dyskinesia syndrome. *Advances in Biochemistry and Psychopharmacology, 24,* 565–568.

Burke RE, Fahn S, Jankovic J, Marsden CD, Lang AE, Gollomp S, Ilson J, 1982: Tardive dystonia: Late onset and persistent dystonia caused by antipsychotic drugs. *Neurology, 32,* 1335–1346.

Caligiuri MP, Lohr JB, 1990: Fine force instability: A quantitative measure of neuroleptic-induced dyskinesia in the hand. *Journal of Neuropsychiatry Clinical Neurosciences, 2,* 395–398.

Casey DE, 1985: Spontaneous and tardive dyskinesia: Clinical and laboratory studies. *Journal of Clinical Psychiatry, 46*(4, Sec 2):42–47.

Casey DE, Hansen TE, 1984: Spontaneous dyskinesia. In: *Neuropsychiatric movement disorders,* edited by DV Jeste, RJ Wyatt. Washington, DC: American Psychiatric Press.

Davidson M, Harvey PD, Bergman RL, Powchik P, Kaminsky R, Losonczy MF, Davis KL, 1990: Effects of the D_1 agonist SKF-38393 combined with haloperidol in schizophrenic patients. *Archives of General Psychiatry, 47,* 190–191.

Elkashef AM, Ruskin PE, Bacher N, Barrett D, 1990: Vitamin E in the treatment of tardive dyskinesia. *American Journal of Psychiatry, 147,* 505–506.

Gardos G, Casey DE, 1984: *Tardive dyskinesia and affective disorders.* Washington, DC: American Psychiatric Press.

Glazer WM, 1989: Noradrenergic function and tardive dyskinesia. *Psychiatric Annals, 19,* 297–301.

Glazer WM, Moore DC, Schooler NR, Brenner LM, Morgenstern H, 1980: Tardive dyskinesia: A discontinuation study. *Archives of General Psychiatry, 41,* 623–627.

Gordon JH, Borison RL, Diamond BI, 1980: Estrogen in experimental tardive dyskinesia. *Neurology, 30,* 551–554.

Jeste DV, Linnoila M, Fordis CM, 1982: Enzyme studies in tardive dyskinesia, III: Noradrenergic hyperactivity in a subgroup of dyskinetic patients. *Journal of Clinical Psychopharmacology, 2,* 318–320.

Jeste DV, Linnoila M, Wagner RL, Wyatt RJ, 1982: Serum neuroleptic concentrations and tardive dyskinesia. *Psychopharmacology, 76,* 377–380.

Jeste DV, Lohr JB, Kaufmann CA, Wyatt RJ, 1986: Pathophysiology of tardive dyskinesia: Evaluation of supersensitivity theory and alternative hypotheses. In: *Tardive dyskinesis and neuroleptics: From dogma to reason,* edited by D Casey, G Gardos. Washington, DC: American Psychiatric Press.

Jeste DV, Lohr JB, Clark K, Wyatt RJ, 1988: Pharmacological treatments of tardive dyskinesia in the 1980s. *Journal of Clinical Psychopharmacology, 8,* 385–485.

Jeste DV, Wyatt RJ, 1982a: Therapeutic strategies against tardive dyskinesia—Two decades of experience. *Archives of General Psychiatry, 39,* 803–816.

Jeste DV, Wyatt RJ, 1982b: *Understanding and treating tardive dyskinesia.* New York: Guilford Press.

Jeste DV, Wyatt RJ, 1987: Aging and tardive dyskinesia. In: *Schizophrenia and aging,* edited by NE Miller, GD Cohen. New York: Guilford Press.

Kane JM, Woerner M, Lieberman J, 1985: Tardive dyskinesia: Prevalence, incidence and risk factors.

In: *Dyskinesia: Research and treatment,* edited by DE Casey, TN Chase, AV Christensen, J Gerlach. Berlin: Springer-Verlag.

Kidger T, Barnes TRE, Trauer T, Taylor PJ, 1980: Sub-syndromes of tardive dyskinesia. *Psychological Medicine, 10,* 513–520.

Koller WC, 1983: Edentulous orodyskinesia. *Annals of Neurology, 13,* 97–99.

Lieberman J, 1989: Dopamine pathophysiology in tardive dyskinesia. *Psychiatric Annals, 19,* 289–296.

Lieberman J, Kane JM, Woerner M, Weinhold P, Basavaraju N, Kurucz J, Bergmann K, 1984: Prevalence of tardive dyskinesia in elderly samples. *Psychopharmacology Bulletin, 20,* 382–386.

Lohr JB, Bracha HS, 1988: Association of psychosis and movement disorders in the elderly. *Psychiatric Clinics of North America, 11,* 61–82.

Lohr JB, Cadet JL, Lohr MA, Larson L, Wasli E, Wade L, Hylton R, Vidoi C, Jeste DV, Wyatt RJ, 1988: Vitamin E in the treatment of tardive dyskinesia: The possible involvement of free radical mechanisms. *Schizophrenia Bulletin, 14,* 291–296.

Lohr JB, Jeste DV, 1988: Neuroleptic-induced movement disorders: Tardive dyskinesia and other tardive syndromes. In: *Psychiatry,* edited by JO Cavenar, Jr. Philadelphia: Lippincott.

Lohr JB, Wisniewski A, 1987: *Movement disorders: A neuropsychiatric approach.* New York: Guilford Press.

Lohr JB, Wisniewski A, Jeste DV, 1986: Neurological aspects of tardive dyskinesia. In: *Handbook of schizophrenia, vol. 1, neurology of schizophrenia,* edited by H Nasrallah, DR Weinberg. Amsterdam: Elsevier.

Marsden CD, 1976: Blepharospasm-oromandibular dystonia syndrome (Breughel's syndrome). *Journal of Neurology, Neurosurgery, and Psychiatry, 39,* 1204–1209.

Mukherjee S, Wisniewski A, Bilder R, Sackeim HA, 1985: Possible association between tardive dyskinesia and altered carbohydrate metabolism. *Archives of General Psychiatry, 42,* 205.

Nguyen JA, Thaker GK, Tamminga CA, 1989: Gamma-aminobutyric acid (GABA) pathways in tardive dyskinesia. *Psychiatric Annals, 19,* 302–309.

Schooler N, Kane JM, 1982: Research diagnostic criteria for tardive dyskinesia. *Archives of General Psychiatry, 39,* 486–487.

Schonecker M, 1957: Ein Eigentumliches syndrom im oralen bereich bei megaphen applikation. *Nervenarzt, 28,* 35.

Schwartzmann J, 1950: Chorea minor: Review of 175 cases with reference ↔ etiology, treatment and sequelae. *Rheumatism, 6,* 89–95.

Sutcher HD, Underwood RB, Beatty RA, Sugar O, 1971: Orofacial dyskinesia: A dental dimension. *Journal of the American Medical Association, 216,* 1459–1463.

Thaker GK, Nguyen JA, Strauss ME, Jacobson R, Kaup BA, Tamminga CA, 1990: Clonazepam treatment of tardive dyskinesia: A practical GABA mimetic strategy. *American Journal of Psychiatry, 147,* 445–451.

Thaker GK, Tamminga CA, Alphs LD, Lafferman J, Ferraro TN, Hare TA, 1987: Brain gamma aminobutyric acid abnormality in tardive dyskinesia: Reductions in cerebrospinal fluid GABA levels and therapeutic response to GABA agonist treatment. *Archives of General Psychiatry, 44,* 522–529.

Todd R, Lippman S, Manshadi M, Chang A, 1983: Recognition and treatment of rabbit syndrome, an uncommon complication of neuroleptic therapies. *American Journal of Psychiatry, 140,* 1519–1520.

Villeneuve A, Langlier P, Bedard P, 1978: Estrogens, dopamine and dyskinesias. *Canadian Psychiatric Association Journal, 23,* 68–70.

Wirshing WC, Freidenberg DL, Cummings JL, Bartzokis, G, 1989: Effects of anticholinergic agents on patients with tardive dyskinesia and concomitant drug-induced parkinsonism. *Journal of Clinical Psychopharmacology, 9,* 407–411.

11

Neuroleptic Malignant Syndrome

Gerard Addonizio

Neuroleptic malignant syndrome (NMS) is a potentially fatal disorder that can occur following the use of antipsychotic medication. The syndrome's main characteristics are extrapyramidal symptoms (EPS) and elevated temperature. Frequently associated features include agitation, confusion, diaphoresis, leukocytosis, elevated creatine phosphokinase (CPK), tachycardia, and elevated or low blood pressure (Addonizio, Susman, & Roth, 1987). Originally described in the French literature (Delay, 1960), NMS has become increasingly recognized and discussed in the English language literature. For many years the literature on NMS has been based largely on published case reports and analytic reviews of these cases. More recently there has been an expansion of knowledge based on systematic retrospective and prospective studies. The result of this work has been to alter many long-held beliefs about NMS while validating others. Various treatment modalities have been tried with some success, but no treatment has been invariably effective in ameliorating the symptoms of this serious disorder. The pathophysiology underlying NMS remains unclear, although several hypotheses have been discussed but not clearly validated.

The psychiatric community's increased awareness of NMS has probably led to earlier recognition and consequently lower morbidity (Pearlman, 1986). On the other hand, heightened sensitivity about NMS may have also led to excessive fear, and consequently premature termination of antipsychotic therapy in cases that might have benefited from continued treatment. Associated with this problem has been the inclination of some authors of diagnosing NMS with vague and loose criteria, thereby creating undue panic and obfuscating the pursuit of a clearer understanding of this disorder. This chapter will attempt to provide an overview of NMS, clarifying what is known and identifying areas of ambiguity.

EPIDEMIOLOGY

Reviews of NMS have fairly consistently reported that NMS occurs more frequently in men than in women (Addonizio et al., 1987). Reasons for this are unclear but may be related to the use of larger doses of antipsychotics and higher potency antipsychotics in men. It had often been reported that NMS largely occurred in young adults, but more recently this idea has been revised (Addonizio et al., 1987). NMS has been reported from childhood through late elderly years. In one review of 115 cases of NMS, only 51% of the patients were under 40 years old (Addonizio et al., 1987). In addition, cases occurring with NMS patients over the age of 60 have become much more frequently reported in the literature (Addonizio et al., 1987). The primary psychiatric diagnoses of the majority of patients with NMS have been schizophrenia and bipolar, manic disorder. Some authors have suggested that mania itself may be a risk factor for NMS. Organic brain disease and retardation have also been suggested as risk factors for the development of NMS. In one review of 115 cases of NMS, 5% of the patients had mental retardation as a primary or secondary diagnosis (Addonizio et al., 1987).

MEDICATIONS

Most of the reported cases of NMS have occurred in patients on high-potency antipsychotics such as haloperidol (Levenson, 1985). Although it makes intuitive sense that the most potent dopamine receptor blockers would most likely cause NMS, this assumption has not been definitively substantiated. Other factors such as frequency of prescribing a particular antipsychotic and the tendency to use higher doses of high potency antipsychotics need to be considered before clearly establishing high-potency antipsychotics as the main culprit. High doses of antipsychotic drugs, especially when rapidly increased, are more likely to cause NMS (Shalev, Hermesh, & Munitz, 1986). There is also evidence that parenteral administration of antipsychotics will more likely cause NMS than oral administration (Keck, Pope, Cohen, McElroy, & Nierenberg, 1989).

Some investigators have suggested that lithium may be a risk factor for NMS (Keck, Pope, & McElroy, 1987). In 1974, several cases were reported in which the lithium-haloperidol combination appeared to cause a devastating syndrome similar to NMS (Cohen & Cohen, 1974). A follow-up study of a large series of cases treated with this combination did not substantiate that the lithium-haloperidol combination was toxic (Baastrup, Hollnagel, Sorenson, & Schou, 1976). On the other hand, several lines of evidence suggest that the lithium-antipsychotic combination may enhance the risk of developing both EPS and NMS. In some individuals, lithium has been shown to potentiate EPS when added to a stable antipsychotic regimen (Addonizio, 1985; Addonizio, Roth, Stokes, & Stoll, 1988). In several cases of resolved NMS, lithium alone has precipitated a reoccurrence of the syndrome (Susman & Addonizio, 1987). Further clarification of this issue requires controlled, prospective studies.

A syndrome identical to NMS has been described in patients who have not received any antipsychotic but who have been receiving dopaminergic agents for Parkinson's disease (Friedman, Feinberg, & Feldman, 1985). When these medicines were abruptly discontinued, a florid NMS-like syndrome developed, in some cases with fatal consequences. These cases provide further substantiation for the idea that NMS is the result of a sudden decrease in dopaminergic function in susceptible individuals.

PATHOPHYSIOLOGY

The precise nature of the pathophysiological mechanisms underlying NMS is not clear. What is particularly mysterious is why some patients develop NMS, whereas others seem to be relatively immune even at high doses of antipsychotic. It is generally assumed that one component of NMS involves hypodopaminergic functioning in the striatum and possibly in the hypothalamus (Addonizio et al., 1987). There are several lines of evidence that suggest this hypothesis. EPS, a prominent aspect of NMS, can be caused by dopaminergic blockade in the striatum. The fact that some patients with Parkinson's disease can develop a florid, NMS-like syndrome when their dopaminergic agents are suddenly stopped also supports this notion. Bromocriptine, a dopamine agonist, can dramatically ameliorate the symptoms of NMS in some patients (Zubenko & Pope, 1983). Autonomic dysfunction in NMS may be related to impaired dopaminergic functioning in the hypothalamus. Even though muscular contraction itself may generate heat, some authors have proposed that the elevated temperature in NMS also involves a disorder of central thermal regulation (Kurlan, Hamill, & Shoulson, 1984). One model of thermoregulation indicates that the major integration of thermal afferents occurs in the preoptic-anterior hypothalamus, which then correlates this input to a set point in the posterior hypothalamus (Kurlan et al., 1984). Dopamine is an important mediator within this system. When chlorpromazine is injected into the rostral hypothalamus or third ventricle of the rat, hyperthermia is produced (Abbot & Loizou, 1986). Heat-dissipating mechanisms such as vasodilation may also be impaired (Weinberg & Twersky, 1983) as they are in Parkinson's disease (Sechi, Tanda, & Mutani, 1984).

Other attempts to explain the etiology of NMS have tried to correlate similar pathophysiological links with malignant hyperthermia (MH) (Caroff, Rosenberg, Fletcher, Heinman-Patterson, & Mann, 1987). Several investigators have used tests for MH in patients with NMS in an attempt to show a similar muscle abnormality in patients with NMS. The test is performed by exposing muscle biopsy specimens in vitro to halothane or caffeine, or both of these agents, and then examining for increased muscle tension. Based on this type of study, some investigators have found that NMS patients may be at risk for developing MH (Araki, Takagi, Higuchi, & Sugita, 1988). On the other hand, there is evidence from other studies that does not find the same susceptibility (Krivosic-Horber, Adnet, Guevant, Theunynck, & Lestavel, 1987). To date there is no definitive answer to a potential pathophysiological link between MH and NMS. Reasons for these discrepant results are unclear but may be related to variance in technique in muscle biopsy studies. Further study is required to elucidate this issue.

Other pathophysiological hypotheses include possible imbalances in various catecholamine systems, deficiencies in gamma-aminobutyric acid transmission, and problems in calcium metabolism. To date there are very little data to substantially support these interesting possibilities.

CLINICAL AND LABORATORY FEATURES

In general there is a fairly strong consensus that elevated temperature and EPS are essential features for making the diagnosis of NMS. The range of temperature elevation varies from mild increases to extremely high levels. It is extremely important in making the diagnosis of NMS that nonantipsychotic related causes of fever be ruled out such as febrile states secondary to infection. Although it is true that many patients with NMS have medical problems that can cause fever (Levinson & Simpson, 1986), in most cases patients develop an elevated temperature before developing these problems. The EPS seen in NMS usually takes the form of severe rigidity and tremors with some patients also developing dystonic reactions. Most patients become tachycardic (Levenson, 1985). Many patients develop elevated systolic and diastolic blood pressure, whereas others develop a labile or low blood pressure. Many patients become confused, agitated, and diaphoretic, and some develop incontinence and dehydration. In fact, prior dehydration and agitation may be risk factors for the development of NMS (Itoh et al., 1977).

The most common laboratory abnormality in NMS is elevated CPK (muscle fraction) with a range extending from minor elevations to dramatically high levels (Harsch, 1987). Other causes of increased CPK such as intramuscular injections, use of restraints, and muscle trauma must be kept in mind. Patients admitted in a psychotic state may also have mild to moderate elevations in CPK (Meltzer, Ross-Stanton, & Schlessinger, 1980). Myoglobinuria secondary to rhabdomyolysis may also develop and should be monitored closely as this could lead to renal failure and death. Leukocytosis develops in many patients, sometimes reaching very high levels (Harsch, 1987). As NMS progresses, it must be remembered that a rising white blood cell count may also be the result of a superimposed infection. In cases of NMS, CT scans of the head, electroencephalograms, and analysis of cerebrospinal fluid are generally normal. To date, no specific findings on any of these tests have been correlated with NMS. Nevertheless, these tests may provide critical information in ruling out other disorders that can simulate NMS.

CLINICAL COURSE AND OUTCOME

Although it is true that NMS can occur at any point during antipsychotic drug treatment, most cases seem to occur within the first 2 weeks of treatment (Addonizio et al., 1987). Although many cases develop full blown symptoms within hours, many cases progressively evolve over days and do not necessarily occur in a fulminant way. Once antipsychotics have been discontinued, resolution of NMS occurs within a mean duration of approximately 2 weeks, whereas resolution of symptoms may take 1 month after depot antipsychotic preparations (Addonizio et al., 1987). Medical complications of NMS include pneumonia, renal failure, cardiac arrest, seizures, sepsis, pulmonary embolism, and pulmonary edema. Fatality rates have been estimated to be 10–20%, but these rates probably reflect the reporting biases of published cases (Addonizio et al., 1987). As NMS has gained wider recognition, the fatality rate in published cases has decreased (Pearlman, 1986). Large prospective studies with strict diagnostic criteria will be necessary to determine actual fatality rates.

DIFFERENTIAL DIAGNOSIS

Various disorders may simulate NMS and need to be considered when patients present with its symptoms. One of the most important tasks in diagnosis is distinguishing NMS from psychogenic catatonia. There were numerous reports in the preantipsychotic era of patients who developed EPS, elevated temperature, autonomic dysfunction, and confusional states (Mann et al., 1986). Many of these cases developed catastrophic medical complications that resulted in death. Various names have been used to describe this condition, but the one that is currently used most frequently is lethal catatonia. Making this differential diagnosis can be critical because continuing antipsychotics in a patient who has NMS may have fatal consequences.

Much has been written about the clinical and potential pathophysiological similarities between MH and NMS, but clinically differentiating the two disorders should not be difficult (Addonizio et al., 1987). MH is a genetic disorder usually associated with the use of halogenated inhalational anesthetics and the depolarizing muscle relaxant succinylcholine that results in a hypermetabolic state of skeletal muscle (Nelson & Flewellen, 1983). Patients exhibit hyperpyrexia, hypertonicity, tachycardia, and elevated CPK. Unlike NMS, MH clearly has a genetic basis, a much more fulminant onset, and a much higher mortality rate. Neuroleptic malignant syndrome usually evolves over days, whereas MH may occur within minutes of starting anesthesia. Succinylcholine and general anesthesia have been administered to patients with NMS without toxic effects (Addonizio & Susman, 1987). In addition, there are no reports of antipsychotic-induced NMS in patients who have had clear episodes of MH. Also, patients who are susceptible to MH have successfully had antipsychotic analgesia (Lotstra, Linkowski, & Mendelwicz, 1983). Phenothiazines have actually been used to enhance temperature fall in patients with MH. Whereas curare and pancuronium cause flaccidity in patients with NMS, patients with MH do not have the same effect (Guze & Baxter, 1985).

Heat stroke is sometimes seen in patients on antipsychotics who are in a hot, humid environment. This disorder can usually be differentiated from NMS by a lack of rigidity and diaphoresis (Caroff, 1980). Other disorders that need to be considered include central nervous system infections, akinetic mutism "locked-in syndrome," tetany, thyrotoxicosis, pheochromocytoma, intermittent acute porphyria, and tetanus. These disorders can usually be distinguished from NMS by the additional presence of various physical and neurological features not usually associated with NMS. Patients with Parkinson's disease who abruptly discontinue their antiparkinsonian medication can develop a reaction virtually identical to NMS (Toru, Matsuda, Makiguchi, & Sugano, 1981). Use of other medications and use of illicit drugs may also simulate NMS. Drugs sometimes associated with this type of reaction include monoamine oxidase inhibitors, lithium toxicity, large doses of anticholinergic medication, amphetamines, fenfluramine, cocaine, and phencyclidine (PCP).

TREATMENT AND PREVENTION OF RECURRENCE

The mainstay of care in the management of a patient with NMS is immediate cessation of antipsychotic treatment and supportive medical care. Close attention must be paid to hydration and to the potential development of medical problems such as renal failure, infection, and cardiovascular problems. Many patients will have a remission of symptoms simply by stopping the antipsychotic, whereas others will demand a more vigorous approach. Benzodiazepines can be useful in ameliorating symptoms of NMS (Lew & Tollefson, 1983) while simultaneously calming an agitated psychotic patient who is no longer receiving the tranquilizing effects of antipsychotics. There have been a number of case reports demonstrating an apparent efficacy of bromocriptine (Addonizio et al., 1987). Based on its usefulness in MH, dantrolene has also been used successfully in case reports (Addonizio et al., 1987). In spite of the success reported in these cases, a more recent study has called into question the efficacy of these pharmacological interventions (Rosebush & Stewart, 1989). Electroconvulsive therapy (ECT) has been used in some patients with NMS with an amelioration of psychosis and symptoms of NMS, although cardiovascular complications have occurred in some patients (Shalev, Hermesh, & Munitz, 1986). This modality of treatment requires close monitoring of cardiac function. ECT is particularly helpful in patients in whom there is a problem in diagnosis between lethal catatonia and NMS, as ECT can be extremely beneficial in lethal catatonia and continuing antipsychotics in a patient with NMS can be very dangerous. Others have tried L-dopa and amantadine with mixed results.

The efficacy of specific pharmacological interventions remains to be determined as various patients may have individualistic differences in response to treatment. Another problem is that most reports of efficacy are based on case reports. This is a problem when evaluating response to treatment with a disorder that is often self-limited. It can be difficult to know whether improvement is coincidental with pharmacological management or whether the course of the illness is truly affected by the use of specific medication. Large, controlled, prospective studies are necessary to answer these questions.

Following an episode of NMS, reintroduction of antipsychotic drugs should be undertaken with caution and only after the episode has resolved. An interval of at least 2 weeks between termination of symptoms and reintroduction of an antipsychotic is probably most prudent (Rosebush, Stewart, & Gelenberg, 1989). Low-potency antipsychotics are probably safer and should be started at low doses with very gradual increases. Parenteral administration of antipsychotics should be avoided. Some patients will have a recurrence (Susman & Addonizio, 1988). Other treatment modalities may be considered. Lithium may be used, but it must be kept in mind that lithium has been reported to reinduce NMS in the post-NMS period (Susman & Addonizio, 1987). ECT may be useful in the patient who has recovered from NMS but who continues to be psychotic (Addonizio & Susman, 1987). Clozapine is another option, but even with this agent there have been a couple of reports of NMS (Pope, Cole, Choras, & Fulwiler, 1986; Muller, Becker, & Fritze, 1988). Continuing psychosis may be as devastating as NMS, and some patients who have had NMS may safely use antipsychotics in the future. With appropriate caution, antipsychotics may be reintroduced when the potential benefits clearly outweigh the risks.

REFERENCES

Abbott RJ, Loizou LA, 1986: Neuroleptic malignant syndrome. *British Journal of Psychiatry, 148,* 47–51.
Addonizio G, 1985: Rapid induction of extrapyramidal side effects with combined use of lithium and neuroleptics. *Journal of Clinical Psychopharmacology, 5,* 296–298.
Addonizio G, 1987: Neuroleptic malignant syndrome in elderly patients. *Journal of the American Geriatric Society, 35,* 1011–1012.
Addonizio G, Roth SD, Stokes PE, Stoll PM, 1988: Increased extrapyramidal symptoms with addition of lithium to neuroleptics. *Journal of Nervous and Mental Disease, 176,* 682–685.
Addonizio G, Susman VL, 1987: ECT as a treatment alternative for patients with symptoms of neuroleptic malignant syndrome. *Journal of Clinical Psychiatry, 48,* 102–105.
Addonizio G, Susman VL, Roth SD, 1987: Neuroleptic malignant syndrome: Review and analysis of 115 cases. *Biological Psychiatry, 22,* 1004–1020.
Araki M, Takagi A, Higuchi I, Sugita H, 1988: Neuroleptic malignant syndrome: Caffeine contracture of single muscle fibers and muscle pathology. *Neurology, 38,* 297–301.

Baastrup PC, Hollnagel P, Sorensen R, Schou M, 1976: Adverse reactions in treatment with lithium carbonate and haloperidol. *Journal of the American Medical Association, 236,* 2645–2646.

Caroff SN, 1980: The neuroleptic malignant syndrome. *Journal of Clinical Psychiatry, 41,* 79–83.

Caroff SN, Rosenberg H, Fletcher JE, Heiman-Patterson TD, Mann SC, 1987: Malignant hyperthermia susceptibility in neuroleptic malignant syndrome. *Anesthesiology, 67,* 20–25.

Cohen WJ, Cohen NH, 1974: Lithium carbonate, haloperidol, and irreversible brain damage. *Journal of the American Medical Association, 230,* 1283–1287.

Delay J, Pichot P, Lemperiere T, Elissalde B, Peigne F, 1960: Un neuroleptique majeur non phenothiazinique et non reserpinique, l'haloperidol, dans le traitement des psychoses. *Annales Medico Psychologique, 118,* 145–152.

Friedman JH, Feinberg SS, Feldman RG, 1985: A neuroleptic malignant-like syndrome due to levodopa therapy withdrawal. *Journal of the American Medical Association, 254,* 2792–2795.

Guze BH, Baxter LR Jr, 1985: Neuroleptic malignant syndrome. *New England Journal of Medicine, 313,* 1292–1293.

Harsch HH, 1987: Neuroleptic malignant syndrome: Physiological and laboratory findings in a series of nine cases. *Journal of Clinical Psychiatry, 48,* 328–333.

Itoh H, Ohtsuka N, Ogita K, Yagi G, Miura S, Koga Y, 1977: Malignant neuroleptic syndrome—Its present status in Japan and clinical problems. *Folia Psychiatrica et Neurologica Japonica, 31,* 565–576.

Keck PE Jr, Pope HG Jr, McElroy SL, 1987: Frequency and presentation of neuroleptic malignant syndrome: A prospective study. *American Journal of Psychiatry, 144,* 1344–1346.

Keck PE, Jr, Pope HG Jr, Cohen BM, McElroy SL, Nierenberg AA, 1989: Risk factors for neuroleptic malignant syndrome: A case-control study. *Archives of General Psychiatry, 46,* 914–918.

Krivosic-Horber R, Adnet P, Guevart E, Theunynck D, Lestavel P, 1987: Neuroleptic malignant syndrome and malignant hyperthermia. *British Journal of Anesthesiology, 59,* 1554–1556.

Kurlan R, Hamill R, Shoulson I, 1984: Neuroleptic malignant syndrome. *Clinical Neuropharmacology, 7,* 109–120.

Levenson JL, 1985: Neuroleptic malignant syndrome. *American Journal of Psychiatry, 142,* 1137–1145.

Levinson DF, Simpson GM, 1986: Neuroleptic-induced extrapyramidal symptoms with fever. *Archives of General Psychiatry, 43,* 839–848.

Lew TY, Tollefson G, 1983: Chlorpromazine-induced neuroleptic malignant syndrome and its response to diazepam. *Biological Psychiatry, 18,* 1441–1446.

Lotstra F, Linkowski P, Mendlewicz J, 1983: General anesthesia after neuroleptic malignant syndrome. *Biological Psychiatry, 18,* 243–247.

Mann SC, Caroff SN, Bleier HR, Welz WK, Kling MA, Hayashida M, 1986: Lethal catatonia. *American Journal of Psychiatry, 143,* 1374–1381.

Meltzer HY, Ross-Stanton J, Schlessinger S, 1980: Mean serum creatine kinase activity in patients with functional psychoses. *Archives of General Psychiatry, 37,* 650–655.

Muller T, Becker T, Fritze J, 1988: Neuroleptic malignant syndrome after clozapine plus carbamazepine. *Lancet, 2,* 1500.

Nelson TE, Flewellen EH, 1983: Current concepts. The malignant hyperthermia syndrome. *New England Journal of Medicine, 309,* 416–418.

Pearlman CA, 1986: Neuroleptic malignant syndrome: A review of the literature. *Journal of Clinical Psychopharmacology, 6,* 257–273.

Pope HG Jr, Cole JO, Choras PT, Fulwiler CE, 1986: Single case study. Apparent neuroleptic malignant syndrome with clozapine and lithium. *Journal of Nervous and Mental Disease, 174,* 493–495.

Rosebush P, Stewart T, 1989: A prospective analysis of 24 episodes of neuroleptic malignant syndrome. *American Journal of Psychiatry, 146,* 717–725.

Rosebush P, Stewart T, Gelenberg A, 1989: Twenty neuroleptic rechallenges after neuroleptic malignant syndrome in 15 patients. *Journal of Clinical Psychiatry, 50,* 295–298.

Sechi GP, Tanda F, Mutani R, 1984: Fatal hyperpyrexia after withdrawal of levodopa. *Neurology, 34,* 249–251.

Shalev A, Hermesh H, Munitz H, 1986: The role of loading rate in neuroleptic malignant syndrome. *American Journal of Psychiatry, 143,* 1059.

Susman VL, Addonizio G, 1987: Reinduction of neuroleptic malignant syndrome by lithium. *Journal of Clinical Psychopharmacology, 7,* 339–341.

Susman VL, Addonizio G, 1988: Recurrence of neuroleptic malignant syndrome. *Journal of Nervous and Mental Disease, 176,* 234–241.

Toru M, Matsuda O, Makiguchi K, Sugano K, 1981: Neuroleptic malignant syndrome-like state following a withdrawal of antiparkinsonian drugs. *Journal of Nervous and Mental Disease, 169*, 324–327.

Weinberg S, Twersky RS, 1983: Neuroleptic malignant syndrome. *Anesthesiology and Analgesia, 62*, 848–850.

Zubenko G, Pope HG Jr, 1983: Management of a case of neuroleptic malignant syndrome with bromocriptine. *American Journal of Psychiatry, 140*, 1619.

12

Akathisia

K. N. Roy Chengappa and Patrick Flynn

At the turn of the century, Haskovec (1901) described akathisia (Greek: *a kathisia*—the inability to remain seated) in a patient with hysteria and in another with neurasthenia. Sicard (1923) noted the phenomenon in patients with idiopathic and postencephalitic parkinsonism. Sigwald, Grassiard, Duriel, & Dumont (1947) described akathisia in patients being treated with promethazine for Parkinson's disease. After this report of drug-induced akathisia, reports have associated it with chlorpromazine, reserpine, haloperidol, and many other psychotropic and nonpsychotropic drugs (Ayd, 1961, 1963; Barnes, Braude, & Hill, 1982; Brody, Adler, Kim, Angrist, & Rotrosen, 1990; Delay, Denniker, Green, & Morduet, 1957; Freyhan, 1957; Kruse, 1960b; Lipinski, Mallya, Zimmerman & Pope, 1989; Steck, 1954; Van Putten, 1975).

EPIDEMIOLOGY

The wide range of prevalence of drug-induced akathisia reported in the literature (3–75%; Ayd, 1961, 1983; Braude, Barnes, & Gore, 1983; Goldman, 1961; National Institute of Mental Health, 1964; Van Putten, May, & Marder, 1984b) reflects differences in diagnostic criteria, patient populations, drugs used, and lack of awareness of the condition. A commonly accepted figure is that between 20% and 25% of patients on antipsychotics will develop akathisia (Braude et al., 1983). Most patients developing the acute syndrome do so between 5 to 40 days after treatment is begun (Ratey & Salzman, 1984; Van Putten, 1975). Ayd (1983) in his second survey of 5,000 patients on antipsychotics showed that between 1961 and 1981 the prevalence of akathisia increased from 21.2–36.8%. His earlier survey of 3,775 patients (Ayd, 1961) revealed that twice as many women as men had akathisia. Some of the risk groups for akathisia include: females; elderly; mentally retarded patients; alcoholic patients; patients treated with conjugated estrogens; patients with low serum iron levels; patients with recent changes in dosage of antipsychotics; patients experiencing recent withdrawal from antipsychotics or antidepressants; and patients with increased sulcal prominence, cognitive deficits, and brain damage. The elderly are at greater risk (Steinberg, 1985). Risk is also associated with the use of high-potency antipsychotics such as haloperidol, droperidol, and thiothixene. Low levels of serum iron may predispose to the condition (Brown, Glen, & White, 1987). Alcohol and estrogens may worsen or precipitate the condition (Shen, 1984; Krishnan, France, & Ellinwood, 1984). Increased sulcal prominence, preexisting brain damage and cognitive deficits may be risk factors for the development of akathisia (Sandyk & Kay, 1990). Late-onset (tardive) akathisia and persistent forms may occur in chronic patients when antipsychotic drug dosages are changed or when antipsychotics and tricyclics are withdrawn (Dilsaver, 1989; Dufresne & Wagner, 1988). The late-onset form is often seen in association with parkinsonism and tardive dyskinesia, or as a precedent to tardive dyskinesia (Barnes & Braude, 1985; Barnes, Kidger, & Gore, 1983; Braude & Barnes, 1983). Akathisia has been described in mentally handicapped patients (Ganesh, Rao, & Cowie, 1989) in whom the subjective component may be difficult to elicit. Of 1,227 developmentally disabled subjects 13% demonstrated akathisia that was significantly correlated with the use of antipsychotic drugs (Stone, May, Alvarez, & Ellman, 1989). Persistent forms of akathisia are noted in patients where the antipsychotic dose needs to be continued at a dosage that stabilizes them clinically but results in some side effects—including akathisia. Here patients experience both the subjective and objective components of the condition.

Pseudoakathisia is often noted in chronic psychiatric patients on antipsychotics. In this form of akathisia, patients either do not experience or do not report inner restlessness (subjective component).

Withdrawal akathisia involves both subjective and objective components and may occur in patients coming off antipsychotic drugs. Generally, it should resolve in a few weeks after the last oral or injected dose.

PATHOLOGY AND PATHOPHYSIOLOGY

Based on animal experiments, Marsden and Jenner (1980) suggest that dopamine receptor blockade in the mesocortical areas causes hyperactivity and that a similar mechanism may be operating in human akathisia (Table 1). Human studies showing the effectiveness of β adrenergic blockers and α_2 noradrenergic agonists in treating akathisia (see below) provide evidence for involvement of the central noradrenergic system. Lipophilic β blockers (propranolol, betaxolol, low-dose metoprolol) are superior to hydrophilic ones (atenolol, nadolol, sotalol) in alleviat-

Table 1 Pathophysiological mechanisms in akathisia

Neurotransmitter/ peptide/compound	Proposed mechanism
Dopaminergic	Postsynaptic dopamine receptor blockade in the mesocortical areas causes hyperactivity in animals. A similar mechanism may be operative in humans.
Central adrenergic β_1, β_2, and α_2	Lipophilic β blockers are effective in treatment of akathisia, as is an α_2 agonist, suggesting a reciprocal relationship between these two systems.
Cholinergic	Muscarinic antagonists are useful in some patients.
Serotonergic	The effectiveness of L-tryptophan in akathisia and methysergide-induced akathisia hint at the involvement of 5-HT mechanisms.
GABA (gamma amino butyric acid)	GABA potentiation by benzodiazepines and baclofen improves symptoms in some patients.
Iron	Low serum iron may induce D2 receptor hypofunction increasing the susceptibility to akathisia in patients on antipsychotic drugs.
Endogenous opoids	Increased opoid activity has been implicated in a few patients.
Melanocyte-stimulating hormone peptides	Increased function of MSH peptides has been proposed as a mechanism in akathisia.

ing symptoms of akathisia (Adler, Angrist, Peselow, Corwin, & Rotrosen, 1985; Adler et al., 1986, 1987b; Kramer, Gorkin, DiJohnson, & Sheves, 1988; Lipinski, Zubenko, Cohen, & Barriera, 1983, 1984; Ratey, Sorgi, & Polakoff, 1985). It appears that nonselective β blockade (i.e., propranolol) is as effective as selective β blockade (β_1 blockade using betaxolol and low-dose metoprolol or β_2 blockade using ICI 118,551) (Adler, Reiter, Angrist, & Rotrosen, 1987c; Derom, Elinck, Buylaert, & Van Der Straeten, 1984; Dupuis, Catteau, Dumon, Libert, & Petit, 1987; Reiter, Adler, Angrist, Corwin, Rotrosen, 1987). Clonidine, an α_2 agonist, has been effective in treating akathisia (Adler, Angrist, Peselow, Reitano, & Rotrosen, 1987a; Zubenko, Cohen, Lipinski, & Jonas, 1984a).

There is some pharmacological evidence for the involvement of cholinergic, serotonergic, and GABA-ergic systems, although the mechanisms are unclear (Bernick, 1988; DiMascio, Bernardo, Greenblatt, & Marder, 1976; Friss, Christensen, & Gerlach, 1982; Gagrat, Hamilton, & Belmatier, 1978; Kramer, DiJohnson, Davis, Dewey, & DiGiambattista, 1990; Van Putten et al., 1984b). Sandyk (1985b, 1989) has suggested that excessive endogenous opioids and melanocyte-stimulating hormone peptides may play a role in the pathophysiology of akathisia. Low serum iron has been associated with akathisia, Ekbom's syndrome, and tricyclic-induced jitteriness (Brown, Glen, & White, 1987; Ekbom, 1960; Yeragani, Pohl, Balon, Kulkarni, & Keshavan, 1989). Reviewing animal and clinical studies, Brown et al. (1987) propose that low serum iron increases the susceptibility to akathisia in patients on antipsychotics via an induced D_2 receptor hypofunction.

CLINICAL FEATURES

Akathisia is characterized by subjective and objective clinical components. In mild cases only the subjective symptoms may be present, whereas in the moderate and severe cases the objective signs described here may be seen. Akathisia's presence commonly causes considerable distress to the patient. Weiden, Mann, Haas, Mattson, & Frances (1987b) noted that clinicians missed 20 of 27 cases of antipsychotic-induced akathisia in the psychiatric wards of a university medical center. Milder forms of the condition were particularly prone to be overlooked in some of these cases. Akathisia was misdiagnosed and attributed to "agitation," "restlessness," and "acting-out." This common error in diagnosis often results in increased antipsychotic dose and worsening of the problem. This study also found that akathisia was often missed when it presented behaviorally (elopement or an incident requiring seclusion), or when the patient was too disorganized, psychotic, or akinetic to complain of akathisia. Akathisia should be considered whenever such behavior of recent onset coincides temporally with increases of antipsychotic drug doses or decreases in patients exposed chronically to antipsychotics.

Subjective Component

Patients often describe (sometimes to leading questions) a sense of unease and restlessness associated with tension and localized parasthesiae in their calf muscles, overlying skin, and other parts of the lower limbs and abdomen. Akathisia must be distinguished from the more generalized sense of tension and restlessness, which may be a nonspecific complaint among acute psychiatric inpatients (Braude & Barnes, 1986). When suspected, inquiry of the patient must often be quite direct. Words often used to describe this feeling include: "pulling," "pins and needles," "ants under the skin and in the muscles," "going crazy," "can't sit down," "shaking inside," and so on. Another factor that may help distinguish akathisia from other forms of restlessness is that patients with akathisia are more troubled by the symptoms while standing in one spot for a few minutes (as in a medication or meal line or while standing in line at a supermarket checkout). Patients often feel a compulsion to move about and are unable to sit in one place for a more than a few minutes. In milder forms of akathisia the presence of akathisia in a patient on antipsychotic drugs may offer an additional aid to diagnosis (Weiden et al., 1987b). Severely disturbed patients may not complain about akathisia.

Objective Component

Rocking from foot to foot or marching on the spot while standing (Braude et al., 1983; Frost & Lal, 1989; Gibb & Lees, 1986) is common. Patients who are seated display crossing and uncrossing of their legs, swinging of legs when crossed, fidgeting in the chair, foot tapping, hand wringing, and wanting to rise out of the chair and pace. In an extreme instance, one of the authors had to conduct an interview by following the patient around the room. This inability to sit down and compulsion to move about has been referred to as tasikinesia (Delay & Deniker, 1968; Sicard, 1923). An objective test for akathisia is finding the presence of a low-frequency (less than 4 Hz), coarse, jerky foot tremor (Braude, Charles, & Barnes, 1984). An additional objective test is to test for cogwheel rigidity by "recruitment." The patient is instructed to perform alternating movements in the wrist or elbow opposite to the one being tested for cogwheel rigidity (Maltbie & Cavenar, 1977).

There are a few rating scales that are helpful in rating akathisia. Barnes (1989) has combined the subjective and objective elements of akathisia into a useful rating scale, which also includes a global clinical assessment. Akathisia items can be extracted from Chouinard's (1980) Extrapyramidal Rating Scale and the Hillside Long Island Jewish Hospital modification of the Simpson-Angus Extrapyramidal Rating Scale (Adler et al., 1989; Simpson & Angus, 1970). In addition to these scales, a new rating scale—the Hillside Akathisia Scale—has been introduced (Fleischhacker et al., 1989).

CLINICAL SIGNIFICANCE

Akathisia has been implicated in medication refusal, noncompliance, and medication withdrawal (Schmidt et al., 1984; Van Putten, 1974a; Van Putten, May, & Marder 1984a). Studies have associated akathisia with exacerbation of psychosis, increased length of hospital stay in schizophrenics, increased rates of admission, worsening of Tourette's disorder, and dysphoric mood in schizophrenic patients (Galdi & Bonato, 1988; Hermesh, Shalev, & Munitz, 1985; Van Putten et al., 1984a; Van Putten & Marder, 1987; Van Putten, Mutalipassi, & Malkin, 1974b; Weiden & Bruun, 1987a). Akathisia, as noted earlier, has also been linked to suicide, suicide attempts, violence, homicidal ideas, homicide, and "acting out" (Drake & Ehrlich, 1985; Herrera et al., 1988; Keckich, 1978; Schulte, 1985; Shaw et al., 1986; Shear, Frances, & Weiden, 1983; Siris, 1985; Weiden, 1985). In a preliminary observational study of violent adult patients in a special 14-bed unit, using close-circuit television and video recording, Crowner et al. (1990) demonstrated that both victims and assailants were akathisic before half of the assaults, whereas bystanders rarely were akathisic for nine recorded incidents of violence. Ayd (1988) points out that given the 25% incidence of akathisia and the extensive number of patients on antipsychotics, suicide is a rare complication of akathisia. Nevertheless, the individual patient manifesting suicidal and homicidal behavior who in addition is experiencing akathisia must be considered to be potentially at risk to produce injury to him- or herself and others.

DIAGNOSIS

Akathisia Versus Other Causes of Psychomotor Agitation

It is important to distinguish akathisia from psychomotor agitation, since different treatment strategies are used for these two conditions (see Table 2 for characterization). This may be difficult to do in an emergency situation. If immediate management of the patient is critical, a benzodiazepine may do until a better evaluation can be made. Propranolol helps akathisia but not the concomitant subjective anxiety. Restless legs syndrome (Blom & Ekbom, 1961; Ekbom, 1960) is seen in normal individuals (the prevalence is around 5%), pregnancy, iron deficiency, diabetes mellitus, carcinoma, uremia, postgastric surgery (Banerji & Hurwitz, 1980) and chronic pulmonary disease (Spillane, 1970). Tricyclic-induced jitteriness may bear resemblance to akathisia, and reports have linked akathisia with antidepressant use (Lipinski et al., 1989; Zubenko, Cohen, & Lipinski, 1987) and antidepressant withdrawal (Dilsaver, 1989). Some patients with panic disorder and agoraphobia are exquisitively sensitive to low doses of antidepressants, and doses of 10 to 50 mg of imipramine or desipramine have caused patients to exhibit jitteriness and inner restlessness (see also Chapter 13). Opiate withdrawal states sometimes present with features of akathisia; clonidine has been used for its treatment (Charney, Sternber, Kleber, Henninger, & Redmond; Gold, Redmond, & Klieber, 1978; Washton & Resnick, 1981). The increasing use of antiemetics and psychotropic medications for pain management in terminally ill patients may increase the incidence of akathisia in this group of patients.

Akathisia variants such as "marching in place" (Frost, Lal, & Yassa, 1989), pseudoakathisia, and tardive akathisia (Barnes & Braude, 1985; Munetz & Cornes, 1983) are generally described in chronic psychiatric patients and are often seen in association with or as a precedent to tardive dyskinesia and parkinsonism. Patients may not report or experience inner restlessness in pseudoakathisia, which if severe may make the differentiation from severe akathisia particularly difficult. Akathisia should be considered whenever there is a recent onset of behavioral changes such as "agitation," "restlessness," "acting out," or incidents leading to impulsive acts—such as suicidal or assaultive incidents. These may lead to seclusionary measures, and as noted earlier the clue to recognition is often the association of these behaviors with recent changes in antipsychotic doses (Weiden et al., 1987b).

Table 2 Differential diagnoses of akathisia

Condition	Diagnostic features
Psychomotor agitation of psychoses	Increasing the antipsychotic worsens akathisia but may improve psychotic agitation. Decreasing the antipsychotic usually improves akathisia.
Anxiety	Psychopathology of anxiety is different (e.g., autonomic symptoms).
Restless legs syndrome (Ekbom's syndrome)	Unrelated to antipsychotic use; occurs when the patient is relaxed, lying down, or just before retiring to bed. May cause leg pain and insomnia.
Tricyclic jitteriness	Exquisite sensitivity to low doses of antidepressants; mainly subjective symptoms.
Opiate withdrawal	History of recent opiate use preceding onset of restlessness.
Akathisia variants	Marching in place: Like soldiers marking time, chronic patients keep lifting their feet off the ground shifting from one foot to another.
	Pseudoakathisia: Chronic patients who exhibit volitional and repetitive movements of the legs (not unlike mannerisms) that to the observer appear as motor restlessness. However, the patients do not experience inner restlessness and do not report it.
	Tardive akathisia: Characterized by late onset (weeks to years) and may be a precedent to or accompanied by parkinsonism or tardive dyskinesia. Clinical features may be similar to the early form.
	Persistent akathisia: Characterized by both subjective and objective components of the syndrome, it is seen as a persistence of acute akathisia in patients whose clinical condition demands that the antipsychotic needs to be continued at a dosage at which side effects are noted, including akathisia.

INVESTIGATIONS

It is unclear if correction of low serum iron with iron will correct akathisia; however, iron deficiency anemia if present will require treatment. Likewise, in a chronic psychiatric patient who has neglected his diet and has been wandering homeless before admission, vitamin deficiency, electrolyte imbalance, and exposure to cold may need to be ruled out as possible causes of restless legs syndrome. Diabetes mellitus, uremia, chronic obstructive pulmonary disease, malignancy, pregnancy, and a history of gastric surgery will also have to be ruled out.

A history of recent opiate use, physical examination evidence of injection marks, abscesses, thrombosed veins, pupillary changes, and urine analysis for opioids may help detect restless legs associated with this condition. A history of panic disorder and/or agoraphobia and treatment with small doses of tricyclic antidepressants may indicate tricyclic-induced jitteriness.

ETIOLOGY

Drugs known to cause akathisia include antipsychotics, antidepressants (including the newer drugs such as amoxapine and fluoxetine), lithium, reserpine, metoclopramide, buspirone, nifedipine, cinnarizine, flunarizine, and diltiazem, the 5-

HT antagonist methysergide, and carbamazepine. Medical conditions that cause akathisia include idiopathic parkinsonism (Lang & Johnson, 1987), postencephalitic parkinsonism, and head injury (Schwarz, Gosenfeld, Gilderman, Jiwesh, & Ripple, 1986; Stewart, 1989).

TREATMENT

Drug and Dosage Modification

In many cases of acute akathisia, a decrease in the dosage of the antipsychotic may ameliorate akathisia and nothing further may be required (Braude et al., 1983). Sometimes switching from a high-potency antipsychotic (haloperidol) to a low-potency one (thioridazine) may be adequate (Ayd, 1984; Munetz & Cornes, 1983). Attention should be directed to drugs such as metoclopramide, methysergide, conjugated estrogens, and nifedipine, which may cause akathisia. If these are present and alternates can be substituted, no further action may be needed. Drug interactions must be borne in mind; certain drugs (e.g., lithium) may raise antipsychotic levels and induce akathisia.

Drugs Used to Treat Akathisia

Adler et al. (1989) and Fleischhacker, Roth, & Kane (1990) have reviewed this topic in detail. In spite of increased study of the condition, the published literature does not provide consistent guidelines for the treatment of akathisia. The reasons include differences in study designs (open, single blind, double blind, parallel group, crossover), measures used to rate akathisia, antipsychotics under study, patient populations (bipolars, schizophrenics), the presence or absence of other extrapyramidal symptoms, stages of patient's illness (acute, chronic), and the use of the study drug either as the first-line treatment or after the failure of other drugs. No single therapeutic approach has predictable benefit to all or even most patients. Many approaches have been reported to help some patients. Given these caveats, some general conclusions are presented here.

Beta Blockers

The successful use of propranolol in parkinsonian patients with restless legs (Strang, 1967) and the similarity between this syndrome and antipsychotic-induced akathisia led Lipinski to try propranolol for akathisia (Lipinski et al., 1983). Since this positive report, most of the studies have reported good results with β-blockers (Adler et al., 1985, 1986, 1987c; Adler, Angrist, & Rotrosen, 1990; Kramer et al., 1988; Lipinski et al., 1984; Zubenko, Lipinski, Cohen, & Barriera, 1984c). Adler et al. (1990) have demonstrated that D-propranolol (which has no significant β-blocking activity) has no efficacy in treating akathisia, suggesting that it is the β-blockade that contributes to the efficacy of racemic propranolol.

Subjective and objective components of akathisia begin to improve in hours; the improvement may be complete in 2 to 7 days. Bipolar manics achieve almost complete remission as compared to 50% of schizophrenic patients (Adler et al., 1986; Lipinski et al., 1983, 1984; Zubenko et al, 1984c). There is no clear guideline for discontinuing the treatment. One study found that all patients relapsed when propranolol was stopped after 6 months and all responded to another lipophilic β-blocker (Dupuis et al., 1987). Adler et al. (1989a) have treated 15 patients for a year without loss of therapeutic effect and without serious side effects.

If drug or dosage modification fails to influence akathisia, current opinion clearly favors lipophilic β-blockers (such as propranolol 20–80 mg/day) in the treatment of akathisia not complicated by parkinsonian features. At these doses, no major problems with blood pressure or pulse have been observed (Adler et al., 1989a; Lipinski et al, 1984). Before prescribing β-blockers, contraindications to their use (bronchial asthma, left ventricular failure, bradycardia, and Raynaud's disease) will have to be borne in mind. In some instances the selectivity of the β-blocker can be exploited—for example, using $β_1$-blockers (betaxolol 10–20 mg/day; low-dose metoprolol 50–100 mg/day) in an akathisia patient with asthma. In cases of bradycardia, a nonselective β-blocker with intrinsic sympathomimetic activity such as pindolol (5 mg/day) may be useful in treating akathisia.

Anticholinergics

Studies have shown that in some patients, anticholinergic drugs are effective in relieving akathisia (DiMascio et al., 1976; Kruse, 1960b; Neu, DiMascio, & Demirgion, 1972; Van Putten et al., 1984b). It has been reported that a greater number of patients find relief from procyclidine than benztropine (Kruse, 1960a). Another study found that 30 out of 37 patients on thiothixene responded to anticholinergics, whereas less than half of patients on haloperidol responded (Van Putten et al., 1984b). It has been suggested that akathisia accompanied by parkinsonian features is most likely to respond to anticholinergics (Braude et al., 1983).

The World Health Organization (WHO, 1990) recommends that patients should not be routinely started on anticholinergics until they develop features of parkinsonism. It is recommended that other measures such as lowering the dose of the antipsychotic or substituting another antipsychotic that is less prone to induce parkinsonism should be tried first. The need for the anticholinergic agent must be reevaluated at intervals with a view to discontinue it if possible.

Although clinical guidelines suggest that anticholinergic drugs can be withdrawn after about 3 months, actual studies concerning withdrawal from anticholinergics have produced widely disparate results regarding the proportion of patients whose parkinsonian features relapsed (Barnes, 1990). The situation regarding continued use in remitted akathisia is even less clear.

In acute akathisia, when dosage reductions are possible, no further antiakathisia medication may be required. In persistent akathisia, where the clinical state precludes dose reduction, the continued use of the anticholinergics must be weighed against the side effects they are known to cause. Gradual tapering of the medication (over 3 months) might be one way to decide if it needs to be continued. The relapse of the extrapyramidal symptoms and akathisia during the discontinuation phase may suggest that these medications need to be continued for longer periods of time. Again, it is difficult to decide at the discontinuation phase whether the relapsed extrapyramidal syndromes and akathisia are a result of unmasking of the syndrome at lower doses. It may be necessary to wait for a few weeks after discontinuation of the anticholinergic drug to decide whether it needs to be restarted. However, in the individual patient, the severity of the relapse might force the clinician to restart the anticholinergic medication sooner rather than later.

In tardive (late-onset) akathisia, especially when the condition coexists with tardive dyskinesia, a trial of discontinuation of the anticholinergic medication may be warranted, especially as these drugs have been implicated in the pathogenesis of tardive dyskinesia.

Amantadine

Double-blind studies involving small numbers of patients ($N = 11$–13) have shown this antiviral and antiparkinsonian drug to be an effective treatment for akathisia (DiMascio et al., 1976; Merrick & Schmitt, 1973; Stenson et al., 1976) although tolerance to the effect within a week of treatment has been reported (Zubenko, Barriera, Lipinski, 1984b), and the condition has returned.

Benzodiazepines

Benzodiazepines provide effective relief of akathisia in some patients (Donlon, 1973; Gagrat et al., 1978). Diazepam up to 15 mg/day and lorazepam 1 to 5 mg are commonly used. Some members of this group can be used by the intravenous (lorazepam, diazepam) and intramuscular (lorazepam) routes. Benzodiazepines are particularly useful when immediate treatment is required and when the differentiation between psychomotor agitation and akathisia is not clear; they may also help coexisting anxiety. Clonazepam given orally (0.5–3 mg/day) has a long halflife and once-a-day treatment is possible. Both subjective and objective components of the akathisia should improve within a week of starting treatment (Kutcher, Williamson, MacKenzie, Maxton, & Ehrlich, 1989). Although these medications are useful in the short-term, the potential for addiction and abuse limits long-term usage.

Buspirone

One open study involving 3 patients found buspirone (10–15 mg/day) to improve akathisia in 48–72 hours (D'Mello, McNeil, & Harris, 1989), but another open study involving 7 schizophrenic patients found that it worsened akathisia (Brody et al., 1990). Unlike the benzodiazepines, buspirone is not associated with an addiction potential.

Clonidine

Clonidine, an α_2 noradrenergic agonist, decreases central noradrenergic transmission. Given orally (0.15–0.8 mg/day), improvement in subjective symptoms of akathisia begins within 24–48 hours and is maximal in 3–15 days; improvement in objective signs begins in 2–4 days and is maximal in 3–15 days. Clonidine decreases subjective anxiety, whereas propranolol may not. Hypotension and sedation are limiting factors. Results with transdermal clonidine are awaited as this route is believed to produce less sedation and more steady plasma levels (Adler et al., 1987a, 1989a; Zubenko et al., 1984a). There are no reports of the long-term administration of clonidine.

Piracetam

In a double-blind crossover, placebo-controlled trial, the efficacy of IV piracetam in antipsychotic-induced extrapyramidal side effects was confirmed by Kabes et al. (1982). They investigated 40 patients receiving an average of 600-mg chlorpromazine equivalents per day. Patients receiving 4 mg piracetam by IV injection were significantly improved on akathisia ratings as compared to patients receiving placebo. The onset of action was noted to begin 30–60 minutes after infusion with the improvement lasting for at least 2 hours. Although this is an interesting study, the practical use of IV piracetam in day-to-day clinical practice remains uncertain. The authors speculate on the action of this drug on neuronal membrane permeability and energy metabolism.

Amitriptyline

A patient who had failed to respond to trihexyphenidyl improved rapidly when amitriptyline (100 mg/day) was added to treat depression (Danel, Servant, & Goudemand, 1988). No systematic studies are available.

L-Tryptophan

Six schizophrenic patients who were treated with this drug (1 g P. O. q.i.d.) showed improvement in both the objective and subjective symptoms of akathisia. This effect was noted after several days (Kramer et al., 1990; Sandyk, Consroe, & Iacono, 1986).

Baclofen and Clonazepam

Sandyk (1985) used this combination (baclofen 5–10 mg P. O. t.i.d. and loraze-pam 0.5 mg P. O. t.i.d.) to treat a patient whose akathisia had failed to respond to diazepam and anticholinergic drugs. The drug was tolerated well in a follow-up of 6 months without adverse effects.

Cyproheptadine

Bacher, Lewis, & Field (1989) used cyproheptadine (2–6 mg P. O. t.i.d.) to treat 15 male patients with movement disorders who were on antipsychotics and other medications. Patients reported feeling calmer and being able to sleep better. Improvements in akathisia and tardive dyskinesia were also noted.

Treatment of Tardive Akathisia

This condition is more resistant to treatment and often coexists with tardive dyskinesia. Like tardive dyskinesia, it worsens when the antipsychotic is decreased or when anticholinergics are added and improves temporarily when the antipsychotic is increased. In general, anticholinergics are not useful (Braude & Barnes, 1983; Kruse, 1960a; Stein & Pohlman, 1987; Weiner & Luby, 1983; Yassa, Iskandar, & Nastase, 1988). Long-term discontinuation of antipsychotics has been found to be useful in some patients (Shearer, Bownes, & Curran, 1984; Weiner and Luby, 1983). Gardos, Cole, Solomon, & Schniebolk (1987) reported improvement of tardive akathisia with the use of clozapine. In anecdotal reports, chlordiazepoxide, lorazepam, propranolol, the combination of lorazepam and procyclidine, the combination of low-dose thioridazine, alprazolam and ethopropazine, dopamine-depleting drugs, and ECT have been found to be useful (Burke et al., 1989; DeKeyser & D'Haenan, 1986; Kruse, 1960a; Stein & Pohlman, 1987; Yassa et al., 1988; Yassa & Groulx, 1989). Sachdev and Chee (1990) studied one male patient using a variety of pharmacological challenges (IV and oral) to characterize tardive akathisia. They found the patient responded positively to benztropine, bromocriptine, and propranolol and negatively to physostigmine. The patient showed little or no response to discontinuation of antipsychotics and challenges with metoclopramide, metoprolol, atenolol, and clonidine.

PREVENTION

Judicious use of psychotropics and careful attention to nonpsychotropic drugs that induce akathisia may minimize the risk of akathisia. A previous history of akathisia and belonging to a high-risk group of patients should alert the clinician to the development of akathisia. Drug interactions, recent changes in doses of antipsychotics or recent withdrawal from antipsychotics, use of antidepressants, and possibly low serum iron predispose patients to develop akathisia and call for clinical intervention. Once akathisia has been diagnosed, drug or dosage modification, changing from a high-potency to a low-potency antipsychotic, or the use of medications to decrease the symptoms will help minimize consequences such as noncompliance with medications and worsening of impulsive behavior.

CONCLUSION

About 1 in 5 patients on antipsychotic drugs will develop akathisia, especially those on high-potency antipsychotics. Diagnosis is critical, as interventions are available to prevent what might be serious and even fatal consequences for the patient. Although there seem to be many pharmacological subtypes of akathisia, the underlying mechanisms are unclear. Research using the newer rating scales and various pharmacological probes may shed more light on these mechanisms. Since there is no clear guideline as to the length of treatment, it is prudent to review each patient on an individual basis and make a decision based on risks versus benefits as to whether to continue or discontinue the drug treatment for akathisia. The guidelines for the treatment of tardive akathisia await systematic investigations.

REFERENCES

Adler LA, Angrist B, Fritz P, Rotrosen J, Mallya G, Lipinski JF, 1990: Lack of efficacy of propranolol in neuroleptic induced akathisia (abstract). *Biological Psychiatry, 27,* 133A.

Adler L, Angrist B, Peselow E, Corwin J, Maslansky R, Rotrosen J, 1986: A controlled assessment of propranolol in the treatment of neuroleptic-induced akathisia. *British Journal of Psychiatry, 149,* 42–45.

Adler L, Angrist B, Peselow E, Corwin J, Rotrosen J, 1985: Efficacy of propranolol in neuroleptic-induced akathisia. *Journal of Clinical Psychopharmacology, 5,* 164–166.

Adler L, Angrist B, Peselow E, Reitano J, Rotrosen J, 1987a: Clonidine in neuroleptic-induced akathisia. *American Journal of Psychiatry, 144,* 235–236.

Adler L, Angrist B, Reiter S, Rotrosen J, 1989a: Neuroleptic-induced akathisia: A review. *Psychopharmacology, 97,* 1–11.

Adler L, Angrist B, Rotrosen J, 1990: Metoprolol versus propranolol. *Biological Psychiatry, 27,* 673–675.

Adler L, Duncan E, Angrist B, Hemdahl P, Rotrosen J, Slotuick V, 1989: Effects of a specific β-2 receptor blocker in neuroleptic induced akathisia. *Psychiatry Research, 27,* 1–4.

Adler LA, Reiter S, Angrist B, Rotrosen J, 1987c: Pindolol and propranolol in neuroleptic-induced akathisia. *American Journal of Psychiatry, 144,* 1241–1242.

Adler LA, Reiter S, Corwin J, Hemdal P, Angrist B, Rotrosen J, 1987b: Differential effects of benztropine and propranolol in akathisia. *Psychopharmacology Bulletin, 23,* 519–521.

Ayd FJ, 1961: A survey of drug-induced extrapyramidal reactions. *Journal of the American Medical Association, 175,* 1054–1060.

Ayd FJ Jr, 1983: Early onset neuroleptic-induced extrapyramidal reactions: A second survey, 1961–1981. In: *Neuroleptics: Neurochemical, behavioral and clinical perspectives,* edited by JT Coyle and SJ Enna. New York: Raven Press.

Ayd FJ Jr, 1984: High potency neuroleptics and akathisia. *Journal of Clinical Psychopharmacology, 4,* 237.

Ayd FJ Jr, 1988: Akathisia and suicide: Fact or myth? *International Drug Therapy Newsletter, 23,* 37–39.

Bacher NM, Lewis HA, Field PB, 1989: Cyproheptadine in movement disorders. *American Journal of Psychiatry, 146,* 557–558.

Banerji NK, Hurwitz LJ, 1970: Restless legs syndrome, with particular reference to its occurence after gastric surgery. *British Medical Journal, 4,* 774–775.

Barnes TRE, 1989: A rating scale for drug induced akathisia. *British Journal of Psychiatry, 154,* 672–676.

Barnes TRE, 1990: Comment on the WHO consensus statement. *British Journal of Psychiatry, 156,* 413–414.

Barnes TR, Braude WM, 1985: Akathisia variants and tardive dyskinesia. *Archives of General Psychiatry, 42,* 874–878.

Barnes TRE, Braude WM, Hill DJ, 1982: Acute akathisia after oral droperidol and metoclopramide pre-operative medication. *Lancet, 2,* 48–49.

Barnes TR, Kidger T, Gore SM, 1983: Tardive dyskinesia: A 3 year follow-up study. *Psychological Medicine, 13,* 71–81.

Bernick C, 1982: Methysergide-induced akathisia. *Clinical Neuropsychopharmacology, 11,* 87–89.

Blom S, Ekbom KA, 1961: Comparison between akathisia developing on treatment with phenothiazine derivatives and the restless leg syndrome. *Acta Medica Scandinavica, 170,* 684–694.

Braude WM, Barnes TR, 1983: Late onset akathisia—an indicant of covert dyskinesia: Two case reports. *American Journal Psychiatry, 136,* 611–612.

Braude WM, Barnes T, 1986: Akathisia or not sitting. *British Medical Journal, 292,* 1393.

Braude WM, Barnes TRE, Gore SM, 1983: Clinical characteristics of akathisia. A systematic investigation of acute psychiatric inpatient admissions. *British Journal of Psychiatry, 143,* 139–150.

Braude WM, Charles IP, Barnes TRE, 1984: Coarse, jerky foot tremor: Tremographic investigation of an objective sign of acute akathisia. *Psychopharmacology, 82,* 95–101.

Brody D, Adler LA, Kim T, Angrist B, Rotrosen J, 1990: Effects of buspirone in seven schizophrenic patients. *Journal of Clinical Psychopharmacology, 10,* 68–69.

Brown KW, Glen SE, White T, 1987: Low serun iron status and akathisia. *Lancet, 1,* 1234–1236.

Brown P, 1988: Review: Drug induced akathisia in medical and surgical patients. *International Journal of Psychiatry in Medicine, 18,* 1–15.

Burke RE, Kang UJ, Jankovic J, Miller LG, Fahn S, 1989: Tardive akathisia: An analysis of clinical features and response to open therapeutic trials. *Movement Disorders, 4,* 157–175.

Charney DS, Sternber DE, Kleber HD, Henninger GR, Redmond DE, 1981: The clinical use of clonidine in the abrupt withdrawal from methadone. *Archives of General Psychiatry, 38,* 1273–1277.

Chouinard G, Ross-Chouinard A, Annable L, Jones BD, 1980: Extrapyramidal rating scale. *Canadian Journal of Neurological Sciences, 7,* 233.

Crowner ML, Douyon R, Convit A, Gaztanaga P, Volavka J, Bakall R, 1990: Akathisia and violence. *Psychopharmacology Bulletin, 26,* 115–117.

Danel T, Servant D, Goudemand M, 1988: Amitryptiline in the treatment of neuroleptic induced akathisia. *Biological Psychiatry, 23,* 186–188.

DeKeyser J, D'Haenan H, 1986: Disappearance of akathisia following electroconvulsive therapy. *Clinical Neuropharmacology, 9,* 563–565.

Delay J, Deniker T, 1968: Drug induced extrapyramidal syndromes. In: *Diseases of the basal ganglia, handbook of clinical neurology,* Volume 6, edited by PJ Vinken and GW Bruyn. Amsterdam: North Holland Publishing.

Delay J, Denniker P, Green A, Morduet M, 1957: Le syndrome exitomoteur provoque pat les medicaments neuroleptiques [A syndrome of psychomotor excitation provoked by neuroleptic medications]. *Presse Medicale, 65,* 1771–1774.

Derom E, Elinck W, Buylaert W, Van Der Straeten M, 1984: Which beta-blocker for the restless leg? *Lancet, 1,* 857.

Dilsaver SC, 1989: Antidepressant withdrawal syndromes: Phenomenology and pathophysiology. *Acta Psychiatrica Scandinavica, 79,* 113–117.

DiMascio A, Bernardo DL, Greenblatt D, Marder JE, 1976: A controlled trial of amantadine in drug-induced extrapyramidal disorders. *Archives of General Psychiatry, 33,* 599–602.

D'Mello D, McNeil JA, Harris W, 1989: Buspirone supression of neuroleptic-induced akathisia: Multiple case reports. *Journal of Clinical Psychopharmacology, 9,* 151–152.

Donlon P, 1973: The therapeutic use of diazepam for akathisia. *Psychosomatics, 14,* 222–225.

Drake RE, Ehrlich J, 1985: Suicide attempts associated with akathisia. *American Journal of Psychiatry, 142,* 499–501.

Dufresne RL, Wagner Rl, 1988: Antipsychotic-withdrawal akathisia versus antipsychotic-induced akathisia: Further evidence for the existence of tardive dyskinesia. *Journal of Clinical Psychiatry, 49,* 435–438.

Dupuis B, Catteau J, Dumon JP, Libert C, Petit H, 1987: Comparison of propranolol, sotalol, and betaxolol in the treatment of neuroleptic-induced akathisia. *American Journal of Psychiatry, 144,* 802–805.

Ekbom KA, 1960: Restless leg syndrome. *Neurology, 10,* 868–873.

Fleischhaker WW, Bergman KJ, Perovich R, Pestreich LK, Borenstein M, Lieberman JA, Kane JM, 1989: The Hillside Akathisia Scale: A new rating instrument for neuroleptic-induced akathisia. *Psychopharmacology Bulletin, 25,* 222–226.

Fleischhaker WW, Roth SD, Kane JM, 1990: The pharmacologic treatment of neuroleptic-induced akathisia. *Journal of Clinical Psychopharmacology, 10,* 12–21.

Freyhan Fa, 1957: Psychomotility and parkinsonism in treatment with neuroleptic drugs. *Archives of Neurology and Psychiatry, 78,* 465–472.

Friss T, Christensen TR, Gerlach J, 1982: Sodium valproate and biperiden in neuroleptic-induced akathisia, parkinsonism and hyperkinesia: A double-blind cross-over study with placebo. *Acta Psychiatrica Scandinavica, 67,* 178–187.

Frost L, Lal S, Yassa R, 1989: Neuroleptic-induced marching-in-place. *Acta Psychiatrica Scandinavica, 79,* 48–51.

Gagrat D, Hamilton J, Belmatier R, 1978: Intravenous diazepam in the treatment of neuroleptic-induced dystonia or akathisia. *American Journal of Psychiatry, 135,* 1232–1233.

Galdi J, Bonato RR, 1988: Relationship of adverse drug reactions to length of hospital-stay in genetically subgrouped schizophrenics. *Canadian Journal of Psychiatry, 33,* 816–818.

Ganesh S, Rao JM, Cowie VA, 1989: Akathisia in neuroleptic medicated mentally handicapped subjects. *Journal of Mental Deficiency Research, 33,* 323–329.

Gardos G, Cole JO, Solomon M, Schniebolk S, 1987: Clinical forms of severe tardive dyskinesia. *American Journal of Psychiatry, 144,* 895–902.

Gibb WRG, Lees AJ, 1986: The clinical phenomenon of akathisia. *Journal of Neurology, Neurosurgery and Psychiatry, 49,* 861–866.

Gold MS, Redmond DE, Kleiber HD, 1978: Clonidine blocks the acute opiate withdrawal syndrome. *Lancet, 2,* 403–405.

Goldman D, 1961: Parkinsonism and related phenomena from administration of drugs: Their production and control under clinical conditions and possible relation to therapeutic effect. *Revue Canadienne de Biologie Experimental, 20,* 549–560.

Haskovec L, 1901: L'akathisie. *Revue Neurologique* (Paris), *9,* 1107–1109.

Hermesh H, Shalev A, Munitz H, 1985: Contribution of adverse drug reaction to admission rates in an acute psychiatric ward. *Acta Psychiatrica Scandinavica, 72,* 104–110.

Herrera JN, Sramek JJ, Costa JF, Roy S, Heh CW, Nguyen BN, 1988: High potency neuroleptics and violence in schizophrenics. *Journal of Nervous and Mental Disease, 76,* 558–561.

Jeste DV, Wyatt RJ, 1982: *Understanding and treating tardive dyskinesia.* New York: Guilford Press.

Kabes J, Sikora J, Pisvejc J, Hanzlicek L, Skondia V, 1982: Effect of piracetam on extrapyramidal side effects induced by neuroleptic drugs. *International Pharmacopsychiatry, 17,* 185–192.

Keckich WA, 1978: Violence as a manifestation of akathisia. *Journal of the American Medical Association, 240,* 2185.

Kramer MS, DiJohnson C, Davis P, Dewey DA, DiGiambattista S, 1990: L-tryptophan in neuroleptic-induced akathisia. *Biological Psychiatry, 27,* 671–672.

Kramer MS, Gorkin RA, DiJohnson C, Sheves P, 1988: Propranolol in the treatment of neuroleptic-induced akathisia (NIA) in schizophrenics: A double blind, placebo-controlled study. *Biological Psychiatry, 24,* 823–827.

Krishnan KRR, France RD, Ellinwood EH Jr, 1984: Tricyclic-induced akathisia in patients taking conjugated estrogens. *American Journal of Psychiatry, 141,* 696–697.

Kruse W, 1960a: Treatment of drug-induced extrapyramidal symptoms. *Diseases of the Nervous System 21,* 79–81.

Kruse W, 1960b: Persistent muscular restlessness after phenothiazine treatment. Report of three cases. *American Journal of Psychiatry, 117,* 152–153.

Kutcher S, Williamson P, MacKenzie S, Maxton P, Ehrlich M, 1989: Successful clonazepam treatment of neuroleptic-induced akathisia: A double-blind, place-controlled study. *Journal of Clinical Psychopharmacology, 9,* 403–406.

Lang AE, Johnson K, 1987: Akathisia in idiopathic Parkinson's disease. *Neurology, 37,* 477–481.

Lipinski JF, Zubenko GS, Cohen BM, Barriera PJ, 1983: Propranolol in the treatment of neuroleptic induced akathisia. *Lancet, 2,* 685–686.

Lipinski JF, Zubenko GS, Cohen BM, Barreira PJ, 1984: Propranolol in the treatment of neuroleptic-induced akathisia. *American Journal of Psychiatry, 141,* 412–415.

Lipinski JF, Mallya G, Zimmerman P, Pope H, 1989: Fluoxetine-induced akathisia: Clinical and theoretical implications. *Journal of Clinical Psychiatry, 50,* 339–342.

Maltbie AA, Cavenar JO, 1977: Akathisia diagnosis: An objective test. *Psychosomatics, 18,* 36–39.

Marsden CD, Jenner P, 1980: The pathophysiology of extrapyramidal side-effects of neuroleptic drugs. *Psychological Medicine, 10,* 55–72.

Marsden CD, Tarsy D, Baldessarini RJ, 1975: Spontaneous and drug-induced movement disorders in psychotic patients. In: *Psychiatric aspects of neurological disease,* edited by DF Benson, D Blumer. New York: Grune and Stratton.

Merrick EM, Schmitt PP, 1973: A controlled study of the clinical effects of amantadine hydrochloride (Symmetrel). *Current Therapy Research, 15,* 552–558.

Munetz MR, Cornes CL, 1983: Distinguishing akathisia and tardive dyskinesia: A review of the literature. *Journal of Clinical Psychopharmacology, 3,* 343–350.

National Institute of Mental Health, 1964: Psychopharmacology survey center collaborative study group. Phenothiazine treatment in acute schizophrenia. *Archives of General Psychiatry, 10,* 246–261.

Neu C, DiMascio A, Demirgian E, 1972: Antiparkinsonian medication in the treatment of extrapyramidal side-effects: Single or multiple doses? *Current Therapy Research, 4,* 246–251.

Ratey JJ, Salzman C, 1984: Recognizing and managing akathisia. *Hospital and Community Psychiatry, 35,* 915–917.

Ratey JJ, Sorgi P, Polakoff S, 1985: Nadolol as a treatment for akathisia. *American Journal of Psychiatry, 142,* 640–642.

Reiter S, Adler L, Angrist B, Corwin J, Rotrosen J, 1987: Atenolol and propranolol in neuroleptic-induced akathisia. *Journal of Clinical Psychopharmacology, 6,* 390.

Sachdev P, Chee KY, 1990: Pharmacological characterization of tardive akathisia. *Biological Psychiatry, 28,* 809–818.

Sandyk R, 1985a: Successful treatment of neuroleptic-induced akathisia with baclofen and clonazepam. *European Neurology, 24,* 286–288.

Sandyk R, 1985b: The endogenous opioid system in neurological disorders of the basal ganglia. *Life Sciences, 37,* 1655–1663.

Sandyk R, 1989: Neuroleptic-induced akathisia: A role for MSH peptides. *Psychopharmacology, 99,* 134–135.

Sandyk R, Consroe PF, Iacono RP, 1986: L-tryptophan in drug-induced movement disorders with insomnia. *New England Journal of Medicine, 314,* 1257.

Sandyk R, Kay SR, 1990: Sulcal size and neuroleptic induced akathisia. *Biological Psychiatry, 27,* 466–467.

Schmidt LG, Grohmann R, Helmchen H, Langscheid-Schmidt K, Miller-Oerlinghausen B, Poser W, Ruther E, Scherer J, Strauss A, Wolf B, 1984: Adverse drug reactions: An epidemiological study at psychiatric hospitals. *Acta Psychiatrica Scandinavica, 70,* 77–89.

Schulte JL, 1985: Homicide and suicide associated with akathisia and haloperidol. *American Journal of Forensic Psychiatry, 6,* 3–7.

Schwarcz G, Gosenfeld L, Gilderman A, Jiwesh J, Ripple RE, 1986: Akathisia associated with carbamazepine therapy. *American Journal of Psychiatry, 143,* 1190–1191.

Shaw ED, Mann JJ, Weiden P, Sinsheimer LM, Bruun RD, 1986: A case of suicidal and homicidal ideation and akathisia in a double blind neuroleptic crossover study. *Journal of Clinical Psychopharmacology, 6,* 196–197.

Shear K, Frances A, Weiden P, 1983: Suicide associated with akathisia and depot fluphenazine treatment. *Journal of Clinical Psychopharmacology, 3,* 235–236.

Shearer RM, Bownes IT, Curran P, 1984: Tardive akathisia and agitated depression during metoclopramide therapy. *Acta Psychiatrica Scandinavica, 70,* 428–431.

Shen W, 1981: Akathisia: An overlooked distressing but treatable condition. *Journal of Nervous and Mental Disease, 169,* 599–600.

Sicard JA, 1923: Akathisie et tasikinesie [Akathisia and taskinesia]. *La Presse Medicale* (Paris), *23,* 265–266.

Sigwald J, Grossiord A, Duriel P, Dumont G, 1947: Le traitment de la maladie de Parkinson et des manifestations extra pyramidales par le diethylaminoethyl-N-thiodiphenylamine (2987 RP). Resultats d'une annee d'application [Results of the treatment of the extrapyramidal manifestations of Parkinson's disease with diethylaminoethyl-N-thiodiphenylamine (2967 RP)]. *Revue Neurologique* (Paris), *79,* 683–687.

Simpson GM, 1977: Neurotoxicity of major tranquilizers. In: *Neurotoxicology,* edited by L Roezin H Shiroki and N Grcevic. New York: Raven Press.

Simpson GM, Angus JWS, 1970: A rating scale for extrapyramidal side-effects. *Acta Psychiatrica Scandinavica, 212* (suppl), 11–19.

Siris SG, 1985: Three cases of akathisia and "acting out." *Journal of Clinical Psychiatry, 46,* 395–397.

Spillane JD, 1970: Restless legs syndrome in chronic pulmonary disease. *British Medical Journal 4,* 796–798.

Steck H, 1954: Le syndrome extrapyramidal et diencephalique au cours des traitement au largactil et au Serpasil [An extrapyramidal and diencephalic syndrome during the course of treatment with largactil and serpasil]. *Annales Medico-Psychologiques, 112,* 737–744.

Stein MB, Pohlman ER, 1987: Tardive akathisia associated with low-dose haloperidol use. *Journal of Clinical Psychopharmacology, 7,* 202–203.

Steinberg SK, 1985: Drug-induced extrapyramidal symptoms in the elderly. *Modern Medicine of Canada, 40,* 473–482.

Stenson RL, Donlon PT, Mayer JE, 1976: Comparison of benztropine mesylate and amantadine hydrochloride in neuroleptic-induced extrapyramidal symptoms. *Comprehensive Psychiatry, 17,* 763–768.

Stewart JT, 1989: Akathisia following traumatic brain injury: Treatment with bromocriptine. *Journal of Neurology, Neurosurgery and Psychiatry, 52,* 1200–1201.

Stone RK, May JE, Alvarez WF, Ellman G, 1989: Prevalence of dyskinesia and related movement disorders in a developmentally disabled population. *Journal of Mental Deficiency Research, 33,* 41–53.

Strang RR, 1967: The symptom of restless legs. *Medical Journal of Australia, 24,* 1211–1213.

Van Putten T, 1974: Why do schizophrenic patients refuse to take their drugs? *Archives of General Psychiatry, 31,* 67–72.

Van Putten T, 1975: The many faces of akathisia. *Comprehensive Psychiatry, 16,* 43–47.

Van Putten T, Marder SR, 1987: Behavioural toxicity of antipsychotic drugs. *Journal of Clinical Psychiatry, 48* (9, suppl), 13–19.

Van Putten T, May PR, Marder SR, 1984a: Response to antipsychotic medication: The doctor's and the consumer's view. *American Journal of Psychiatry, 141,* 16–19.

Van Putten T, May PRA, Marder SR, 1984b: Akathisia with haloperidol and thiothixene. *Archives of General Psychiatry, 41,* 1036–1039.

Van Putten T, Mutalipassi LR, Malkin MD, 1974: Phenothiazine induced decompensation. *Archives of General Psychiatry, 30,* 102–105.

Washton AM, Resnick RB, 1981: Clonidine in opiate withdrawal: Review and appraisal of clinical findings. *Pharmacotherapy, 1,* 140–146.

Weiden P, 1985: Akathisia from prochlorperazine. *Journal of the American Medical Association, 253,* 635.

Weiden P, Bruun R, 1987a: Worsening of Tourette's disorder due to neuroleptic-induced akathisia. *American Journal of Psychiatry, 144,* 504–505.

Weiden PJ, Mann J, Haas G, Mattson M, Frances A, 1987b: Clinical nonrecognition of neuroleptic-induced movement disorders: A cautionary study. *American Journal of Psychiatry, 144,* 1148–1153.

Weiner WJ, Luby ED, 1983: Tardive akathisia. *Journal of Clinical Psychiatry, 44,* 417–419.

World Health Organization, Consensus Statement 1990: Prophylactive use of anticholinergic patients on long-term neuroleptic treatment. *British Journal of Psychiatry, 156,* 412.

Yassa R, Groulx B, 1989: Lorazepam in the treatment of lithium induced akathisia. *Journal of Clinical Psychopharmacology, 9,* 70–71.

Yassa R, Iskandar H, Nastase C, 1988: Propranolol in the treatment of tardive akathisia. *Journal of Clinical Psychopharmacology, 8,* 283–285.

Yeragani VK, Pohl R, Balon R, Kulkarni A, Keshavan M, 1989: Low serum iron levels and tricyclic-induced jitteriness. *Journal of Clinical Psychopharmacology, 9,* 447–448.

Zubenko GS, Barreira P, Lipinski JF, 1984b: Development of tolerance to the therapeutic effect of amantadine on akathisia. *Journal of Clinical Psychopharmacology, 4,* 218–219.

Zubenko GS, Cohen BM, Lipinski JF, 1987: Antidepressant related akathisia. *Journal of Clinical Psychopharmacology, 7,* 254–257.

Zubenko GS, Cohen BM, Lipinski JF, Jonas JM, 1984a: Use of clonidine in treating neuroleptic-induced akathisia. *Psychiatry Research 13,* 253–259.

Zubenko GS, Lipinski JF, Cohen BM, Barriera PJ, 1984c: Comparison of metoprolol and propranolol in the treatment of akathisia. *Psychiatry Research, 11,* 143–148.

13

Tricyclic Antidepressant-Induced Jitteriness

Vikram K. Yeragani, Robert Pohl, and Richard Balon

Tricyclic antidepressants (TCAs) produce an acute jitteriness syndrome in some panic disorder patients (Pohl, Yeragani, Balon, & Lycaki, 1988; Zitrin, Klein, & Woerner, 1980). This syndrome is characterized by jitteriness, restlessness, trouble sitting still, and increased anxiety. Zitrin, Klein, and Woerner (1978) have described this as an exquisite sensitivity to imipramine with an excitatory or stimulant effect. Patients also experience insomnia characterized by both difficulty in falling asleep and repeated awakening during sleep, irritability, and unusual energy.

EPIDEMIOLOGY

In the study by Zitrin et al. (1978), 18% of patients receiving imipramine showed this effect on doses ranging from 5–75 mg/day. The patients in this study included agoraphobics, mixed phobics, and simple phobics. A few patients were never able to tolerate more than 10 mg/day. Others were able to tolerate higher doses when the dosage was gradually and cautiously increased. Zitrin et al. (1978) have speculated that there may be a basic physiological difference between the patients who develop this side effect compared to those who do not.

Zitrin, Klein, and Woerner (1980), in another report on treatment effects of imipramine in 67 agoraphobic patients, found that 20% were exquisitely sensitive to imipramine and developed insomnia, jitteriness, irritability, and unusual energy while receiving 25 mg of imipramine per day. Again, a small group of patients were unable to tolerate more than 10 mg/day, and some patients tolerated it better when the dosage was cautiously increased. Aronson (1987) also has reported that a sizable number of panic disorder patients experienced a stimulant effect of imipramine.

TCA-induced jitteriness has been examined in a retrospective study on 158 patients with panic attacks and 22 with other psychiatric diagnoses (Pohl, Yeragani, Balon, & Lycaki, 1988). All these patients received antidepressants as a first treatment for panic disorder, major depressive disorder, bulimia, obsessive compulsive disorder, or some combination of these. Jitteriness developed in 49 of the 180 patients. Age and sex distribution did not have a significant association with this side effect. None of the 22 patients without a history of panic attacks had jitteriness. Thus, there was a very significant difference in the incidence of jitteriness between patients with and without a history of panic attacks. A prior history of jitteriness with tricyclics was significantly associated with the current development of jitteriness. Jitteriness occurred at a mean dose of 50 mg of the tricyclic antidepressant per day and typically during the first week of treatment. Desipramine was associated with a much higher frequency of jitteriness than was imipramine.

PATHOPHYSIOLOGY

The pathophysiology of TCA-induced jitteriness is unknown. There is some evidence that implicates serum iron changes and alterations in biogenic amines. Iron-deficiency states may produce symptoms similar to antipsychotic-induced akathisia (Ekbom, 1960), and akathisia may be associated with low serum iron levels (Brown, Glen, & White, 1987). Because of the phenomenological similarity between akathisia and jitteriness, Yeragani, Pohl, Balon, Kulkarni, & Keshavan, (1989) have studied serum iron levels in 57 panic disorder patients with and without jitteriness. The mean serum iron level in patients who developed jitteriness was significantly lower than in patients who did not. Patients with a lower iron level also developed jitteriness at a relatively lower mean dose of TCAs.

These findings, if confirmed by prospective studies, may have important theoretical implications. Iron is involved in the synthesis of monoamines at the step of tyrosine hydroxylase (Cooper, Bloom, & Roth, 1978). A deficiency of iron may therefore be associated with low levels of dopamine and norepinephrine. On the other hand, iron deficiency may be associated with low monoamine oxidase activity, thus enhancing monoaminergic transmission (Youdim, Grahame-Smith, & Woods, 1976). Excess serotonin has been associated with restlessness and autonomic symptoms (Insel, Roy, Cohen, & Murphy, 1982). Gorman et al. (1987) have reported jitteriness-like symptoms during treatment with fluoxetine, a relatively selective serotonin reuptake blocker. Iron deficiency produces an increase in serotonin and 5-hydroxy indole compounds (Mackler, Person, Miller, Inamdar, & Finch, 1978), and TCA-induced jitteriness thus may partly be related to altered serotonin function.

Noradrenergic mechanisms may be involved in the pathogenesis of this syndrome. TCAs increase noradrenergic activity by inhibition of uptake of norepinephrine into the presynaptic nerve ending. This acute effect appears to coincide with the occurrence of jitteriness during the first week of treatment; desipramine, which is more frequently associated with jitteriness, also inhibits norepinephrine uptake more than imipramine. These factors suggest a noradrenergic mechanism for the jitteriness syndrome.

CLINICAL PICTURE

There are several similarities between phenothiazine-induced akathisia and TCA-induced jitteriness (Yeragani, Pohl, & Balon, 1988). Although akathisia appears to be seen in about one fifth of patients treated with antipsychotics (see Chapter 12), jitteriness occurs in at least 18% of panic disorder patients treated with tricyclics. The symptoms "trouble sitting still" and "shakiness inside" are frequently reported in both conditions. Like akathisia, jitteriness may be mediated through noradrenergic mechanisms as desipramine is more frequently associated with jitteriness than imipramine (Pohl et al., 1988). Clonidine and propranolol have been reported to be effective in treating akathisia (Adler, Angrist, & Peselow, 1986). The response of jitteriness to anticholinergic drugs is not known. However, jitteriness may respond to low doses of perphenazine, an antipsychotic drug (Pohl, Yeragani, Ortiz, Rainey, & Gershon, 1986), which suggests different mechanisms for antipsychotic-induced akathisia and TCA-induced jitteriness, even though there are phenomenological similarities.

Zubenko, Cohen, and Lipiski (1987) have described antidepressant-related akathisia in some depressed patients. One patient in this study had a history of panic attacks. Thus there may be a relationship between this rare symptom of akathisia associated with tricyclics in some depressed patients and the more common syndrome of jitteriness in panic disorder patients.

TREATMENT AND PREVENTION

Clinicians need to be sensitive to the jitteriness syndrome when treating any patient with panic attacks. Patients should be warned of jitteriness as a possible effect, as it is often frightening to these already anxious patients. It is wise to start all panic disorder patients on low doses of TCAs (i.e., 10 mg the first day and increase the dosage by not more than 10 mg every day at least for the first 7–10 days). Tolerance usually occurs to this side effect. Patients who cannot tolerate even 10 mg can be started on a smaller dose in an oral concentrate form. Blocking this side effect with other drugs may prove useful in the treatment of some patients. One report suggests diazepam may be effective (Klein, Gittelman, Quitkin, & Rifkin, 1980), but there are no systematic studies on this. The reported effectiveness of perphenazine to block jitteriness (Pohl et al., 1986) may be more of a theoretical interest because of the serious side effects associated with the use of phenothiazines.

REFERENCES

Adler LA, Angrist B, Peselow E, 1986: Noradrenergic mechanisms in akathisia. In: *Abstracts of the 139th Annual Meeting of the American Psychiatric Association.* Washington, DC: American Psychiatric Association.

Aronson TA, 1987: A naturalistic study of imipramine in panic disorder and agoraphobia. *American Journal of Psychiatry, 144,* 1014–1019.

Brown KW, Glen SE, White T, 1987: Low serum iron status and akathisia. *Lancet, i,* 1234–1236.

Cooper JR, Bloom FE, Roth RH, 1978: *The biochemical basis of neuropharmacology.* New York: Oxford University Press.

Ekbom KA, 1960: Restless leg syndrome. *Neurology, 10,* 868–873.

Gorman JM, Liebowitz MR, Fyer AJ, Goetz D, Campeas RB, Fyer MR, Davies SO, Klein DF, 1987: An open trial of fluoxetine in the treatment of panic attacks. *Journal of Clinical Psychopharmacology, 7,* 329–332.

Insel TR, Roy BF, Cohen RM, Murphy DL, 1982: Possible development of the serotonin syndrome in man. *American Journal of Psychiatry, 139,* 954–955.

Klein DF, Gittelman R, Quitkin F, Rifkin A, 1980: *Diagnosis and drug treatment of psychiatric disorders: Adults and children,* 2nd edition. Baltimore: Williams and Wilkins.

Mackler B, Person R, Miller LR, Inamdar AR, Finch CA, 1978: Iron deficiency in the rat: Biochemical studies of brain metabolism. *Pediatric Research, 12,* 217–220.

Pohl R, Yeragani VK, Balon R, Lycaki H, 1988: The jitteriness syndrome in panic disorder patients treated with antidepressants. *Journal of Clinical Psychiatry, 49,* 100–104.

Pohl R, Yeragani VK, Ortiz A, Rainey JM, Gershon S, 1986: Response of tricyclic-induced jitteriness to a phenothiazine in two patients. *Journal of Clinical Psychiatry, 47,* 427.

Yeragani VK, Pohl R, Balon R, 1988: Tricyclics, akathisia, and jitteriness. *Journal of Clinical Psychopharmacology, 4,* 295.

Yeragani VK, Pohl R, Balon R, Kulkarni A, Keshavan M, 1989: Low serum iron levels and tricyclic antidepressants-induced jitteriness. *Journal of Clinical Psychopharmacology, 6,* 447–448.

Youdim MBH, Grahame-Smith DG, Woods HF, 1976: Some properties of human platelet monoamine oxidase in iron deficiency anemia. *Clinical Science and Molecular Medicine, 50,* 479–485.

Zitrin CM, Klein DF, Woerner MG, 1978: Behavior therapy, support psychotherapy, imipramine and phobias. *Archives of General Psychiatry, 35,* 307–316.

Zitrin CM, Klein DF, Woerner MG, 1980: Treatment of agoraphobia with group exposure in vivo and imipramine. *Archives of General Psychiatry, 37,* 63–72.

Zubenko GS, Cohen BM, Lipiski JF, 1987: Antidepressant-related akathisia. *Journal of Clinical Psychopharmacology, 7,* 254–257.

14

Anticholinergic Drug-Induced Dysfunction

Joseph P. McEvoy

ETIOLOGY

Many drugs that psychiatrists prescribe block receptors for acetylcholine in the brain. Anticholinergic antiparkinson drugs, long known to exert beneficial effects on the manifestations of primary extrapyramidal disorders, are now also utilized successfully in the treatment of the extrapyramidal side effects of antipsychotic drugs. Unfortunately, the actions of these anticholinergic agents are not restricted to motor circuitry, but also include additional unwanted effects on cholinergic neurotransmission in other areas of the brain.

Certain antipsychotic drugs (e.g., chlorpromazine or thioridazine), and many of the tricyclic antidepressant drugs (e.g., amitriptyline or imipramine), have substantial intrinsic anticholinergic potencies, and these anticholinergic effects also are nonspecific.

Subtle, unwanted anticholinergic effects on the brain begin well within the usual clinically prescribed dose ranges of these drugs (McEvoy, 1987). Unwanted effects become more obvious with increasing doses. Patients may be prescribed doses of an anticholinergic drug that, given their individual sensitivities, prove excessive for them. However, perhaps more commonly it is the cumulative effects of several different prescribed medications taken together, each with some anticholinergic activity, that prove toxic. Occasionally patients will abuse drugs with anticholinergic potency in search of euphoria or hallucinatory experiences (see Chapter 19). Excessive intake of drugs with anticholinergic potency, for whatever reason, can cause brain dysfunction.

PATHOPHYSIOLOGY

Cholinergic neurons extend from certain brainstem nuclei (e.g., the pedunculopontine and lateral dorsal tegmental nuclei) to innervate thalamic way-stations, which connect incoming sensory information to the cerebral cortex (McCormick, 1989). Acetylcholine released from these neurons enhances the efficiency of transfer of specific incoming sensory data through the thalamus to the appropriate cortical receptive fields. McCormick notes:

The thalamus is critical for the generation of certain types of forebrain rhythmic activity and serves as an intermediary between the external world and the neocortex. Indeed, many of the alterations that occur in the forebrain processing state (reflected by changes in the EEG) represent mode of generation of action potentials in thalamic neurons, which in turn is under the control of modulatory neurotransmitters from the brainstem and basal forebrain.

Electroencephalographic (EEG) activity recorded from the cerebral cortex varies with the state of arousal. During drowsiness and sleep, consistent rhythmic oscillations in neuronal activity dominate the tracing. With increasing alertness, as subjects attend more specifically to particular sensory information, the EEG tracing becomes desynchronized as individually crafted neuronal activity for the particular situation becomes predominant. Cholinergic agonists increase EEG desynchronization.

By altering the amplitude of specialized potassium currents in thalamic and cortical neurons, acetylcholine . . . can block the generation of thalamocortical rhythms and promotes a state of excitability that is consistent with cognition. (McCormick, 1989)

In contrast, anticholinergic drugs induce synchronized, rhythmic thalamocortical activity, associated with drowsiness and sleep.

Large cholinergic neurons are distributed through the basal forebrain, clustering in the medial septal nuclei, the diagonal band of Broca, and the basal nucleus of Meynert. Axonal projections from the medial septal nuclei and diagonal band of Broca terminate in the hippocampus, a structure known to be critical for learning and memory (Salamone, 1986). In fact, sectioning of these hippocampal projections in laboratory animals has been shown to produce impairment on tests of new learning.

Neurons from the basal nucleus of Meynert extend cholinergic projections throughout the cerebral cortex and amygdaloid complex. Application of acetylcholine to cortical neurons within primary sensory areas enhances the responsiveness of these neurons to incoming sensory stimuli, especially when rewards are associated with stimulus identification (Richardson & DeLong, 1988). Thus evidence exists that normal functioning of cholinergic neurons may be required for the optimal modulation of arousal and attention, the efficient transfer of incoming sensory data to the cortex, and the recording of these data into memory. Excessive doses of anticholinergic drugs will interfere with all of these important brain functions.

CLINICAL PICTURE

The earliest detectable toxic central nervous system (CNS) effects of anticholinergic drugs appear to be effects on the acquisition of new learning. Performance on tests of immediate recall (e.g., digit span) or on tests of retrieval of previously learned material from remote memory (e.g., naming types of sports or vegetables) is not impaired at low clinical doses of anticholinergic drugs. However, tests of ability to store new material beyond the span of immediate attention reveal significant impairment within the usual clinical dose range (McEvoy et al., 1987a; Van Putten et al., 1987).

If anticholinergic doses increase further, more obvious impairments in attention and cognitive function become apparent, proceeding through delirium to stupor and coma. Patients who become delirious usually are agitated (but may be subdued) and preoccupied with hallucinatory percepts in several sensory modalities. They are lost in space and time (Ullman & Groh, 1972).

Two principal factors appear to routinely interact in clinical situations to produce the unwanted CNS effects of anticholinergic drugs: (1) Individuals suffering from underlying temporary and/or permanent organic CNS disorders are at increased risk to develop anticholinergic toxicity. (2) The likelihood and severity of anticholinergic toxicity increase progressively with increasing dose and plasma level of anticholinergic drugs.

Sunderland et al. (1987) compared the cognitive and behavioral effects of three intravenous doses of scopolamine (.1, .25, and .5 mg) and placebo in 10 patients with Alzheimer's disease and 10 matched elderly subjects. The Alzheimer's disease patients, but not the normal control subjects, showed significant impairment on tests of new learning at the .25-mg scopolamine dose. Although the normal control subjects did show some mild impairment on these tests, the impairment of the Alzheimer's patients was profound at the .5-mg dose. These findings are in keeping with postmortem studies of the brains of patients with Alzheimer's disease, which reveal excessive loss of basal forebrain cholinergic neurons, relative to age matched controls.

Serum levels of anticholinergic drug activity have been found to be inversely related to capacity for self-care in demented nursing home residents (Rovner et al., 1988). Patients with Parkinson's disease and associated dementia are at significantly greater risk for delirium when treated with anticholinergic drugs than are parkinsonian patients without dementia (DeSemet et al., 1982).

Even patients without fixed organic impairment are at risk for toxicity from anticholinergic drugs when their CNS is temporarily affected by physiological stress. The occurrence of postoperative delirium (Tune et al., 1981) and of delirium following electroconvulsive therapy (Mondimore, Damlouji, Folstein, & Tune, 1983) has been found to be significantly related to high anticholinergic blood levels.

In a study involving normal volunteers given scopolamine 5, 8, or 10 μg/kg intravenously, Petersen (1977) found that the 10 μg/kg dose produced significantly greater impairment on tests of new learning than did the 5 μg/kg dose. Both Tune et al. (1982) and Perlick, Stastry, Katz, Mayer, & Mattis, (1986) found significant inverse correlations between the performance of stabilized chronic schizophrenic patients on tests of verbal learning and the patients' serum anticholinergic drug activity (i.e., higher maintenance anticholinergic levels were associated with worse performance).

McEvoy and Freter (1989) have studied a group of stable distressed or defective schizophrenic patients maintained on fluphenazine decanoate and anticholinergic drugs who were given additional intramuscular challenge injections of two anticholinergic agents 1 week apart in a random sequence, double-blind design. One agent penetrated the CNS (benztropine), but the other did not (glycopyrrolate). The intramuscular challenge injections were repeated until patients reported increases in dry mouth or blurred vision. The primary purpose of the study was to assess the effects on distress or defect features of temporarily pushing anticholinergic dose into a mildly uncomfortable range. Performance on tests of memory function was also assessed in a subgroup of these patients. Significantly greater impairment in memory function occurred following the benztropine injections than following the glycopyrrolate injections.

These studies provide compelling evidence that the toxic effects of anticholinergic drugs increase with increasing dose. Clinicians treating Parkinson's disease know that the therapeutic effects of anticholinergic drugs are limited, even as dose is pushed into a clearly toxic range. McEvoy and Freter's (1989) challenge injection studies pushed benztropine dose into a range where clear, discomforting dry mouth or blurred vision became apparent, but provided minimal additional benefit over standard anticholinergic maintenance treatment in terms of further relief of extrapyramidal side effects or subjective distress. Thus, although the deleterious effects of anticholinergic drugs on memory function continue to increase as dose is pushed into a range where peripheral toxicity is apparent, the therapeutic effects of these drugs may have already reached a plateau.

DIAGNOSIS

The diagnosis of central anticholinergic toxicity can most easily be arrived at by looking for evidence of peripheral anticholinergic toxicity (Table 1). Anticholinergic drugs act as competitive inhibitors of acetylcholine at muscarinic cholinergic receptors involved in the innervation of smooth and cardiac muscles and exocrine glands. Evidence of peripheral toxicity occurs in a relatively predictable order with increasing anticholinergic doses and blood levels (Weiner, 1980). First, the secretion of saliva and of sweat is diminished, leading to dry mouth and warm, dry skin through which heat dissipation is inefficient. Subsequently, pupil size increases and accommodation is impaired; photophobia and changes in visual acuity occur. Heart rate increases in healthy young adults as vagal effects are blocked, but this is less prominent in older individuals. Ultimately, the parasympathetic innervation of the detrusor muscle of the bladder is blocked, and difficulties in initiating urination are reported. The tone and motility of the gastrointestinal tract diminish; bowel sounds decrease and severe constipation occurs.

Patients can readily describe the early symptoms of peripheral anticholinergic toxicity. Even in patients so delirious as to be unable to provide useful historical information about their recent medication intake, signs of peripheral anticholinergic toxicity can quickly be identified with a brief examination.

If necessary, after an initial evaluation to assure that the patient is medically stable, physostigmine (1 mg) may be injected subcutaneously to confirm the anticholinergic etiology of CNS toxicity. Unless salivary flow and sweating increase

Table 1 Diagnostic features of anticholinergic syndromes

Symptoms	Signs
Dry mouth	Dry mouth and tongue
Changes in visual acuity	Large, hyporesponsive pupils
Hot, dry skin	Hot, dry skin
Difficulty initiating urination	Bladder distention
Increased speed or forcefulness of pulse	Tachycardia
Constipation	Decreased bowel sounds
Subjective confusion or memory impairment	Impaired learning
	(e.g., 5 objects after 5 minutes)

and intestinal hyperactivity occurs following physostigmine, anticholinergic toxicity is present.

At the dose by which dry mouth is produced, some central toxicity is present. In delirious patients, peripheral evidence of anticholinergic toxicity is usually readily apparent.

TREATMENT

In the vast majority of cases, episodes of central anticholinergic toxicity are best treated by simply discontinuing or markedly reducing the doses of the drugs and waiting for the toxic effects to gradually clear over the hours to days required. Gentle containment and assistance in activities of daily living will be required for confused patients during these periods.

When extreme agitation is present that may lead to accidental injury or exhaustion, or when hyperthermia occurs (usually in children), consideration can be given to the use of physostigmine to rapidly reverse central anticholinergic toxicity (Duvoisin & Katz, 1988). Repeated doses of physostigmine (1–2 mg) may be given intravenously every 15–30 minutes, until the patient shows clinical improvement or cholinergic toxicity appears (bradycardia, hypersalivation, emesis, or defecation). It is important to recall that physostigmine is metabolized more rapidly than most anticholinergic drugs. Thus, signs of anticholinergic toxicity may reappear within 45–120 minutes and repeated doses of physostigmine may be required.

Heiser and Gillin (1971) have noted the following contraindications to the use of physostigmine: " . . . a history of allergy or sensitivity to the drug, the presence of renal hypertension, hyperthyroidism, coronary artery disease, a history of cardiac arrhythmia other than chronic atrial fibrillation, peptic ulcer disease, colitis, bronchitis or asthma, diabetes mellitus, gangrene, mechanical obstruction of the intestines or urogenital tract, glaucoma, myotonia atrophica or congenita, pregnancy, or any vagotonic state." However, Granacher and Baldessarini (1975) state that "probably the most serious acute complications of excessive effect of a single dose of physostigmine would be provocation of an acute asthmatic attack or heart block, but the most common acute toxic responses are nausea and vomiting."

Most episodes of anticholinergic toxicity can be dealt with by simply waiting. A conscious benefit/risk decision must be made before the use of physostigmine is considered.

PREVENTION

Use of the lowest antipsychotic doses that produce maximum available antipsychotic benefit should be the initial step in controlling extrapyramidal side effects. Higher antipsychotic doses offer no further therapeutic benefit for the great majority of patients, but produce more severe and distressing extrapyramidal side effects. The higher anticholinergic drug doses prescribed in association with higher antipsychotic doses do not relieve these extrapyramidal side effects completely, but produce more severe central and peripheral anticholinergic side effects. Strategies for prevention of anticholinergic syndromes include:

1. Use of the lowest possible neuroleptic doses for treatment of psychoses.

2. Adjustment of anticholinergic drug doses based on frequent inquiries and examinations for anticholinergic side effects.

3. Awareness of cumulative anticholinergic effects across all medications that the patient is receiving.

4. Avoidance of pharmacotherapeutic regimens that produce a greater anticholinergic burden than mild dry mouth.

5. Awareness of transient or persistent CNS dysfunction that predisposes patients to anticholinergic toxicity.

6. Trials of dopaminergic antiparkinsonian agents as an alternative therapy for patients at high risk for anticholinergic toxicity.

Whenever a drug with anticholinergic potency is prescribed, clinicians should question and examine patients regularly regarding the central and peripheral toxic effects. This may be especially important when two classes of drugs (e.g., an antipsychotic and tricyclic antidepressant) with additive anticholinergic potency are prescribed together. The clinician who does not increase dose beyond the point at which mild dry mouth first appears will rarely or never see severe central anticholinergic toxicity (McEvoy, 1983).

Identification of patients with preexisting organic mental syndromes, or with histories of abuse of mind-altering drugs, will alert the prescribing clinician to proceed with care.

Some, but not all, patients will have favorable antiparkinson responses to amantadine, a drug that seems to operate primarily through dopaminergic mechanisms. An argument can be made to try amantadine as initial treatment for extrapyramidal side effects (EPSE) in elderly patients, particularly those with dementia who are so exquisitely susceptible to anticholinergic toxicity. It would also certainly be desirable to treat young patients engaged in school, vocational rehabilitation, psychotherapy, or other new learning tasks with amantadine rather than an anticholinergic whenever possible. Unfortunately, amantadine alone proved inadequate in controlling the EPSE of more than half the patients we switched from anticholinergic to amantadine maintenance (McEvoy, McCue, & Freter, 1987).

REFERENCES

DeSemet Y, Ruberg M, Serdaru M, Dubois B, Lhermitte F, Agid Y, 1982: Confusion, dementia and anticholinergics in Parkinson's disease. *Journal of Neurology, Neurosurgery, and Psychiatry, 45,* 1161–1164.

Duvoisin RC, Katz R, 1988: Reversal of central anticholinergic syndrome in man by physostigmine. *Journal of the American Medical Association, 206,* 1963–1965.

Granacher RP, Baldessarini RJ, 1975: Physostigmine—its use in acute anticholinergic syndrome with antidepressants and antiparkinson drugs. *Archives of General Psychiatry, 32,* 375–380.

Heiser JF, Gillin JC, 1972: The reveral of anticholinergic drug induced delirium and coma with physostigmine. *American Journal of Psychiatry, 127,* 1050–1054.

McCormick DA, 1989: Cholinergic and nonadrenergic modulation of thalamocortical processing. *Trends in Neuroscience, 12,* 215–221.

McEvoy JP, 1983: The clinical use of anticholinergic drugs as treatment for extrapyramidal side effects of neuroleptic drugs. *Journal of Clinical Psychopharmacology, 3,* 288–302.

McEvoy JP, 1987: A double-blind crossover comparison of antiparkinson drug therapy: Amantadine versus anticholinergics in 90 normal volunteers, with an emphasis on differential effects on memory function. *Journal of Clinical Psychiatry, 48* (9, Suppl), 20–23.

McEvoy JP, Freter S, 1989: The dose-response relationship for memory impairment by anticholinergic drugs. *Comprehensive Psychiatry, 30,* 135–138.

McEvoy JP, McCue M, Spring B, Mohs RC, Lavori PW, Farr RM, 1987a: Effects of amantadine and trihexyphenidyl on memory in elderly normal volunteers. *American Journal of Psychiatry, 144,* 573–577.

McEvoy JP, Freter S, McCue M, Spring B, Mohs RC, Lavori PW, Farr RM, 1987b: Replacement of chronically administered anticholinergic drugs by amantadine in outpatient management of chronic schizophrenia. *Clinical Therapeutics, 9,* 429–433.

Mondimore FM, Damlouji N, Folstein MF, Tune L, 1983: Post-ECT confusional states associated with elevated serum anticholinergic levels. *American Journal of Psychiatry, 140,* 930–931.

Perlick D, Stastry P, Katz I, Mayer M, Mattis S, 1986: Memory deficits and anticholinergic levels in chronic schizophrenia. *American Journal of Psychiatry, 143,* 230–232.

Petersen RC, 1977: Scopolamine-induced learning failures in man. *Psychopharmacology, 52,* 283–289.

Richardson RT, Delong MR, 1988: A reappraisal of the functions of the nucleus basalis of Meynert. *Trends in Neuroscience, 11,* 264–267.

Rovner BS, David A, Lucas-Blaustein MJ, Conklin B, Filipp L, Tune L, 1988: Self-care capacity and anticholinergic drug levels in nursing home patients. *American Journal of Psychiatry, 145,* 107–109.

Salamone JD, 1986: Behavioral functions of nucleus basalis magnocellularis and its relationship to dementia. *Trends in Neuroscience, 9,* 256–258.

Sunderland T, Tariot PN, Cohen RM, Weingartner H, Mueller EA, Murphy DL, 1987: Anticholinergic sensitivity in patients with dementia of the Alzheimer type and age-matched controls. *Archives of General Psychiatry, 44,* 418–426, 1987.

Tune LE, Damlouji N, Holland A, Gardner TJ, Folstein MF, Coyle JT, 1981: Postoperative delirium is associated with elevated serum anticholinergic levels. *Lancet, 1,* 651–652.

Tune LE, Strauss ME, Lew MF, Breitlinger E, Coyle JT, 1982: Serum levels of anticholinergic drugs and impaired recent memory in chronic schizophrenic patients. *American Journal of Psychiatry, 139,* 1460–1462.

Ullman KC, Groh RH, 1972: Identification and treatment of psychotic states secondary to the usage of over-the-counter sleeping preparations. *American Journal of Psychiatry, 128,* 1244–1248.

VanPutten T, Gelenberg AJ, Lavori PW, Falk WE, Marder SR, Spring B, Mohs RC, Brotman AW, 1987: Anticholinergic effects on memory: Benztropine vs. amantadine. *Psychopharmacology Bulletin, 23,* 26–29.

Weiner N, 1980: Atropine, scopolamine, and related antimuscarinic drugs. In: *The pharmacologic basis of therapeutics,* 6th edition, edited by AF Gilman, LS Goodman, and A Gilman. New York: Macmillan.

15

Drug-Induced Affective Syndromes

Jules Angst

Bonhoeffer's handbook article (1912) on symptomatic psychoses was a milestone in psychiatric classification. He described the so-called acute exogenous reaction type that embraces a variety of psychopathological syndromes as the consequence of acute damage of the brain functions that comes with all sorts of medical diseases. The described syndromes included not only changes of consciousness, confusional states, delirious states, paranoid or catatonic syndromes, but also mania and depression. Psychotropic drugs can in principle induce all these syndromes—for instance, states of agitation, confusion, delirium, or changes of consciousness. Specific drug-induced affective syndromes are drug-induced hypomania/mania and drug-induced depression. This review focuses only on these two phenomena, induced by psychotropic drugs. Numerous other drugs have been considered in the literature and reviewed (Ananth & Ghadirian, 1980; Chevalier & Ginested, 1979; Gangat, Simpson, & Naidoo, 1986; Whitlock, 1982).

METHODOLOGICAL CONSIDERATIONS

Wehr and Goodwin (1987a) stress that "it is generally believed that antidepressant treatments can cause mania." They mention Heinroth (1818): "He argued that depression should be treated with drugs and procedures that have a stimulating effect on the organism, but cautioned that overzealous application of such treatments might have the undesirable effect of causing an overshoot into mania. Too rigorous treatment of mania with calming agents could in turn cause an overshoot into depression, he believed."

Since monoamine oxidase inhibitors (MAOIs) and tricyclic antidepressants (TCAs) were introduced as antidepressants, investigators believed that the occurrence of hypomania during a drug treatment would be drug-induced. In early drug studies the observation of a switch from depression to hypomania was even understood as an indicator for a true antidepressant potency of a drug. In numerous studies with antidepressants, the occurrence of hypomania was reported and ascribed to the treatment. In a retrospective analysis of the literature on drug-induced mania, out of 246 journal articles or book chapters, 124 articles contained 169 individual case descriptions, but only 30 articles reported case series or prevalence information concerning drug-induced mania associated with a particular agent (Sultzer & Cummings, 1989).

This fact points to some serious methodological problems in the field. It is evident that single case reports, which dominate the field, can only be taken as hints for a causal relationship. Also uncontrolled series of cases are biased because negative series are not included and published. The main source of error is selective reporting of cases observed. Even prevalence rates are not conclusive as long as it is not shown that the prevalence of hypomania/mania under drugs is higher than the spontaneous prevalence rate without treatment or with the placebo.

Another source of error is the diagnosis, especially the lack of a breakdown into uni- and bipolar affective disorders. Early studies with antidepressants were carried out under diagnostic conditions that would be unacceptable today. Either the studies were focusing on "depressive syndromes," without any subclassification, or they were referring to *DSM-II* or *ICD* diagnoses, which in the 1950s and 1960s were still dominated by the Kraepelinian concept of a homogeneous "manic-depressive insanity." Today there is no doubt that the dichotomy between uni- and bipolar affective disorders is essential for the analysis of switches. Modern researchers, therefore, distinguish carefully between the two subtypes of affective disorders when they discuss drug-induced hypomania (see, for instance, Angst, 1985; Krauthammer & Klerman, 1978; Kupfer, Carpenter, & Frank, 1988; Lewis & Winokur, 1982; Wehr & Goodwin, 1987a). Following this distinction, we have to separate drug-induced hypomania in bipolar patients from drug-induced hypomania in unipolar (nonbipolar) depressives.

Studies on the switch rate are full of pitfalls. The results are also highly dependent on the selection of the sample studies—for instance, selecting patients for certain drug trials: acute treatment studies versus maintenance studies over 2 years, studies devoted to unipolar depressives only (excluding all bipolars), or studies excluding bipolar I (synonymous with *DSM-III* bipolar disorder) and including either recurrent depressives and bipolar II cases (a term used to refer to cases with depression and hypomanic, not manic episodes) (Kupfer et al., 1988).

HYPOMANIA/MANIA IN BIPOLAR PATIENTS TREATED WITH ANTIDEPRESSANTS

Bipolar disorders are characterized by the spontaneous occurrence of hypomania or mania. Antidepressants can hypothetically change the spontaneous course by: increasing the rates of hypomanic/manic syndromes compared to the spontaneous rate; shortening the time span from the onset of a depressive episode to the switch to hypomania; abbreviating the cycle length of affective episodes by shortening the depressive episodes; or shortening the cycle length by abbreviating interepisode intervals, turning the case into a rapid cycler, or even shortening the cycle length by eliminating such intervals, turning a case into a continuous cycler. There is clinical evidence that antidepressant treatment of bipolar illness may decrease cycle length or even induce rapid cycling between mania and depression (Tondo, Laddomada, Serra, Minnai, & Kukopulos, 1981). The literature in support of this was summarized carefully by Wehr and Goodwin (1987a, b).

More controversial is the question whether antidepressants increase the spontaneous rate of hypomania/mania or not. A causal relationship between antidepressant treatment and the occurrence of mania can be shown in several ways: (1) if, in placebo-controlled drug trials, antidepressants induce mania in bipolar patients more frequently than the placebo does; (2) if the switch from depression to hypomania/mania occurs earlier under drugs than spontaneously or under the placebo; (3) if we can show that antidepressants induce mania more frequently than it occurs spontaneously.

Representative placebo-controlled drug studies of bipolar patients would certainly be most convincing. Unfortunately, they do not exist (Wehr & Goodwin, 1987b). The study of Prien, Klett, and Caffey (1973) on 2 years of maintenance treatment with imipramine, lithium carbonate, and placebo was carried out in a specifically selected group of patients. From the fifth month on through 24 months of the study, mania occurred in 6 of 9 imipramine cases and in 3 of 9 placebo cases. Such small figures are not conclusive (Wehr & Goodwin, 1987a).

Another study of a 2-year treatment compared lithium, imipramine, or a combination of both (Prien et al., 1984), and a third 2-year study compared lithium plus imipramine with lithium alone (Quitkin, Kane, Rifkin, Ramos-Lorenzi, & Nayak, 1981). The two studies do not agree in their results. Quitkin et al. found an incidence of mania that was more than twice as high with lithium plus imipramine (25%) compared with lithium alone (11%). Prien and associates (1984) found 28% of switches on lithium plus imipramine versus 26% on lithium alone. On the other hand, the incidence of mania under imipramine alone was 53%. The reasons for the inconsistent findings of the two studies are unclear and were discussed by Wehr and Goodwin (1987a) in detail. The results can be interpreted in two ways: (1) imipramine (either given alone or given combined with lithium) would increase the incidence or mania or (2) the antimanic effect of lithium lowers the rate of switches from depression to mania.

Kupfer et al. (1988) prospectively studied a group of bipolar II patients at high risk for recurrence (selected by a high number of previous depressive episodes). The authors did not observe any increase in switch rates. In one of 33 bipolar II depressive patients, they observed hypomania compared to five cases of the 197 unipolar depressives. In the total sample of 230 patients only 6 individuals (2.6%) developed hypomania, representing 0.9% of those in the acute phase and 2.5% of those in the continuation phase of drug treatment. This study shows that even selected, highly recurrent bipolar II patients may not be at high risk for developing hypomania under a TCA medication. In this study four of the six switches to hypomania even occurred when imipramine was discontinued. The question of whether or not only the application but also the withdrawal of an antidepressant drug may induce biological changes including hypomania is of great theoretical interest and needs further research. It would support Dilsaver and Gredens's (1984) hypothesis that a manic episode can result from dysfunction of mechanisms that maintain balance between opposing transmitter systems. In that case, both the application and the withdrawal of a drug would create an imbalance of the system and increase the probability of a change. This hypothesis is less specific than certain speculative neurotransmitter hypotheses (Bunney et al., 1977; Pickar, Cowdry, Zis, Cohen, & Murphy, 1984).

THE SPONTANEOUS SWITCH RATE
FROM DEPRESSION TO MANIA IN BIPOLAR DISORDER

If drug-induced mania exists, the incidence should be higher on drugs than spontaneously. But what is the spontaneous switch rate? Studies devoted to this question are extremely rare even though bipolar illness commonly manifests itself as biphasic episodes starting either with mania and switching to depression or starting with depression and switching spontaneously to hypomania or mania.

There are two retrospective chart reviews on the question of drug-induced mania in series of hospitalized bipolar patients. The first was published by Lewis and Winokur (1982). The authors concluded "that the so-called switch effect due to tricyclic antidepressants reported in the past, probably represents random manifestations of bipolar illness" and "is not greater than what one would expect from the natural history of the illness itself." The advantage of this study was that it was based on a representative sample of hospital admissions for major depression at Iowa City Psychiatric Hospital.

Another landmark study was carried out in Zurich (Switzerland) (Angst, 1985, 1987a, 1987b, 1988). This author started to study all admissions for endogenous depression to a university hospital in Zurich over the century to examine switch rates to hypomania as well as depression before the introduction of electroconvulsive therapy (ECT) and antidepressants. It was based on material collected by several investigators. Six hundred records of depressives were investigated independently and blindly by two investigators and, in cases of doubt, two other experts made a consensus diagnosis of hypomania. This study has the advantage that it provides data on large numbers of patients before the introduction of modern treatments. But it has also disadvantages because the quality of the records, the rates of admissions, or the catchment area as well as diagnostic habits may change over decades. Furthermore, some mild hypomanic states may not have been recorded or may have been interpreted by some doctors as normal mood swings compensating for a depression.

The results of this study are nevertheless astonishing. The switch rate from depression to hypomania/mania in bipolar patients is unchanged over all decades of this century. The spontaneous rate of about 30% is independent of sex, age of onset, age, and number of previous episodes in bipolar disorder. The switch occurs with a median on day 125 of a depressive episode. Before the introduction of ECT or drug treatment the day of switch (median) was 143 and since the introduction of the treatments it was 120, the difference being not significant (Angst, 1987a). Based on this data, the Zurich group concluded that there is no evidence for an increased incidence of switches or for earlier switches under treatment compared to the natural course of the disorder. This conclusion is based on comparisons of groups and does not refer to special cases of bipolar disorders, for instance, rapid cyclers. We do not know whether the conclusion drawn from the study carried out in Zurich is valid also for specific subgroups of bipolars.

Highly selected, rapid-cycling bipolar patients may have a higher switch rate on drugs than spontaneously (Wehr & Goodwin, 1987b). However, the evidence is inconclusive. There is some evidence, again inconclusive, that a TCA medication may shorten the cycle length of bipolar patients to rapid cyclers (Tondo et al., 1981).

HYPOMANIA/MANIA IN TREATED AND UNTREATED UNIPOLAR DEPRESSED PATIENTS

In a well-known review of 80 publications (Bunney, 1978), 9.5% of 3,923 patients experienced mania or hypomania when given TCA or MAOI. This rate is similar to the 9% switch observed in 12 prospective placebo-controlled studies mentioned by Wehr and Goodwin (1987a). These rates are misleading, because they refer to a heterogeneous population of patients suffering from bipolar or unipolar affective disorders.

The available studies on long-term maintenance treatment of pure unipolar depressives are biased by the selection of highly recurrent unipolars who may be less prone to develop hypomania than a nonselected group (Kupfer et al., 1988; Prien et al., 1973, 1984). But one can conclude that highly recurrent unipolar depressive patients are not at high risk to develop hypomania on antidepressants. Kupfer et al. observed a switch in only 2.5% (5/197) of unipolar depressives.

The retrospective chart study of Zurich (Angst, 1987a) gives a 3.7% rate of switch from depression to hypomania in unipolar depressives over this century. The figures for the first decade before the introduction of modern treatments are 2.7% (5/185) and not significantly lower than the 4.0% rate (24/602) observed later, after the introduction of ECT and antidepressants. The authors therefore conclude that there is no clear increase of the switch rate resulting from modern antidepressants.

This conclusion does not exclude the existence of single cases with special sensitivity, which is best tested by intermittent treatments to reproduce the effect. But the overall conclusion is negative. Modern antidepressants do not switch unipolar to bipolar disorder to a substantial degree. The few percent of switches that are observed are probably a result of hidden bipolars with a specific genetic predisposition.

DRUG-INDUCED DEPRESSION IN SCHIZOPHRENIA

Soon after the introduction of reserpine and chlorpromazine, a number of investigators reported the occurrence of depression during this treatment (Faucett, 1958; Fellner, 1958) and numerous case reports followed. Some papers referred also to long-term medication (e.g., Booth, Forrest, & Mackay, 1962). The observations were usually made in schizophrenic patients receiving an antipsychotic medication.

There are several possible relationships between depression and schizophrenia; Knights and Hirsch (1981) distinguish among pharmacogenic, akinetic, and postpsychotic depression, depression as an integral part of schizophrenic illness, and coexisting depressive illness with schizophrenia.

Depressive syndromes as an integral part of schizophrenic psychoses have been reported by Bleuler (1911). Gruhle (1932) mentioned the existence of so-called "hypophases" with depressive symptoms in the spontaneous course of schizophrenia, and Weitbrecht (1949) described a special kind of affective relapse syndrome. Depressive symptoms can occur before, during, and after a schizophrenic episode or process (Angst, Stassen, & Woggon, 1989). Depression in schizophrenia may frequently be overlooked and not investigated well enough during drug trials. Depression is frequently noticed only after the psychotic symptoms have been removed by successful treatment. This kind of depressive symptoms was called morbogenic (Helmchen, 1969; Helmchen & Hippius, 1969). In the context of drug treatments, von Baeyer (1951) interpreted the depressive symptoms as residual symptoms of the psychosis after successful treatment with antipsychotic drugs.

This interpretation is close to that of Bohacek (1965). He assumed that in schizophrenia the paranoid-hallucinatory syndrome would be superimposed on an underlying depression and that the drug treatment would eliminate the more superficial symptoms, unmasking the depressive syndrome (Bohacek, 1966, 1967).

Drug-induced depressive symptoms also play a certain role in the concept of a "postremissive exhaustion syndrome" described by Heinrich (1967). He described a drug-induced emotional decrease of reactivity and activity, which could create a reactive depressive mood in addition to psychodynamic factors in the remission period. These changes are reversible and not symptoms of a schizophrenic defect. They depend on an adequate dose and on an adequate psychotherapeutic and sociotherapeutic intervention.

Postpsychotic depression (Goplerud & Depue, 1979; McGlashan & Carpenter, 1976a, b) is a psychological response to the awareness of illness, fear of relapse, and implications of long-term treatment, as well as difficulties of readaptation to meet the challenge of everyday life, loss of self-esteem with difficulties to accept the sick role, and so forth. This psychological reaction was first described extensively by Mayer-Gross (1920) before the introduction of modern somatic treatments of schizophrenia. Psychodynamic mechanisms were described later—for instance, again by Mackinnon (1977) without referring to Mayer-Gross's work.

Akinetic depression was probably first mentioned by van Putten and May (1978), but the phenomenon was described carefully earlier by many other authors. The co-occurrence of depression with extrapyramidal symptoms was interpreted as drug-induced, supported by the fact that after cessation of the treatment the depressive symptoms disappeared (Helmchen & Hippius, 1969). On the other hand, this close association may be interpreted as symptoms occurring as part of a Parkinson syndrome and therefore not being a form of true independent depression.

It is interesting that with clozapine, which is free of Parkinson side effects, the occurrence of depression has not been described and even an antidepressant effect has been mentioned. Indeed, numerous drug studies show an antidepressant effect of antipsychotic drugs. A review of 34 double-blind studies was given by Robertson and Trimble (1982). In a number of studies, some using the placebo, the consistent trend emerged that antipsychotics possess some antidepressant effects. The drugs mentioned especially were thioridazine, thioxanthenes, and flupenthixol. The authors concluded that postpsychotic depression after antipsychotic therapy is likely to be part of the underlying illness and not drug-induced.

In this context, the history of the depressogenic effect of reserpine is remarkable. Originally Faucett (1958) described the effect. Goodwin, Ebert, and Bunney (1972) ascribed this depression to the serotonin depletion. Goodwin and Bunney (1971) suggested that reserpine, alone or in combination with other factors such as stress, may precipitate depression in predisposed individuals rather than actually cause depression de novo. In this context, studies on the previous family history of depression suggesting a precipitation have become important (Whitlock, 1982).

New prospective data have emerged over the past years on the course of depressive symptoms during antipsychotic treatment of schizophrenics. Strong evidence against drug-induced depression was put forward by Hirsch and coworkers (Hirsch, 1983; Hirsch & Knights, 1982; Knights & Hirsch, 1981). They confirmed the decrease of depressive symptoms under antipsychotic drugs as, for instance, shown by Woggon and Angst (1975) and by Hucker, Woggon, & Angst

(1976) in several groups of schizophrenic patients treated over 3 and 6 months. These observations are at variance with the assumption of an increase of depression during antipsychotic treatment. Compatible are the results of the studies of Moeller and von Zerssen in Munich (1981a, b). Studying 280 acute schizophrenic inpatients, they found a depressive syndrome at admission in 48%, and at discharge in 17%. Most of the latter group had suffered from depression already at admission. During the hospital treatment, 56% ($n = 237$) had suffered from long-lasting depressive syndromes. Only 14% of the 237 patients developed depression during the hospital treatment. The interpretation of this phenomenon is open, and the authors stress that morbogenic and psychoreactive factors have to be considered apart from the antipsychotics.

The conclusion of Roy (1984) seems to be justified: ". . . Neuroleptics play no role—or at most a minimal role—in the causation of depressive disorder in chronic schizophrenic patients." This statement should be extended to acute schizophrenics in face of the previously mentioned results reported by Moeller and von Zerssen.

CONCLUSION

This review is restricted to hypomania induced by antidepressants and to depression induced by antipsychotic drugs. Both phenomena are mentioned in the literature. Since these drugs were marketed, numerous case reports and papers on series of cases were published. Most authors assume a well-established causal relationship, and the terms *drug-induced depression* and *drug-induced hypomania* were accepted into text books. Most of the authors do not discuss the question of the spontaneous course or try to control for this. It is obvious that hypomania in affective disorder and depression in schizophrenic disorder can occur spontaneously. In practice, it has been almost impossible to control for these spontaneous mood changes. There is no conclusive study based on a large representative sample with a group on a placebo and a breakdown of patients by the presence of hypomania/mania or depression in the previous history.

Based on the available data, the following conclusions may be drawn:

1. In bipolar illness the spontaneous switch rate of an untreated depressive episode is about 30%; there is no study showing a more frequent occurrence under drugs. It is possible, however, that highly selected, rapid-cycling bipolar patients may show a drug-induced increase in switch rate. On the other hand, there is some evidence that a medication may shorten the cycle length of bipolar patients to rapid cyclers. Highly selected recurrent bipolar II patients seem to be at very low risk of switching from depression to hypomania under tricyclic medication.

2. Up to now there is no drug trial showing, compared to the placebo, an elevation of the switch risk to hypomania in unipolar depressive patients. The slight increase in spontaneous switch rate during this century is too small to be significant or practically relevant. Therefore, there is no convincing evidence that modern antidepressants would switch unipolar depressed patients to hypomania to a substantial degree.

3. There is no convincing drug trial showing a more frequent occurrence of depression under an antipsychotic drug than under the placebo. On the other hand there is a substantial number of studies showing a considerable improvement of

depression during antipsychotic treatment of schizophrenic disorders. Several prospective studies show a clear significant decrease of depression during antipsychotic treatments.

All these conclusions are based on statistical analyses of groups of patients. They do not exclude the existence of single patients who may behave differently and may show reproducible, drug-induced affective syndromes.

REFERENCES

Affleck JW, Booth JCD, Forrest AD, Mackay KJ, 1962: The effect of thioproperazine administered by a continuous method on long-term schizophrenic patients. *Journal of Mental Science, 108,* 862–864.

Ananth J, Ghadirian AM, 1980: Drug induced mood disorders. *International Pharmacopsychiatry, 15,* 59–73.

Angst J, 1985: Switch from depression to mania. A record study over decades between 1920 and 1982. *Psychopathology, 18,* 140–154.

Angst J, 1987a: Switch from depression to mania, or from mania to depression. *Journal of Psychopharmacology, 1,* 13–19.

Angst J, 1987b: Switch from depression to mania, or from mania to depression: Role of psychotropic drugs. *Psychopharmacology, 23,* 66–67.

Angst J, 1988: Recurrent brief depression. A new concept of mild depression. In: Abstracts of XVIth CINP Congres., Munich 1988. *Psychopharmacology, 96*(suppl), 123.

Angst J, Stassen HH, Woggon B, 1989: Effect of neuroleptics on positive and negative symptoms and the deficit state. *Psychopharmacology, 99,* S41–S46.

Baeyer, von, W, 1951: *Die moderne psychiatrische Schockbehandlung* [Shock treatment in modern psychiatry]. Thieme: Stuttgart.

Bleuler E, 1911: Dementia praecox oder Gruppe der Schizophrenien. In: *Handbuch der Psychiatrie,* edited by G. Aschaffenburg, spez. Teil, 4. Abt., I. Hälfte. Deuticke: Leipzig Wien.

Bohacek N, 1965: Discussion working group 4. In: *Neuropsychopharmacology,* vol. 4, edited by D Bente and PB Bradley. Amsterdam, London and New York: Elsevier.

Bohacek N, 1966: Pharmakogene depressive Verschiebung. In: *Proceedings of the Vth International Congress of the Collegium International Neuropsychopharmacologicum.* Excerpta Medica International Congress Series No. 129, Washington, DC, pp. 1080–1082.

Bohacek N, 1967: "Depresivni pomak" u toku lijecenja schizofrenih psihoza nekim fenotijazinima [Depressive shift in the course of treatment of schizophrenic psychoses with some phenothiazines]. *Neuropsihijatrija* (Zagreb), *15,* 97–103.

Bonhoeffer K, 1912: Die symptomatischen Psychosen im Gefolge akuter Infektionen [Symptomatic psychoses in the course of acute infections], Allgemeinerkrankungen und innerer Krankheiten. In: *Handbuch der Psychiatrie,* 3. Abt., 1., Hälfte, edited by G Aschaffenburg. Deuticke: Leipzig Wien.

Bunney WE Jr, 1978; Psychopharmacology of the switch process in affective illness. In: *Psychopharmacology: A generation of progress,* edited by MA Lipton, A DiMascio, and KF Killam, pp. 1249–1259. New York: Raven Press.

Bunney WE Jr, Wehr TA, Gillin JC, Post RM, Goodwin FK, Van Kammen DP van, 1977: The switch process in manic depressive psychosis. *Annals of Internal Medicine, 87,* 319–335.

Chevalier JF, Ginestet D, 1979: Les depressions iatrogenes. *Encephale, 5,* 567–578.

Dilsaver SC, Greden JF, 1984: Antidepressant withdrawal induced activation (hypomania and mania): Mechanisms and theoretical significance. *Brain Research, 319,* 29–48.

Faucett RL, 1958: Induced depressions: Pharmacologic effects. *American Journal of Psychiatry, 115,* 247–248.

Fellner CH, 1958: A clinical note on drug induced depression. *American Journal of Psychiatry, 115,* 547–548.

Gangat AE, Simpson MA, Naidoo LR, 1986: Medication as a potential cause of depression. *South African Medical Journal, 70,* 224–226.

Goodwin FK, Bunney WE Jr, 1971: Depressions following reserpine: A reevaluation. *Seminars in Psychiatry, 3,* 435–448.

Goodwin FK, Ebert MH, Bunney WE Jr, 1972: Mental effects of reserpine in man: A review. In: *Psychiatric complications of medical drugs*, edited by RI Shader, pp. 73–101. New York: Raven Press.

Goplerud E, Depue RA, 1979: Affective symptoms schizophrenia, and the conceptual ambiguity of postpsychotic depression. *Schizophrenia Bulletin, 5,* 554–559.

Gruhle HW, 1932: Die Psychopathologie. In: *Handbuch der Geisteskrankheiten* [Psychopathology. In: *Manual of mental disorders*], Band IX/5, edited by O Bumke. Berlin: Springer.

Heinrich K, 1967: Zur Bedeutung des postremissiven Erschöp-pfungs-Syndromes fur die Rehabilitation Schizophrener [The significance for rehabilitation of an exhaustion syndrome in remitted schizophrenics]. *Nervenarzt, 38,* 487–491.

Heinroth DFCA, 1818: Lehrbuch der Störungen des Seelenlebens oder der Spelenstörungen und iher Behandlung. Von rationalen standpunkt aus entworfen [Textbook on the disturbances of the soul or psychological disorders and their treatment, sketched from the rational viewpoint]. Leipzig: Vogel.

Helmchen H, 1969: Psychische Störungen durch Arzneimittel. *Dtsch Aerztebl, 66,* 3537–3541.

Helmchen H, Hippius H, 1969: Erscheinungsweise depressiver Syndrome unter der Therapie mit Neuroleptika. In: *Pharmaco-psychiatrische Probleme in Klinik und Praxis*, edited by K Heinrich, (pp. 61–67). Symposium, Bad Dürkheim. New York: Schattauer.

Hirsch SR, 1983: The causality of depression in schizophrenia. *British Journal of Psychiatry, 142,* 624–625.

Hirsch SR, Knights A, 1982: Gibt es die pharmakogene Depression wirklich? Beweismaterial aus zwei Prospektiven Untersuchungen. In: *Ergebnisse psychiatrischer Therapieforschung* [Do pharmacogenic depressions really exist? Proofs from two prospective studies. In: *Results of research on psychiatric therapy]*, edited by K Kryspin-Exner, H Hinterhuber, and H Schubert. New York: Schattauer, Stuttgart.

Hucker H, Woggon B, Angst J, 1976: Schweizerische Studie über die Behandlung mit Depotneuroleptika. II. Präparatspezifische Ergenbnisse der Auswertung [A Swiss study on treatment with "depot"-neuroleptics: drug specific results of evaluation]. In: *Schweizerische Studiueber die Behandlung mit Depotneuroleptika, Rundtischgespräch Bern 1975*, edited by J Angst and M Burner (pp. 26–59). Zurich: Squibb.

Knights A, Hirsch SR, 1981: "Revealed" depression and drug treatment for schizophrenia. *Archives of General Psychiatry, 38,* 806–811.

Krauthammer C, Klerman GL, 1978: Secondary mania: Manic syndromes associated with antecedent physical illness or drugs. *Archives of General Psychiatry, 35,* 1333–1339.

Kupfer DJ, Carpenter LL, Frank E, 1988: Possible role of antidepressants in precipitating mania and hypomania in recurrent depression. *American Journal of Psychiatry, 145,* 804–808.

Lewis JL, Winokur G, 1982: The induction of mania: A natural history study with controls. *Archives of General Psychiatry, 39,* 303–306.

McGlashan TH, Carpenter WT Jr, 1976a: An investigation of the postpsychotic depressive syndrome. *American Journal of Psychiatry, 133,* 14–19.

McGlashan TH, Carpenter WT Jr, 1976b: Postpsychotic depression in schizophrenia. *Archives of General Psychiatry, 33,* 231–239.

Mackinnon BL, 1977: Postpsychotic depression and the need for personal significance. *American Journal of Psychiatry, 134,* 427–429.

Mayer-Gross W, 1920: Ueber die Stellungnahme zur abgelaufenen akuten Psychose. Eine Studiueber verständliche Zusammenhänge in der Schizophrenie [The attitude towards past acute psychosis. A study on the intelligible context of schizophrenia]. *Z Gesamte Neurol Psychiatr, 60,* 160–212.

Moeller HJ, von Zerssen D, 1981a: Depressive Symptomatik im stationoren Behandlungsverlauf von 280 schizophrenen Patienten [Depressive symptoms during the treatment of 280 schizophrenic in-patients]. *Pharmacopsychiatry, 14,* 172–179.

Moeller HJ, von Zerssen D, 1981b: Depressive Symptomatik bei Aufnahme und Entlassung stationär behandelter schizophrener Patienten [Depressive symptoms at admission and discharge of schizophrenic in-patients]. *Nervenarzt, 52,* 525–530.

Pickar D, Cowdry RW, Zis AP, Cohen RM, Murphy DL, 1984: Mania and hypomania during antidepressant pharmacotherapy: Clinical and research implications. In: *Neurobiology of mood disorders*, edited by RM Post and JC Ballenger. Baltimore: Williams and Wilkins. (Frontiers of Clinical Neuroscience, vol. 1) pp. 836–845.

Prien RF, Klett CJ, Caffey EM Jr, 1973: Lithium carbonate and imipramine in prevention of affective episodes. A comparison in recurrent affective illness. Report of the Veterans Administration and

National Institute of Mental Health Collaborative Study Group. *Archives of General Psychiatry, 29,* 420–425.

Prien RF, Kupfer DJ, Mansky PA, Small JH, Tuason VB, Voss CB, Johnson WE, 1984: Drug therapy in the prevention of recurrences in unipolar and bipolar affective disorders. Report of the NIMH Collaborative Study Group comparing lithium carbonate, imipramine, and a lithium carbonate-imipramine combination. *Archives of General Psychiatry, 41,* 1096–1104.

Putten, van, T, May PRA, 1978: "Akinetic depression" in schizophrenia. *Archives of General Psychiatry, 35,* 1101–1107.

Quitkin FM, Kane J, Rifkin A, Ramos-Lorenzi JR, Nayak DV, 1981: Prophylactic lithium carbonate with and without imipramine for bipolar I patients: A double-blind study. *Archives of General Psychiatry, 38,* 902–907.

Robertson MM, Trimble MR, 1982: Major tranquilizers used as antidepressants. A review. *Journal of Affective Disorders, 4,* 173–193.

Roy A, 1984: Do neuroleptics cause depression? *Biological Psychiatry, 19,* 777–781.

Sultzer DL, Cummings JL, 1989: Drug induced mania—causative agents, clinical characteristics and management. A retrospective analysis of the literature. *Medical Toxicology and Adverse Drug Experiences, 4,* 127–143.

Tondo L, Laddomada P, Serra G, Minnai G, Kukopulos A, 1981: Rapid cyclers and antidepressants. *International Pharmacopsychiatry, 16,* 119–123.

Wehr TA, Goodwin FK, 1987a: Can antidepressants cause mania and worsen the course of affective illness? *American Journal of Psychiatry, 144,* 1403–1411.

Wehr TA, Goodwin FK, 1987b: Do antidepressants cause mania? *Psychopharmacology Bulletin, 23,* 61–65.

Weitbrecht HJ, 1949: Studie zur Psychopathologie krampfbehandelter Psychosen [Study on the psychopathology of psychoses under shock treatment]. Thieme: Stuttgart.

Whitlock FA, 1982: Drugs and depression. In: *Symptomatic affective disorders. A study of depression and mania associated with physical disease and medication,* edited by FA Whitlock. (pp. 99–119). Sydney, New York, London: Academic Press.

Woggon B, Angst J, 1975: Einzelne Aspekte der Behandlung mit Depotneuroleptika. In: *Therapie, Rehabilitation und Prävention schizophrener Erkankungen* [Some aspects of treatment with "depot"-neuroleptics. In: *Therapy, rehabilitation and prevention of schizophrenic disorders*], edited by G Huber (pp. 191–200). 3 Weissenauer Schizophreniesymposion [3rd symposium on schizophrenia at Weissenau], Lübeck-Travemunde. New York: Schattauer, Stuttgart.

16

Iatrogenic Dysfunction and Electroconvulsive Therapy

B. N. Gangadhar and Chittaranjan Andrade

Electroconvulsive therapy (ECT), introduced by Cerletti and Bini in 1938, is the only somatic therapy in psychiatry to creditably survive the advent of psychopharmacological agents. No therapy is free of adverse consequences, and ECT is no exception. Unfortunately, perhaps because of the use of electricity, the resultant convulsion (both suggesting "electric chair" treatment to lay minds) and inaccurate portrayal by sensationalistic mass media, iatrogenic dysfunction with ECT tends to be disproportionately highlighted. Many clinicians are now discernibly reluctant to use ECT except when illness is very severe or drug-resistant; certain places (e.g., California) have legal restrictions against the use of ECT.

In this overview, we reevaluate ECT-induced iatrogenic dysfunction with a view to provide both a rational perspective of the problem and strategies for its containment. The focus will be on new issues and gray areas in research rather than on conventional descriptions, on which adequate literature already exists (Abrams, 1988; Abrams & Essman, 1982; Endler & Persad, 1988; Fink, 1979).

CLINICAL ISSUES

Cognitive Changes

Cognition is impaired in depression, and ECT produces improvements in such cognitive impairment in depression (e.g., Mackenzie, Price, Tucker, & Culver, 1985). However, ECT itself impairs cognition (Abrams, 1988; Fink, 1979; Price, 1982a,b; Squire, 1986; & Weiner, 1984).

Anterograde Amnesia and Retrograde Amnesia

The obtunded new learning with ECT decreases across time after each ECT but cumulates during the ECT course; baseline levels are attained weeks to months after stopping ECT.

Retrograde amnesia is characterized by loss of acquired data. It is also characterized by a temporal gradient that increases in density with proximity in time to the ECT course and that extends further back in time with successive ECTs. Patchy loss of memory may also be seen; recovery generally occurs weeks to months after stopping ECT.

Both verbal and nonverbal memory are affected. Although on objective assessment memory normalizes in most cases, memory for certain events occurring during and around the ECT course may be permanently lost. Memories of lesser emotional impact and less related to habit are more easily obliterated. About 0.5% of ECT-treated patients experience severe retrograde amnesia (for personal and other memories, for one or more years antedating the ECT course), which does not normalize. Permanent anterograde amnesia has not been described.

Nonmemory Cognitive Functions

These cognitive functions that are often impaired by depression improve with ECT, but in certain respects may deteriorate with cumulative treatment. Normalization, weeks after ECT is discontinued, is the rule.

Reversible Dementia

This syndrome is often produced by regressive ECT, a technique that has been discarded as unscientific (Abrams, 1982; Consensus Conference 1985; Gangadhar, Andrade, & Janakiramaiah, 1990). Irreversible dementia is very rare and may result from hypoxia as a result of a variety of drugs (e.g., muscle relaxants), anesthesia, and procedure-related causes—in vulnerable populations.

Post-ECT Delirium

This is largely unpredictable, and its occurrence and recurrence in individuals known to experience this side effect may be prevented by routine intravenous diazepam after each seizure (Abrams, 1982). A milder syndrome, post-ECT confusion, is often seen. Although usually short-lived, more severe (accompanied by excitement) and prolonged (lasting an hour or longer) confusional states may result from bilateral ECT, high-energy stimuli, sinusoidal waveforms, and overly frequent treatments (Consensus Conference, 1985). Right hemispheric mechanisms were suggested (Sackeim et al., 1983) but are disputed (Leechuy, Abrams, & Kohlaas, 1988) to underlie emergent delirium. No predictors for the development of post-ECT excitement (confusion, with excitement as the major symptom) are demonstrable (Devanand, Briscoe, & Sackeim, 1989).

Subjective Cognitive Changes

Some patients (in some studies, in excess of 50%) may report subjective memory impairment persisting for many months (or longer) after ECT. In the absence of objective findings, one must conclude either that the conventional tests are insufficiently sensitive to detect subtle, subjectively apparent impairment, or that ECT is being blamed for forgetfulness within the normal ambit (Squire, 1986). Cognitive deficit may also result from residual depression, concurrent maintenance drugs (Calev et al., 1989), or patient or rater bias to the patient's having received true, as opposed to sham, ECT (Andrade, 1990).

Remedial Strategies

Cognitive dysfunction with ECT, although mild, innocuous, and transient in the majority of cases, is the single adverse effect responsible for the bulk of the criticism of ECT. Many strategies are suggested to limit the problem (American Psychiatric Association, 1990; Andrade, 1990).

Electrode placement. Unilateral ECT may be as effective as bilateral ECT (at least in depression) and unequivocally relatively spares verbal memory function (Weiner, 1986a); further, bilateral ECT may impair personal memory beyond 6 months post-ECT (Weiner, Rogers, Davidson, & Squire, 1986a). Confirmation of the therapeutic equivalence of unilateral and bilateral ECT would hence indicate unilateral ECT as the technique of choice; until then, the clinician should weigh the choice between the claimed therapeutic advantage with bilateral ECT and the definite cognitive advantage with unilateral ECT (Freeman et al., 1989).

Of note, although higher current densities result in and around the interelectrode axis with unilateral as compared with bilateral ECT (Weaver & Williams, 1982), the fear that these currents are unacceptably high and predispose to brain damage (Breggin, 1986) has not been substantiated.

Stimulus wave form and dose. Sinusoidal wave (which delivers a high electrical dose) may have no therapeutic superiority over brief-pulse (which delivers a low electrical dose) ECT (Andrade, 1990; Weiner & Coffey, 1989). Moderately suprathreshold pulse stimuli produce less cognitive dysfunction than sinusoidal wave stimuli at least acutely (over weeks, the difference disappears) with equivalent therapeutic benefit (Weiner et al., 1986a). Brief-pulse ECT may therefore be preferable. By the same token, avoidance of unnecessarily high electrical doses (irrespective of stimulus waveform) is important. Bilateral sinusoidal wave ECT carries the maximum risk for cognitive adverse effects (Weiner et al., 1986a; Weiner, Rogers, Davidson, & Kahn, 1986b).

Seizure duration. Where incomplete/missed seizures are a frequent problem, remedial measures suggested by Fink (1987) and Freeman et al. (1989) are advisable. If these fail, chemical prolongation of seizures using caffeine may be preferable to increasing the electrical stimulus dose (Coffey, Figiel, Weiner, & Saunders, 1990a). However, unnecessarily prolonged seizures may compromise cognition (Miller, Faber, Hatch, & Alexander, 1985).

Spacing of ECT. McAllister, Perri, Jordan, Rauscher, & Sattin (1987) found ECT given twice a week to be as effective and efficient as thrice weekly ECT, as well as to produce less cognitive deficit. Unfortunately, these promising results have not been confirmed by Shapira, Kindler, & Lerer (1989).

Anesthetic medication. Large doses of anesthetic medications may compromise cognition (Miller et al., 1985). The dose of anesthesia should be reduced as appropriate for light level of anesthesia. However, too light an anesthesia may result in incomplete loss of consciousness and increased arousal during ECT (American Psychiatric Association, 1990).

Concomitant medications. Yohimbine (Sachs, Pollack, Bratman, Farhadi, & Gelenberg, 1986) and possibly concurrent antidepressant pharmacotherapy (Nelson & Benjamin, 1989; but not Haskett, 1982) may hasten recovery, thus decreasing ECT requirement and hence ECT-induced cognitive dysfunction. Other drugs, such as piracetam (Ezzat, Ibraheem, & Mukhawy, 1985), possibly vasopressin (Mattes, Pettinati, Stephens, Robin, & Willis, 1990), and ergoloid mesylates (Sachs et al., 1989), may protect against ECT-induced cognitive impairment; ACTH (Fredericksen, D'Elia, & Holstein, 1985), naloxone (Nasrallah, Varney, Coffman, Bayless & Chapman, 1986), and glycopyrrolate substitutions for atropine in ECT premedication (Sommer, Satlin, & Friedmann, 1989) have no protective effect.

There is a need to identify patients who are at greater risk for ECT-induced cognitive dysfunction, and those who, by virtue of responding slowly to treatment, may require more treatments and thereby experience greater (cumulative) cognitive adverse effects. There is, however, no consensus in the available literature on the subject (Andrade, 1990; Andrade, Gangadhar, Subbakrishna, Channaba-savanna, & Pradhan, 1988b; Price, Mackenzie, Tucker, & Culver, 1978; Rich, Spiker, Jewell, Neil, & Black, 1984a). ECT is considered safe in the elderly (e.g., Zorumski, Rubin, & Burke, 1988) and has been administered without untoward effect in patients with coexisting central nervous system pathology including de-mentia (e.g., Fried & Man, 1988; Hsiao, Messenheimer, & Evans, 1987; Price & McAllister, 1989); however, special precautions are necessary, not only in regard to the electricity, but also in relation to the anticholinergic premedication and anesthesia.

Affective States

Mania and Organic Euphoria

Fewer than 10% of patients treated with ECT experience new affective symp-toms, and a small minority develop a manic syndrome. ECT facilitates do-paminergic neurotransmission by autoreceptor down regulation (Gangadhar, Pradhan, & Mayanil, 1987) and by postsynaptic receptor upregulation (Gangadhar et al., 1989). These may explain development of mania with ECT, in the light of a hyperdopaminergic hypothesis for mania (Swerdlow & Koob, 1987); however, this is only one of many possible explanations.

ECT-induced mania has been suggested to represent a switch phenomenon in bipolar illness (Bunney, 1978; Lewis & Nasrallah, 1986), but the causal role of ECT (as opposed to a spontaneous switch) is difficult to establish. Mania has also been suggested to result as a side effect of ECT, lasting for a few days and remitting spontaneously, and occurring either as depression lifts or in mid-depression; in the latter instance, rechallenge with ECT (after mania has given way to depression) may or may not reelicit the mania. No patient or ECT-related variables are identified as risk factors (Andrade, Gangadhar, & Channabasavanna, 1987; Andrade, Gangadhar, Swaminath, & Channabasavanna, 1988c).

Elation, along with confusion, has been described following ECT (Devanand, Sackeim, Decina, & Prudic, 1988a). Although strict guidelines are unavailable, from the evidence it appears best to stop ECT if either mania or organic euphoria supervenes. The reaction, if treated symptomatically with benzodiazepines, may disappear over a few days. ECT may be resumed if depression reemerges. Antidepressant/lithium continuation pharmacotherapy may be an adequate alterna-tive. If resumption of ECT reelicits the manic reaction, ECT should be withdrawn in favor of antidepressant drug therapy. In case mania persists beyond a week to 10 days, a "switch" should be considered and appropriate pharmacotherapy should be instituted.

ECT-Induced Anxiety

Anxiety, with accompanying autonomic arousal, is occasionally seen. The symptoms mount with successive ECTs. The vulnerability factors to this state are unclear; reassurance before and after treatment, and perhaps concomitant benzo-diazepines, alleviate the complaints. Rarely is it necessary to stop ECT.

Movement Disorders

Although the pathophysiology of tardive dyskinesia (TD) is unclear, it is generally accepted that facilitation or inhibition of dopaminergic neurotransmission respectively augments or diminishes the syndrome (Borison & Diamond, 1987; Gerlach & Casey, 1988). Since ECT, as discussed earlier, increases dopaminergic activity, it may be expected to precipitate, reactivate, or worsen TD, as indeed it sometimes does (e.g., Flaherty, Naidu, & Dysken, 1984; Holcomb, Sternberg, & Henninger, 1983; Roth, Mukherjee, & Sackheim, 1988). Yet, ECT has paradoxically been observed to ameliorate TD (e.g., Chacko & Root, 1983; Gosek & Weller, 1988; Malek-Ahmadi & Weddige, 1988). It is difficult to reconcile these disparate observations unless one accepts that different schedules of ECT may elicit different dopaminergic (or other) effects (Andrade & Gangadhar, 1989), or that TD is a heterogeneous syndrome (Sackeim & Mukherjee, 1989). The results of prospective, controlled trials are awaited.

Although ECT is considered by many to be valuable for the management of catatonia, ECT-induced catatonia has been reported (Pandey & Sharma, 1988). No explanation for this paradox is apparent.

Other Adverse Effects

Death

Mortality with ECT occurs perhaps once in 25,000–40,000 treatments. When death occurs, it happens most often immediately after the seizure or during the recovery state, and is mainly caused by cardiovascular complications.

Fractures, Dislocations, Visceral Trauma, etc.

These are rare with modified ECT. Headaches, nausea, and muscle soreness are common after ECT and respond well to symptomatic treatment.

Adverse Effects Resulting from Anesthesia, Muscle Relaxant, or Anticholinergic Premedications

These usually evolve on a background of preexisting cardiovascular or other disease. For example, excessive rise in blood pressure during ECT may cause conjunctival hemorrhage, peptic ulcer bleeds, stroke, or cardiac failure—particularly in the setting of diseases of the respective organ systems.

Prolonged Apnea

Patients with deficiency of pseudocholinesterase are at an increased risk for this complication. A screening assay is available in such patients; relaxation for ECT can be obtained by very low doses of succinylcholine or alternative agents like atracurium.

Miscellaneous

These include prolonged and "tardive" seizures and status epileptics (Daniel, 1985; Scott & Riddle, 1989) and yawning (D'Mello, Vincent, & Lerner, 1988). Prolonged seizures (greater than 3 minutes) can be terminated pharmacologically using either barbiturates (e.g., methohexitol) or intravenous benzodiazepines (e.g., diazepam 5-10 mg or midazolam 1-2 mg) (American Psychiatric Association, 1990). Failure to terminate such seizures within 3-5 minutes may result in worsening of post-ECT confusion. Tardive seizures (seizures occurring following the ECT seizures) are very rare and may not be accompanied by motor manifestations. Electroencephalographic (EEG) monitoring of the seizures is therefore important.

Drug Interactions

ECT is generally compatible with other therapies (drug or otherwise) in psychiatry; exceptions include use of: (1) drugs that raise the seizure threshold (e.g., benzodiazepines and carbamazepine; the higher currents hence required to induce an adequate convulsion predispose to greater cognitive adverse effects); (2) drugs such as xanthine alkaloids that lower the seizure threshold and could cause status epilepticus (Devanand, Decina, Sackheim, & Prudic, 1988b); and (3) drugs that could increase risk of neurotoxicity, like lithium (El Mallakh, 1988; also see Chapter 3). It is therefore important to carefully review the patient's medication regimen before instituting ECT.

PHYSIOLOGICAL CORRELATES

ECT induces a number of changes in neurotransmitter system functioning, neuroendocrine regulation, and regional cerebral blood flow. It is unclear whether such physiological effects are related to the mechanism of action of ECT, are indices of brain dysfunction, or are unrelated epiphenomena of the seizure. Nevertheless, certain effects are more likely to represent untoward actions of ECT and are briefly discussed.

Neurological Function

ECT does not significantly compromise neurological function (Weiner, 1984). Kriss, Blumhardt, Halliday, and Pratt (1978) observed minor neurological asymmetries with unilateral ECT, resolved within 20 minutes of treatment. Taylor and Abrams (1985) obtained no differences in soft neurological signs either before or after ECT or between unilateral and bilateral treatment.

Electroencephalographic Changes

ECT-induced EEG changes are largely acute. The seizure is followed by transient suppression of background activity characterized as ranging from low-amplitude slow waves to electrocerebral silence. This postictal EEG suppression has been suggested to be related to retrograde amnesia with ECT (Daniel, Crovitz, Weiner, Swartzwelder, & Kahn, 1985). Over the ECT course, interictal EEG records show high-amplitude, slow-wave background activity, which increases with successive treatments (Weiner et al., 1986b; Kolbeinsson & Petursson, 1988). The background activity returns to normal 2-6 weeks after the last ECT (Fink, 1979; Kolbeinsson & Petursson, 1988; Weiner et al., 1986b).

Bilateral sinusoidal wave ECT induces the maximum and unilateral brief-pulse ECT the minimum EEG "toxicity" (Weiner et al., 1986b). Left unilateral and bilateral ECT produce greater left-sided EEG slowing, whereas right unilateral ECT produces greater right-sided slowing. The former effect has, however, been linked to therapeutic response and not to adverse effects (Abrams, Swartz, & Vedak, 1989).

Evoked Potentials

Changes in latency and amplitude of visual-evoked potential components, as well as of early components of somatosensory-evoked potentials, occur within 15 minutes of ECT (Kriss, Halliday, & Pratt, 1980a, b); brainstem auditory-evoked potentials are, however, unchanged (Small, Milstein, Kellams, & Small, 1981; Weiner, Erwin, & Wetzel, 1981). Latency prolongation but not amplitude attenuation of the P-300 event-related potential is seen with ECT, more in schizophrenia than in affective disorders, and more at the conclusion of the ECT course than after the first treatment. These changes, present one or more days after ECT, reflect impaired information processing (Rajendra, 1989). The P-300 event-related potential normalizes at 6 months' follow-up (Gangadhar, unpublished data).

Biochemical Changes

Alexopoulos, Kocsis, and Stoker (1978) found CSF protein to rise after ECT, possibly indicating a breach in blood-brain barrier, as is known to occur with epileptic seizures (Bolwig, Hertz, Paulson, Spotoft, & Rafaelson, 1977). Escape into circulation of brain-specific isoenzyme creatinine phosphokinase-B is an index of brain injury; this does not occur after ECT (Webb, O'Donnell, Draper, Horner, & Phillips, 1984; Rajendra, 1989). Likewise, serum myelin basic protein is not elevated after ECT (Hoyle, Pratt, & Thomas, 1984).

Morphological Changes

Animal studies reveal that ECT-induced seizures, unlike epileptic seizures, even when excessive in number, evoke no gross or histopathological evidence of brain damage (Dam, 1986). Autopsies in cases of acute death following ECT often yield morphological abnormalities, but no interpretation is possible as many uncontrolled and prejudicial variables are invariably present (Weiner, 1984). Interestingly, a case has been reported of absence of neuropathological abnormalities after 1250 ECTs (Selected Staff, 1985). CT scan (e.g., Kolbeinsson, Arnaldsson, Petursson, & Skulason, 1986) and magnetic resonance imaging (e.g., Pande, Grunhaus, & Aisen, 1990) studies are largely reassuring; of note, there is a possibility that subjects referred for ECT—especially the elderly—may have preexisting brain abnormality (Coffey, Figiel, Djang, & Weiner, 1990b).

ECT FOR IATROGENIC CONDITIONS

ECT is effective in many iatrogenic disorders. Its dopaminergic facilitatory effect benefits both antipsychotic-induced parkinsonism (Gangadhar, Chaudhary, & Channabasavanna, 1983; Goswami, Dutta, Kuruvilla, & Perenyi, 1989) and the neuroleptic malignant syndrome (e.g., Hermesh, Aizenberg, & Weisman, 1987). Its paradoxical benefit in certain TD patients has already been discussed. ECT is effective in drug-induced psychoses (e.g., Grover, Yeragani, & Keshavan, 1986), in drug-induced depressions (Rich, Spiker, Jewell, & Neill, 1984b), and possibly in drug-induced mania as well. Although ECT may be effective in other medical/ neurological conditions (Weiner & Coffey, 1988), there is no report on the use or efficacy of ECT when such conditions are iatrogenic.

CONCLUSION

Virtually every patient currently prescribed ECT has already received one or more psychopharmacological treatments for weeks or longer. The extent to which such agents augment or diminish the profile of ECT-induced side effects merits study. At present, available evidence suggests that optimization of the ECT technique considerably enhances its safety. Nevertheless, the incidence, extent, and profile of iatrogenic morbidity with ECT, and strategies for its reduction require further investigation, especially vis-a-vis iatrogenic morbidity with psychotropic drugs. This is essential if the credibility of a highly useful but much maligned therapy in psychiatry is to be redeemed.

REFERENCES

Abrams R, 1982: The technique of electroconvulsive therapy. In: *Electroconvulsive therapy: Biological foundations and clinical applications,* edited by R. Abrams and WB Essman. Lancaster: MTP Press Limited.

Abrams R, Essman WB, 1982: *Electroconvulsive therapy: Biological foundations and clinical applications.* Lancaster: MTP Press.

Abrams R, 1988: *Electroconvulsive therapy.* New York: Oxford University Press.

Abrams R, Swartz CM, Vedak E, 1989: Antidepressant effect of right versus left unilateral ECT and the lateralization theory of ECT action. *American Journal of Psychiatry, 146,* 1190–1192.

Alexopoulos GS, Kocsis JH, Stoker PE, 1978: Increase in CSF protein in association with ECT. *Journal of Neurology, Neurosurgery and Psychiatry, 41,* 1145–1146.

American Psychiatric Association, 1990; *Task force report. The practice of electroconvulsive therapy.* Washington, DC: Author.

Andrade C, Gangadhar BN, Channabasavanna SM, 1987: Mania associated with electroconvulsive therapy. *Journal of Clinical Psychiatry, 48,* 303–304.

Andrade C, Gangadhar BN, Subbakrishna DK, Channabasavanna SM, Pradhan N, 1988a: A double-blind comparison of sinusoidal wave and brief-pulse electroconvulsive therapy in endogenous depression. *Convulsive Therapy, 4,* 297–303.

Andrade C, Gangadhar BN, Subbakrishna DK, Channabasavanna SM, Pradhan N, 1988b: Clinical prediction of rate of response of endogenous depression to electroconvulsive therapy. *Indian Journal of Psychiatry, 30,* 381–387.

Andrade C, Gangadhar BN, Swaminath G, Channabasavanna SM, 1988c: Mania as a side effect of electroconvulsive therapy. *Convulsive Therapy, 4,* 81–83.

Andrade C, Gangadhar BN, 1989: *Electroconvulsive shock and dopamine post-synaptic receptors: clinical implications of time-dependent change.* Paper presented at the 41st Annual Conference of the Indian and Psychiatric Society, Cuttack, India.

Andrade C, 1990: Psychobiological frontiers of electroconvulsive therapy in depression: Evaluation of strategies for rational prescription and reduction in morbidity. *Indian Journal of Psychiatry, 32,* 109–130.

Andrade C, Gangadhar BN, Channabasavanna SM, Pradhan N, 1990: *Subjective side effects of electroconvulsive therapy in endogenous depression.* Paper presented at the 42nd Annual Conference of the Indian Psychiatric Society, Chandigarh.

Bolwig TG, Hertz MM, Paulson DB, Spotoft H, Rafaelson OJ, 1977: The permeability of the blood brain barrier during electrically induced seizures in man. *European Journal of Clinical Investigations, 7,* 87–93.

Borison RL, Diamond BI, 1987: Neuropharmacology of the extrapyramidal system. *Journal of Clinical Psychiatry, 48*(9, suppl), 7–12.

Breggin PR, 1986: Brain damage from non-dominant ECT. *American Journal of Psychiatry, 143,* 1320–1321.

Bunney WE, 1978: Psychopharmacology of the switch process. In: *Psychopharmacology: A generation of progress,* edited by MA Lipton, A DiMascio, and KF Killam. New York: Raven Press.

Calev A, Ben-Tzvi E, Shapira B, Drexler H, Carasso R, Lerer B, 1989: Distinct memory impairments following electroconvulsive therapy and imipramine. *Psychological Medicine, 19,* 111–119.

Chacko R, Root L, 1983: ECT and tardive dyskinesia: Two cases and a review. *Journal of Clinical Psychiatry, 44,* 265–266.

Coffey CE, Figiel GS, Weiner RD, Saunders WB, 1990a: Caffeine augmentation of electroconvulsive therapy. *American Journal of Psychiatry, 147,* 579–585.

Coffey CE, Figiel GS, Djang WT, Weiner RD, 1990b: Subcortical hyperintensity on magnetic resonance imaging: A comparison of normal and depressed elderly subjects. *American Journal of Psychiatry, 147,* 187–189.

Consensus Conference (NIMH-NIH), 1985: Electroconvulsive therapy: *Journal of the American Medical Association, 254,* 2103–2108.

Dam AM, 1986: Quantitative neuropathology in electrically induced generalized convulsions. *Psychopharmacology Bulletin, 22,* 479–482.

Daniel WF, 1985: Spontaneous seizures after ECT. *British Journal of Psychiatry, 146,* 100–101.

Daniel WF, Crovitz HF, Weiner RD, Swartzwelder HS, Kahn EM, 1985: ECT-induced amnesia and post-ictal EEG suppression. *Biological Psychiatry, 20,* 344–352.

Devanand DP, Sackeim HA, Decina P, Prudic J, 1988a: The development of mania and organic euphoria during ECT. *Journal of Clinical Psychiatry, 49,* 69–71.

Devanand DP, Decina P, Sackheim HA, Prudic J, 1988b: Status epilepticus following ECT in a patient receiving theophylline. *Journal of Clinical Psychopharmacology, 8,* 153.

Devanand DP, Briscoe KM, Sackeim HA, 1989: Clinical features and predictors of post-ictal excitement. *Convulsive Therapy, 5,* 140–146.

D'Mello DA, Vincent FM, Lerner MP, 1988: Yawning as a complication of electroconvulsive therapy and concurrent neuroleptic withdrawal. *Journal of Nervous and Mental Disease, 176,* 188–189.

Endler NS, Persad E, 1988: Electroconvulsive therapy: The myths and realities. Toronto: Hans Huber Publishers.

El-Mallakh RS, 1988: Complications of concurrent lithium and electroconvulsive therapy. *Biological Psychiatry, 23,* 595–601.

Ezzat DH, Ibraheem MM, Makhawy B, 1985: The effect of piracetam on ECT-induced memory disturbances. *British Journal of Psychiatry, 147,* 720–721.

Fink M, 1979: *Convulsive therapy: Theory and practice.* New York: Raven Press.

Fink M, 1987: New technology in convulsive therapy: A challenge in training (editorial). *American Journal of Psychiatry, 144,* 1195–1198.

Flaherty J, Naidu J, Dysken M, 1984: ECT, emergent dyskinesia and depression. *American Journal of Psychiatry, 141,* 808–809.

Frederiksen SO, D'Elia G, Holstein F, 1985: ECT, ACTH and cognition. *European Archives of Psychiatry and Neurological Sciences, 234,* 291–294.

Freeman C, Crammer JL, Deakin JFW, McClelland R, Mann SA, Pippard J, 1989: *The practical administration of electroconvulsive therapy (ECT).* Report of the ECT sub-committee of the Research Committee of the Royal College of Psychiatrist. London: Gaskell.

Fried D, Mann JJ, 1988: Electroconvulsive treatment of a patient with a known intracranial tumor. *Biological Psychiatry, 23,* 176–180.

Gangadhar BN, Chaudhary JR, Channabasavanna SM, 1983: ECT and drug-induced parkinsonism. *Indian Journal of Psychiatry, 25,* 212–213.

Gangadhar BN, Pradhan N, Mayanil CSK, 1987: Dopamine autoreceptor down-regulation following repeated electroconvulsive shock. *Indian Journal of Medical Research, 86,* 787–791.

Gangadhar BN, Ramadevi G, Andrade C, Pradhan N, 1989: Dopaminergic effects of repeated electroconvulsive shocks. *Convulsive Therapy, 5,* 157–161.

Gangadhar BN, Andrade C, Janakiramaiah N, 1992: Electroconvulsive therapy: Theory and practice. In: *Postgraduate psychiatry,* edited by JN Vyas. New Delhi: B. I. Churchill Livingstone.

Gerlach J, Casey DE, 1988: Tardive dyskinesia. *Acta Psychiatrica Scandinavica, 77,* 369–378.

Gosek E, Weller RA, 1988: Improvement of tardive dyskinesia associated with electroconvulsive therapy. *Journal of Nervous and Mental Disease, 176,* 120–122.

Goswami U, Dutta S, Kuruvilla K, Papp E, Perenyi A, 1989: Electroconvulsive therapy in neuroleptic-induced parkinsonism. *Biological Psychiatry, 26,* 234–238.

Grover D, Yeragana VK, Keshavan MS, 1986: Improvement of phencyclidine-induced psychosis with ECT. *Journal of Clinical Psychiatry, 47,* 477–478.

Haskett RF, 1982: Factors affecting outcome after successful electroconvulsive therapy. *Psychopharmacology Bulletin, 19*(2) 75–78.

Hermesh H, Aizenberg D, Wiezman A, 1987: A successful electroconvulsive treatment of neuroleptic malignant syndrome. *Acta Psychiatrica Scandinavica, 75,* 237–239.

Holcomb HH, Sternberg DE, Henninger GR, 1983: Effects of electroconvulsive therapy on mood, parkinsonism and tardive dyskinesia in a depressed patient: ECT and dopamine systems. *Biological Psychiatry, 18,* 865–873.

Hoyle NR, Pratt RTC, Thomas DGT, 1984: Effect of electroconvulsive therapy on serum myelin basic protein immunoreactivity. *British Medical Journal, 288,* 1110–1111.

Hsiao JK, Messenheimer JA, Evans DL, 1987: ECT and neurological disorders. *Convulsive Therapy, 3,* 121–136.

Kolbeinsson H, Arnaldsson OS, Petursson H, Skulason S, 1986: Computed tomographic scans in ECT patients. *Acta Psychiatrica Scandinavica, 73,* 28–32.

Kolbeinsson H, Petursson H, 1988: Electroencephalographic correlates of electroconvulsive therapy. *Acta Psychiatrica Scandinavica, 78,* 162–168.

Kriss A, Blumhardt LD, Halliday AM, Pratt RTC, 1978: Neurological asymmetries immediately after unilateral ECT. *Journal of Neurology, Neurosurgery and Psychiatry, 41,* 1135–1144.

Kriss A, Halliday AM, Halliday E, Pratt RTC, 1980a: Evoked potentials following unilateral ECT. I. the somatosensory evoked potentials. *Electroencephalography and Clinical Neurophysiology, 48,* 481–489.

Kriss A, Halliday AM, Halliday E, Pratt RTC, 1980b: Evoked potentials following unilateral ECT, II. The flash evoked potential. *Electroencephalography and Clinical Neurophysiology, 48,* 490–501.

Leechuy I, Abrams R, Kohlaas J, 1988: ECT-induced postictal delirium and electrode placement. *American Journal of Psychiatry, 145,* 880–881.

Lewis DA, Nasrallah HA, 1986: Mania associated with electroconvulsive therapy. *Journal of Clinical Psychiatry, 47,* 366–367.

Mackenzie TB, Price TRP, Tucker GJ, Culver CM, 1985: Early change in cognitive performance accompanying bilateral ECT. *Convulsive Therapy, 1,* 183–189.

Malek-Ahmadi P, Weddige RL, 1988: Tardive dyskinesia and ECT. *Convulsive Therapy, 4,* 328–331.

Mattes JA, Pettinati HM, Stephens S, Robin SE, Willis KW, 1990: A placebo-controlled evaluation of vasopressin for ECT-induced memory impairment. *Biological Psychiatry, 27,* 289–303.

McAllister DA, Perri MG, Jordan RC, Rauscher FP, Sattin A: 1987: Effects of ECT given two vs. three times weekly. *Psychiatry Research, 21,* 63–69.

Miller AL, Faber FA, Hatch JP, Alexander HE, 1985: Factors affecting amnesia, seizure duration and efficacy in ECT. *American Journal of Psychiatry, 142,* 692–696.

Nasrallah HA, Varney N, Coffman JA, Bayless J, Chapman S, 1986: Opiate antagonism fails to reverse post-ECT cognitive deficits. *Journal of Clinical Psychiatry, 47*(11), 555–556.

Nelson JP, Benjamin L, 1989: Efficacy and safety of combined ECT and tricyclic antidepressant therapy in the treatment of depressed geriatric patients. *Convulsive Therapy, 5*(4), 321–329.

Pande AC, Grunhaus LJ, Aisen AM, Haskett RF, 1990: A preliminary magnetic resonance imaging study of ECT treated depressed patients. *Biological Psychiatry, 27,* 102–104.

Pandey R, Sharma P, 1988: ECT induced catatonia: A case report. *Indian Journal of Psychiatry, 30,* 105–107.

Price TRP, Mackenzie TB, Tucker GJ, Culver C, 1978: The dose-response ratio to electroconvulsive therapy. *Archives of General Psychiatry, 35,* 1131–1136.

Price TRP, 1982a: Short and long-term cognitive effects of ECT: Part I—Effects on memory. *Psychopharmacology Bulletin, 18*(1), 81–91.

Price TRP, 1982b: Short and long-term cognitive effects of ECT: Part II—Effects on nonmemory associated cognitive functions. *Psychopharmacology Bulletin, 18*(1), 91–101.

Price TRP, McAllister TW, 1989: Safety and efficacy of ECT in depressed patients with dementia: A review of clinical experience. *Convulsive Therapy, 5,* 61–74.

Rajendra PN, 1989: *An investigation into post-ECT cognitive dysfunction using electrophysiological and neurochemical parameters.* Master's thesis. Bangalore: Bangalore University.

Rich CL, Spiker DG, Jewell SW, Neil JF, Black NA, 1984a: The efficiency of ECT: I. Response rate in depressive episodes. *Psychiatry Research, 11,* 167–176.

Rich CL, Spiker DG, Jewell SW, Neill JF, 1984b: DSM III, RDC and ECT: Depression subtypes and immediate response. *Journal of Clinical Psychiatry, 45,* 14–18.

Roth SD, Mukherjee S, Sackeim HA, 1988: Electroconvulsive therapy in a patient with mania, parkinsonism and tardive dyskinesia. *Convulsive Therapy, 4,* 92–97.

Sachs GS, Pollack MH, Brotman AW, Farhadi AM, Gelenberg AJ, 1986: Enhancement of ECT benefit by yohimbine. *Journal of Clinical Psychiatry, 47,* 508–510.

Sachs GS, Gelenberg AJ, Bellinghausen B, Wojcik F, Falk WE, Farhadi AM, Jenike M, 1989: Ergoloid mesylates and ECT. *Journal of Clinical Psychiatry, 50,* 87–90.

Sackeim HA, Decina P, Malitz S, Hopkins N, Yudofsky SC, Provohnik I, 1983: Postictal excitement following bilateral and right unilateral ECT. *American Journal of Psychiatry, 144,* 1449–1455.

Sackeim HA, Mukherjee S, 1989: What are your suggestions for using electroconvulsive therapy (ECT) as a treatment for tardive dyskinesia, and what are the possible contributions of ECT to an understanding of the pathophysiology of tardive dyskinesia? *Journal of Clinical Psychopharmacology, 9,* 156.

Scott AIF, Riddle W, 1989: Status epilepticus after electroconvulsive therapy. *British Journal of Psychiatry, 155,* 119–121.

Selected Staff, University of Louisville School of Medicine, 1985: 1250 electroconvulsive treatments without evidence of brain injury. *British Journal of Psychiatry, 147,* 203–204.

Shapira B, Kindler S, Lerer B, 1989: Treatment schedule and rate of response to ECT (abstract). *Biological Psychiatry, 25,* 106A.

Small JG, Milstein V, Kellams JJ, Small IF, 1981: Auditory brain evoked response in hospitalized patients undergoing drug treatment or ECT. *Biological Psychiatry, 16,* 287–290.

Sommer BR, Satlin A, Friedman L, 1989: Glycopyrrolate versus atropine in post ECT amnesia in the elderly. *Journal of Geriatric Psychiatry and Neurology, 2,* 18–21.

Squire LR, 1986: Memory functions as affected by electroconvulsive therapy. *Annals of the New York Academy of Sciences, 462,* 307–314.

Squire LR, Zouzounis JA, 1986: ECT and memory: Brief pulse versus sine wave. *American Journal of Psychiatry, 143,* 596–601.

Swerdlow NR, Koob GF, 1987: Dopamine, schizophrenia, mania and depression: Toward a unified hypothesis of cortico-striato-pallido-thalamic function. *Behavioral and Brain sciences, 10,* 197–245.

Taylor MA, Abrams R, 1985: Short-term cognitive effects of unilateral and bilateral ECT. *British Journal of Psychiatry, 146,* 308–311.

Weaver LA Jr, Williams RW, 1982: The electroconvulsive therapy stimulus. In: *Electroconvulsive therapy: Biological foundations and clinical applications* (pp. 129–156), edited by R Abrams and WB Essman. Lancaster: MTP Press Limited.

Webb MGT, O'Donnell MP, Draper RJ, Horner B, Phillips JP, 1984: Brain type creatinine phosphokinase serum levels before and after ECT. *British Journal of Psychiatry, 144,* 525–529.

Weiner RD, Erwin CW, Wetzel PA, 1981: Acute effects of electroconvulsive therapy on brain stem auditory evoked potentials. *Electroencephalography and Clinical Neurophysiology, 52,* 202–204.

Weiner RD, 1984: Does electroconvulsive therapy cause brain damage? *The Behavioral and Brain Sciences, 7,* 1–54.

Weiner RD, 1986a: Minimizing therapeutic differences between bilateral and unilateral nondominant ECT. *Convulsive Therapy, 2,* 261–265.

Weiner RD, 1986b: Electrical dosage, stimulus parameters, and electrode placement. *Psychopharmacology Bulletin, 22,* 499–502.

Weiner RD, Coffey CE, 1988: Indications for use of electroconvulsive therapy. In *Review of psychiatry,* vol. 7, edited by AJ Francis and RE Hales. Washington, DC: American Psychiatric Press.

Weiner RD, Coffey CE, 1989: Comparison of brief-pulse and sine wave ECT stimuli. *Convulsive Therapy, 5,* 184–185.

Weiner RD, Rogers HJ, Davidson JR, Squire LR, 1986a: Effects of stimulus parameters on cognitive side effects. *Annals of the New York Academy of Sciences, 462,* 315–325.

Weiner RD, Rogers HJ, Davidson JR, Kahn EM, 1986b: Effects of electroconvulsive therapy upon brain electrical activity. *Annals of the New York Academy of Sciences, 462,* 270–281.

Zorumski CF, Rubin EH, Burke WJ, 1988: Electroconvulsive therapy for the elderly: A review. *Hospital and Community Psychiatry, 39,* 643–647.

17

Drug-Induced Psychotic Disorders

Matcheri S. Keshavan and Asha Keshavan

A wide variety of prescribed and recreational drugs can induce psychotic symptoms. In this chapter, we describe the adverse reactions induced by administration or withdrawal of the drugs used in psychiatric practice. For details of psychoses induced by nonpsychiatric medications and recreational agents, the reader is referred elsewhere (Estroff & Gold, 1986; McNeil & Soreff, 1987; Wood, Harris, Morreale, & Rizos, 1988). Table 1 provides a list of prescribed drugs known to cause psychotic reactions.

DRUGS USED IN PSYCHIATRY

Stimulants

Amphetamines and other central nervous system (CNS) stimulants are often used to treat mild chronic depression, as appetite suppressants, and in the treatment of narcolepsy. Psychotic reactions usually occur with overdose or abuse of amphetamines but may occur less frequently with lower doses. The fact that amphetamines can produce symptoms very similar to paranoid schizophrenia was well recognized as early as 1958 and is described by Connell (1958) in his classic monograph. However, amphetamine psychosis is characterized by intact cognitive function, rapid onset, dreamlike quality of the experiences, hyperalertness, and well-preserved affect (Lishman, 1987). Visual hallucinations are common and thought disorder is rare. Subsequent research (Angrist & Gershon, 1970) has further substantiated Connell's observations and has served as a basis for pathophysiological theories of schizophrenia. Indeed, amphetamine psychosis has been considered one of the best available models for schizophrenia (Snyder, 1973).

A careful history of drug use and abuse and the temporal relationship between drug use and psychosis help in the diagnosis. In doubtful cases, testing urine for amphetamines is helpful. If psychotic symptoms persist for over a week after urinary tests have become negative, another primary psychiatric illness must be considered (Lishman, 1987).

Psychotic reactions of a similar nature have been described during treatment with other CNS stimulants such as methylphenidate (Lucas & Weiss, 1971), pemoline (Polchert & Morse, 1985), phenmetrazine, methamphetamine (Sato, Chen, Akiyama, & Otsuki, 1983) and phentermine (Devan, 1990).

Table 1 Prescribed drugs associated with psychotic disorders

Category	Specific drugs
Analgesics	Pentazocine
Anticancer agents	Asparaginase, methotrexate, vinblastine, vincristine
Anticholinergics	Scopalamine, atropine, trihexyphenidyl, benztropine
Anticonvulsants	Phenytoin, ethosuximide, primidone
Antidepressants	Tricyclics, monoamine oxidase inhibitors
Antiinflammatory agents	Chloroquine, indomethacin, sulindac
Antimicrobials	Amphotericin B, cycloserine, isoniazid, nalidixic acid, thiabendazole, niridazole, chloroquine, quinacrine, dapsone, procaine penicillin, acyclovir
Cardiovascular agents	Propranolol, methyldopa, reserpine, digitalis, lidocaine, disopyramide, procainamide, quinidine
Dopamine agonists	Levodopa, bromocriptine, amantadine
Drug withdrawal	Barbiturates, benzodiazepines, antipsychotics
Gastrointestinal medication	Cimetidine
Hormones	Thyroid hormone, insulin, corticosteroids
Immunosuppressants	Cyclosporine
Over-the-counter medications	Phenylpropanolame, ephedrine, pseudoephedrine
Stimulants	Amphetamine, methylphenidate, pemoline
Vitamins	Vitamin A, vitamin D

For further details, see McNeil and Soreff (1987), Estroff ad Gold (1986), and Medical Letter (1986).

Antidepressants

The question whether tricyclic antidepressants potentiate or precipitate psychotic symptoms is controversial. In a review of 150 patients treated with nortriptyline and imipramine, about 13% of the patients manifested sleep difficulties, poor memory, or illogical thoughts (Davies, Tucker, Harrow, & Detre, 1971). These effects seemed to parallel antidepressant concentrations and were more frequent in the elderly. Antidepressants are known to exacerbate schizophrenia (Nelson, Bomers, & Sweeney, 1975; Siris, Van Kammen, & Docherty,1978). In particular, the antidepressant amoxapine has been described to cause delusions, visual hallucinations, or mania-like symptoms when treated in therapeutic doses (Barnes, 1982). There is some evidence that antidepressants may delay the resolution of psychotic symptoms in schizophrenia and are not beneficial in the treatment of depressive symptoms in acute schizophrenic symptoms (Kramer et al., 1989). Caution should therefore be exercised in using antidepressants as adjunct treatment in schizophrenia.

Psychotic reactions have also been described during treatment with monoamine oxidase inhibitors (Sheehy & Maxman, 1978). The newer antidepressant, bupropion, has been reported to cause excitement, agitation, and psychotic symptoms in about 9% of patients treated with this drug. This may be related to the dopaminergic effects of bupropion (Fleet, Mauberg, & Miller, 1983).

Benzodiazepines

Psychotic reactions have been described during withdrawal from benzodiazepines. Keshavan et al. (1988) have described delusional depression in four patients following benzodiazepine withdrawal. Visual and auditory hallucinations are also common during benzodiazepine withdrawal. Psychosis with delirium (Heritch, Capwell, & Roy-Byrne, 1987), catatonic features (Hauser, Devinsky, DeBellis, & Theodore, 1989), as well as first rank symptoms of schizophrenia (Roberts & Vass, 1986), have also been described during benzodiazepine discontinuation.

Antiparkinsonian Medications

There is some evidence that anticholinergic agents may worsen positive symptoms in schizophrenia (Shader & Greenblatt, 1982). The psychological dysfunction caused by excessive doses of anticholinergic agents is described in Chapter 14.

Other antiparkinsonian drugs such as amantadine, levodopa, and bromocriptine may all result in psychotic symptoms. These latter drugs increase dopaminergic activity; psychoses caused by them is consistent with the dopaminergic theory of schizophrenia. Amantadine acts by releasing dopamine from intact dopaminergic terminals. Levodopa is metabolized directly to dopamine. Bromocriptine is a direct agonist of dopamine receptor in the CNS. Levodopa induces a variety of psychiatric symptoms including delusions and depression (Goodwin, 1972). Typically, amantadine may cause visual hallucinations and agitation in patients after 2–3 weeks of treatment (Postma & Van Tilburg, 1975). Bromocriptine has been reported to cause psychotic symptoms (Parkes, 1980) and exacerbation of schizophrenic symptoms (Frye, Pariser, Kim, & O'Shaughnessy, 1982).

Treatment of psychotic reactions induced by antiparkinsonian drugs often poses a pharmacological challenge, particularly in patients with parkinsonism. Scholz and Dichgans (1985) have reported successful treatment of such patients with the atypical antipsychotic agent, clozapine.

Antipsychotic Drugs

Discontinuation of antipsychotic drugs is often followed by an immediate relapse of psychotic symptoms. Such psychotic relapse often parallels reemergence of tardive dyskinesia (Choinard, 1978; Jawed & Singh, 1989). It has been postulated that this is related to postsynaptic dopaminergic supersensitivity caused by chronic dopaminergic blockade; the term "supersensitivity psychosis" has been coined in this context (Chouinard, Jones, & Annable, 1978). This theory remains speculative.

Anticonvulsant Medications

Use of anticonvulsants is associated with severe adverse behavioral effects, including psychoses. However, evaluation of cause-effect relationships is difficult because of the well-known association between epilepsy and psychoses. Hallucinations, delusions, depression, and confusion can all occur during treatment with commonly used anticonvulsants such as phenytoin (Stores, 1975; Tollefson, 1980). Rare reports exist of worsening of psychosis with carbamazepine (Dalby, 1971; Stores, 1975; Tollefson, 1980).

Disulfiram

Psychotic symptoms, unrelated to the disulfiram-alcohol reaction, have been described during treatment with disulfiram (Hall, 1980; Liddon & Satran, 1967; Rainey, 1977). Hallucinations, delusions, and confusional states may all be seen. The mechanism is unclear but may be related to the effect of disulfiram in inhibiting dopamine beta hydroxylase activity. Antipsychotic drugs may worsen symptoms and should therefore be used with caution (Hall, 1980).

DIAGNOSIS AND MANAGEMENT

A careful history of drug exposure is crucial for the diagnosis of drug-induced psychosis. When history obtained from the patient is unreliable, family, friends, and previous medical records may be helpful. Physical examination may provide some indications: anticholinergic syndrome is associated with dry skin, pupillary dilation, and other features of cholinergic blockade. Psychosis caused by sympathomimetic agents such as amphetamine may be accompanied by signs of sympathetic overactivity such as tachycardia and hypertension. Urine analysis for the suspected drugs (e.g., amphetamines) is also helpful. In difficult cases, stopping the suspected medication and observing the psychopathological state during the drug-free washout period may help resolve the diagnostic question.

Psychotic reactions may often be caused by either the drug or the illness for which the drug is prescribed. For example, patients with lupus cerebritis can have psychosis as a result of either the illness or of the corticosteroid treatment. A careful analysis of the clinical picture is needed in such cases to decide whether to increase or decrease the medication dosage.

Once a specific medication is identified as the offending agent, administration of the drug should be stopped. This frequently results in a clearing of the psychiatric side effects. If the symptoms of an underlying primary psychiatric illness emerge, judicious restarting of an alternative, safer treatment should be considered.

REFERENCES

Angrist BM, Gershon S, 1970: The phenomenology of experimentally induced amphetamine psychosis— preliminary observations. *Biological Psychiatry, 2,* 95–107.

Barnes F, 1982: Precipitation of mania and visual hallucinations by amoxapine. *Comprehensive Psychiatry, 23,* 590.

Borrison R, 1979: Amantadine induced psychosis in geriatric patients with renal disease. *American Journal of Psychiatry, 136*(1), 111.

Chouinard G, Jones BD, Annable L, 1978: Neuroleptic induced supersensitivity psychosis. *American Journal of Psychiatry, 135,* 1409–1410.

Connell P, 1970: *Amphetamine psychosis.* London: Chapman and Hall.

Dalby MA, 1971: Antiepileptic and psychotropic effects of carbamazepine (Tegretol) in the treatment of psychomotor epilepsy. *Epilepsia, 12,* 325–334.

Davies R, Tucker G, Harrow M, Detre TP, 1971: Confusional episodes and antidepressant medications. *American Journal of Psychiatry, 128,* 95.

Devan GS, 1990: Phentermine and psychosis. *British Journal of Psychiatry, 156,* 442–443.

Estroff TW, Gold MS, 1986: Medication induced and toxin induced psychiatric disorders. In: *Medical mimics of psychiatric disorders,* edited by I Extein and MS Gold. Washington, DC: American Psychiatric Press.

Fleet J, Manberg P, Miller L, 1983: Overview of clinically significant adverse reactions of bupropion. *Journal of Clinical Psychiatry, 44,* 191.

Frye PE, Pariser SF, Kim MH, O'Shaughnessy RW, 1982: Bromocriptine associated with symptom exacerbation during neuroleptic treatment of schizoaffective schizophrenia. *Journal of Clinical Psychiatry, 43*(6), 252–253.

Goodwin FK, 1971: Psychiatric side effects of levodopa in man. *Journal of the American Medical Association, 218*, 1915–1920.

Hall RCW, Stickney SK, Gardner ER, 1980: Behavioral toxicity of non-psychiatric drugs. In: *Psychiatric presentations of medical illness: Somatopsychic disorders*, edited by RCE Hall. New York: Spectrum Publications.

Hauser P, Devinsky O, DeBellis M, Theodore WS, 1989: Benzodiazepine withdrawal delirium with catatonic features: Occurrence in patients with partial seizure disorders. *Archives of Neurology, 46*(6), 696–699.

Heritch AJ, Capwell R, Roy-Byrne PP, 1987: A case of psychosis and delirium following withdrawal from triazolam. *Journal of Clinical Psychiatry, 48*(4), 168–169.

Jawed SH, Singh I, 1989: Tardive dyskinesia with schizophrenic relapse. *Journal of Mental Deficiency Research, 33*(4), 331–334.

Keshavan MS, Moodley P, Eales M, Joyce E, Yeragani VK, 1988: Delusional depression following benzodiazepine withdrawal. *Canadian Journal of Psychiatry, 33*, 626–627.

Kramer MS, Vogel WH, Dijohnson C, Dewey D, Sheves P, Cavicchia S, Litle P, Schmidt R, Kimes I, 1989: Antidepressants in "depressed" schizophrenic patterns. *American Journal of Psychiatry, 46*, 922–928.

Liddon SC, Satran R, 1967: Disulfiram (Antabuse) psychosis. *American Journal of Psychiatry, 123*, 1284–1289.

Lishman WA, 1987: *Organic psychiatry*, 2nd edition. Oxford: Blackwell Scientific Publications.

Lucas A, Weiss M, 1971: Methylphenidate hallucinosis. *Journal of the American Medical Association, 217*, 1079.

McNeil GN, Soreff SM, 1987: Psychosis. In: *Handbook of psychiatric differential diagnosis*, edited by SM Soreff and GN McNeil. Littleton, Massachusetts: PSG Publishing.

Medical Letter, 1986: *Drugs that cause psychiatric symptoms, 28*, 81–86.

Nelson C, Bomers MB, Sweeney D, 1974: Exacerbation of psychosis in tricyclic antidepressants in delusional depression. *American Journal of Psychiatry, 136*, 574–579.

Parkes D, 1980: Mechanisms of bromocriptine induced hallucinations. *New England Journal of Medicine, 302*, 1479.

Polchert SE, Morse RM, 1985: Pemoline abuse. *Journal of the American Medical Association, 254*, 946–947.

Postma JU, Van Tilburg W, 1975: Visual hallucinations and delirium during treatment with amantadine. *Journal of the American Geriatric Society, 23*(5), 212.

Rainey JM, 1977: Disulfiram toxicity and carbon disulfide poisoning. *American Journal of Psychiatry, 123*, 1284–1289.

Roberts K, Vass N, 1986: Schneiderian first-rank symptoms caused by benzodiazepine withdrawal. *British Journal of Psychiatry, 148*, 593–594.

Sato M, Chen CC, Akiyama K, Otsuki S, 1983: Acute exacerbation of paranoid psychotic state after long-term abstinence in patients with previous methamphetamine psychosis. *Biological Psychiatry, 18*(4), 429–440.

Scholz E, Dichgans J, 1985: Treatment of drug-induced exogenous psychosis in parkinsonism with clozapine and fluperlapine. *European Archives of Psychiatry, Neurology and Science, 235*(1), 60–64.

Shader RI, Greenblatt DJ, 1972: Belladonna alkaloids and synthetic anticholinergics: Uses and toxicity. In: *Psychiatric complications of medical drugs*, edited by RI Shader. New York: Raven Press.

Sheehy LM, Maxman JH, 1978: Phenlzine induced psychosis. *American Journal of Psychiatry, 135*, 1422.

Siris SG, Van Kammen DP, Docherty JP, 1978: The use of antidepressant drugs in schizophrenia. *Archives of General Psychiatry, 35*, 1368–1377.

Snyder SH, 1973: Amphetamine psychosis: A "model" schizophrenia mediated by catecholamines. *American Journal of Psychiatry, 130*, 61–67.

Stores G, 1975: Behavioral effects of anti-epileptic drugs. *Developmental Medicine and Child Neurology, 17*, 647–658.

Tollefson G, 1980: Psychiatric implications of anticonvulsant drugs. *Journal of Clinical Psychiatry, 41*, 295–302.

Wood KA, Harris MJ, Morreale A, Rizos AL, 1988: Drug induced psychosis and depression in the elderly. *Psychiatric Clinics of North America, 11*(1), 167–193.

18

Adverse Cognitive Effects of Psychotropic Medications

John S. Kennedy and John Kenny

Psychotropic medication properly employed to reverse or to reduce the abnormalities characterizing mental disorders may alter the functioning of brain processes that are operating in a normal or well-compensated fashion. Competent individuals benefit from knowing how their illness is affecting the functioning of their "mind" and knowing the potential effects of treatment. This is also true of individuals who are not competent even while a guardian or the court may ultimately determine the need for therapy.

Cognition (or faculty of knowing) taken in its broadest sense includes sensation-perception, conception, and other associated components of mental operations including memory (*Oxford English Dictionary,* 1971). These functions allow the individual to employ information from and about the environment to adapt to changing demands. Although there are many models of how the brain accomplishes the tasks of organizing and employing information (Kausler, 1990) a detailed discussion of these is beyond the scope of this chapter. Common to most models is the attempt to explain how human beings acquire information via the senses (acquisition-attention and sensory memory); retain information for a brief period and either forget it if it is of insufficient interest or retain it and prepare it for later recollection [retention-short term/working memory (Baddeley, 1986)]; transfer and establish information in long-term store (consolidation); and search for and retrieve the stored information (retrieval).

Psychopharmacological studies evaluating cognition typically employ standardized psychometric measures such as the Wechsler Adult Intelligence Scale-Revised (WAIS-R) or Halsted-Reitan batteries (Trimble, 1987) to report on global cognitive function or to attempt more discrete evaluation of elements of cognitive function by applying measures that have theory-driven applications. The use of differing tests, measuring presumed different functions, produces a complex literature as can be seen in the measures of attention applied in schizophrenia research (Nuechterlein & Dawson, 1984). The advantages of testing selected functions is that such approaches may allow identification of clinically meaningful, adverse consequences—less apparent than when broader global measures are employed. The disadvantages arise when the test selected is not well understood to be sensitive to medication effects and when tests are applied that have poorly understood reliability and validity (Franzen, 1989; Loftus, 1991). Criticisms of the methodology of neuropsychological studies of cognitive impairment in schizophrenia have recently been reviewed (Gur, Saykin, & Gur, 1991), and these criticisms apply equally to many of the reported studies of medication effects in schizophrenia and other neurological and psychiatric patient populations. However, there is sufficient evidence of psychotropic medication effects on cognition in nonpatients, as well as patient populations, to allow for some conclusions about their adverse effects to be drawn.

This chapter reviews the adverse cognitive effects of the most commonly used classes of psychotropic medication including the benzodiazepines, antidepressants, neuroleptics, lithium, and the anticonvulsants carbamazepine and valproate. The adverse cognitive effects of anticholinergic medicines are reviewed elsewhere in this volume (see Chapter 14).

BENZODIAZEPINES

Benzodiazepines and structurally related medications have received the most extensive examination of their effects on cognitive function of all the classes of prescribed medications. The voluminous literature indicates that all these may produce adverse effects on memory. This is made most apparent when a subject is evaluated for anterograde amnesia and demonstrates deficits when asked to learn new information after having taken medication. This type of impairment is most readily observed following acute high-dose intravenous administration and is considered by many physicians an advantage in producing consequent impairment of memory for diagnostic procedures. Older adults are believed to be more sensitive to adverse cognitive effects of benzodiazepines (Lister, 1984).

Differences are observed between drugs from this structural class, particularly when single-dose effects are compared. Differences observed in single-dose studies may be accounted for in part by variation in the time medication is given relative to the presentation of material to be later recalled, the dosage used, and the relationship between the pharmacokinetic and pharmacodynamic duration of action of individual members of this class of medications (Greenblatt, Harmatz, & Engelhardt, & Shader, 1989; Spiegel, 1989).

As reviewed by Lister and File (1984), the principal effect of a benzodiazepine on cognition is impairment of the acquisition of new information. The nature of the deficit is similar but not identical to the type of dysfunction seen in the alcohol amnestic disorder (Korsakoff's syndrome). This observed impairment occurs independent of the extent of sedation (Roache & Griffiths, 1985). Short-term memory functions are thought to be only minimally impaired or unimpaired by the benzodiazepines. Anterograde amnesia is considered to arise because of interference in the brain processes that underlie the ability to consolidate new information being stored in long-term memory (Lister, 1985). The type of long-term memory impairment seen primarily involves episodic memory—the type of memory involved in remembering an episode of personal experience. The episodic memory deficit is apparent in both its free recall (remembering without cues or prompts) and recognition elements (recognition that the subject has been previously exposed to some stimuli and not exposed to others). Benzodiazepines are thought to have no significant effect on the process of retrieval of previously stored memories (Lister, 1985; Sanders & Wauschkuhn, 1988). This is most evident in measures of semantic memory (or factual memory) as is evaluated by tests such as the information subtest of the WAIS-R, which is minimally affected if at all (Brown, Brown, & Bowes, 1983; Ghoneim, Hinrichs, & Mewaldt 1984). The benzodiazepines' effects on cognition have been the subject of several recent extensive reviews (Lister, 1984, 1985; Saunders & Wauschkuhn, 1988; Taylor & Tinklenberg, 1987). The literature is sufficiently vast that the interested reader should refer to these reviews for further discussion.

A significant deficiency in the literature on the amnestic effects of benzodiazepines is the relatively small number of chronic-dosing studies examining the extent to which tolerance develops to the amnestic effects. A few reported studies suggest that tolerance of the adverse effect does not develop fully even after long-term use (Golombok, Maadley, & Lader, 1988; Petursson & Lader, 1982). This is also seen in shorter term use, where after each dose of chronically administered medicines such as diazepam or oxazepam, a brief amnestic period has been observed to follow (Ghoneim, Hinrichs, & Mewaldt, 1986; Lucki & Rickels, 1988). A recently published review (American Psychiatric Association, 1990) concludes that "therapeutic dosages of high-potency, short half-life benzodiazepines impair memory more than comparable therapeutic dosages of the low-potency, short half-life drug oxazepam." Such problems have not been observed in studies of the nonsedating, nonbenzodiazepine anxiolytic buspirone (Lucki & Rickels, 1988).

The effects of the benzodiazepines on psychomotor performance related to skills involved in operating complex machinery such as an automobile have also been recently reviewed (Taylor & Tinklenberg, 1987; APA, 1990), and the reader in search of detailed discussion of this topic should refer to these summaries. Also note the conclusion of the APA Task Force Report, paraphrased as: "Acute dosages of benzodiazepines given to individuals for the first time and especially to the older adult may produce impairment of skills believed to be relevant to driving an automobile or operating machinery. These effects are not consistently and predictably seen between individuals and are often a consequence of dose and other sources of individual variation. Use of the benzodiazepines have not been clearly demonstrated to be causally related to the occurrence of automobile accidents. With chronic dosages, given in appropriate therapeutic amounts, sufficient tolerance appears to develop to the psychomotor impairing effects, that in most individuals automobile related driving skills are not significantly impaired." We agree with Taylor and Tinklenberg's conclusion: "Clinicians are obligated to warn their patients about the increased hazards of driving while taking benzodiazepines. . . ." (Taylor & Tinklenberg, 1987).

ANTIDEPRESSANTS

Antidepressants in use today are drawn from a number of structurally distinct groups of compounds. Each has a relatively unique pattern of acting as an antagonist or agonist at brain and peripheral receptor populations. Although poorly studied for indications other than depression and perhaps panic disorder, in clinical practice, these medicines are reportedly given to the nondepressed to assist in management of problems such as pain, spastic bowel disorder, sleep disorders, or to reduce urinary incontinence. In children, antidepressants have primarily been studied in attention deficit disorder, and for this possible indication, only to a very limited extent. The action of tricyclics studied in children has reportedly resembled the effects of stimulant medications (Werry, 1988). As with many other pharmacotherapies, the older adult patient is thought to be more likely to manifest adverse cognitive effects in response to therapy with these medicines than younger individuals (Branconnier, Harto, Dessain, Spera, & McNiff, 1987; Deptula & Pomara, 1990). The older adult is particularly at risk for side effects such as delirium when antidepressants with greater anticholinergic effects are used (Deptula & Pomara, 1990; Judd, Squire, Butters, Salmons, & Paller, 1987). The cognitive effects of these agents have not been subjected to extensive or systemic investigation (Deptula & Pomara, 1990; Judd et al., 1987). The most studied are the oldest tricyclics: amitriptyline and imipramine. In normal (nondepressed) individuals, amitriptyline's most pronounced effects are seen in immediate memory (short-term memory/working memory) impairment following single dosages (Deptula & Pomara, 1990; Judd et al., 1987). This deficit may result from the acute anticholinergic side effect of this medication (Branconnier, DeVitt, Cole, & Spera, 1982). Similar conclusions based on the current literature may also apply to other significantly anticholinergic antidepressants such as imipramine (Judd et al., 1987).

Although little studied, the effects of chronic dosing in depressed individuals may be different from reported acute effects, as indicated by several studies of amitriptyline (Elwan, Sonief, Hassan, & Allam, 1976; Lamping, Spring, & Gelenberg, 1984; Sternberg & Jarvik, 1976) and imipramine (Glass, Uhlenhuth, Hartel, Matuzas, & Fischman, 1981; Raskin, Freedman, & DiMascia, 1983; Wittenborn, Plante, Burgess, & Maurer, 1962). Cognitive performance has been shown to either remain unchanged or improve over several weeks of therapy. The more recently Food and Drug Administration-approved nontricyclic antidepressants including serotonin reuptake inhibitors and bupropion have been even less studied, but no consistent, significant adverse effects have been observed.

The effects of antidepressant therapies on skilled performance and car driving have also been recently reviewed (Hindmarch, 1988). Typically, studies evaluating performance and driving-related skills have employed standard laboratory methods to characterize the effects of an acute dosage of the antidepressant of interest. Medicines that are either potentially anticholinergic or sedating (amitriptyline, doxepine, imipramine, mianserin, and trazodone) may be more likely in single-dosage use to produce impairment in skills necessary for safe driving and skilled performance. Medicines that have less of these properties (desipramine, bupropion, fluoxetine) may not produce such impairment. The effect of chronic-dosing regimens of amitriptyline and imipramine on skilled performance may be similar to the effects suggested on cognition—adaptation or tolerance may develop to this type of impairment over several weeks of therapy (Seppela, 1977; Hindmarch & Parrott, 1977). However, chronic-dosing effects have been little studied, to our knowledge, leaving such a conclusion premature.

NEUROLEPTICS

Neuroleptics are most commonly prescribed for psychiatric conditions in which cognitive impairment may coexist: bipolar disorder (Johnstone, Owens, Firth, & Calvert, 1985); schizophrenia (Levin, Yurgelin-Todd, & Crafts, 1989), and organic mental disorders. Relatively few studies of cognitive effects of the neuroleptic medications have been conducted in normal individuals (Judd et al., 1987; King, 1990). The medications studied have primarily been the significantly anticholinergic medications, chlorpromazine and thioridazine. Maximal dosages of these medications given to normals (chlorpromazine or thioridazine, 60 mg/day) have generally not exceeded one tenth the amount given for treatment of schizophrenia. These dosages are within the range that is usually given to older adults with organic mental disorders. In most studies of normals, no serious adverse cognitive effects have been noted (King, 1909; Liljequist, Linnoila, & Mattila, 1978; Liljequist, Linnoila, Mattila, Saario, & Seppala, 1975).

In schizophrenia, attentional measures employed to evaluate sensory memory, vigilance, and selective attention, and which are influenced by neuroleptics, generally show improvement in association with reduction in psychoses (Spohn & Strauss, 1989). The influence of high-dosage versus low-dosage therapy on measures of attention has been subjected to limited examination. One study found span of apprehension (a measure of sensory memory) to be impaired in the presence of neuroleptic therapy. This was noted to be present in chronic patients on high dosages (Spohn, Coyne, Lacoursiere, Mazur, & Hayes, 1985). With respect to other elements of cognitive function, such as short- and long-term memory, as well as executive functions, relative to the patient's baseline level of difficulty, most measures are believed to be improved or unaffected by usual chronic dosages (Cassens, Inglis, Appelbaum, & Gutheil, 1990; King, 1990). It should be noted that not all reviewers agree with this view (Medalia, Gold, & Merriam, 1988). Support for the need to maintain dosages of neuroleptics in patients at the lowest necessary and sufficient level to control psychoses is seen in the reports of the association of cognitive impairment and tardive dyskinesia (TD) (Ganguli & Raghu, 1985; Sorokin et al., 1988; Struve & Willner, 1983) and the recent review of evidence linking the presence of neuronal lipopigment (arising from free radical damage) to the presence of psychotropic drugs (Dowson, 1989). It remains unclear whether the association between TD and cognitive impairment is because of preexisting brain damage giving rise to increased risk for TD or whether the factors responsible for TD also produce the cognitive impairment.

Neuroleptic therapy (thioridazine) has been evaluated in at least two studies of driving-related psychomotor performance tests. In young, normal individuals given a single dose of 25 mg of thioridazine, performance impairments were noted in some individuals (Linnoila & Maki, 1974). A second study found that a single dose of 25 mg of thioridazine had more deleterious effects on vigilance than 10 mg of diazepam. In this study, subjects were also evaluated for the effect of 0.5 mg haloperidol, which was also noted to reduce vigilance but less than thioridazine (Linnoila, 1973). The data available suggest that neuroleptics do have the potential to impair driving performance and that physicians should advise patients of this attendant risk of driving when taking neuroleptic medicines.

LITHIUM

Lithium therapy has been studied in both normal individuals and in patient populations. Patients taking lithium chronically frequently complain of feeling less alert and sluggish. The clinician may misinterpret these complaints as reflecting the patient's sense of being less mood elevated or that the patient is entering a depressive phase of their illness. This subjective slowing may be a result of lithium's effect on cognitive processes. Several studies of normal individuals support the view that lithium causes changes in the subject's ability to process information, and this medicine may produce difficulty with retrieval of information from memory (Judd et al., 1987; Weingartner, Rudorfer, & Linnoila, 1985). A recent study suggests that the apparent slowing of cognitive functions is selective to "the translation of physical (visual) stimuli into its verbal meaning" and that lithium may produce a deficit involving the processing of semantic memory (Glue, Nutt, Cowen, & Broadbent, 1987). These same findings of a slowing of the rate of information processing have been noted in lithium-managed patients and are suggested to reduce modestly the ability to learn and memorize (Judd et al., 1987). It is unclear if this is a blood-level related phenomenon.

The effects of chronic lithium therapy in remitted bipolar patients and normal controls on psychomotor performance related to driving have been evaluated in several studies. Lithium has been suggested to produce a modest decrement in skills related to driving, which is most evident in measures of reaction time (Hatcher, Sims, & Thompson, 1990). It is unclear if such changes are likely to prove clinically significant in an otherwise normally functioning patient.

ANTICONVULSANTS

Carbamazepine

Carbamazepine (CBZ) is a tricyclic anticonvulsant (Evans & Gualtieri, 1985). The study of its application in psychiatric disorders has evolved since it was first noted in 1971 to have antimanic and prophylactic effects in bipolar disorder (Takezakl & Hanaoka, 1971).

CBZ's effect on neuropsychological test performance has been examined in a small number of normal volunteers who received CBZ for a 2-week period in a placebo-controlled study. This study found no adverse effects of CBZ on shortterm or longer-term recall or recognition memory (Trimble, Thompson, & Huppert, 1980). In a second, larger study of normal individuals, where blood levels were in the therapeutic range for the management of epilepsy, CBZ was noted to have a minimal effect on performance parameters but no effect on memory functions (Trimble & Thompson, 1983).

At least one controlled study has examined the effects of CBZ compared to lithium in bipolar patients. This study included both untreated normal and medication-free bipolar patient control groups. The concentration of CBZ was maintained at a therapeutic blood level, and lithium blood levels were kept in the range of 0.7 to 0.9 mmol/liter. Comparisons across the four groups on measures of attention, visuomotor function, and memory found no significant differences (Joffe, MacDonald, & Kutcher, 1988). CBZ has been compared to lithium in a small group of bipolar patients who were elderly (Lenzi, 1988). CBZ-related side effects produced large numbers of dropouts and cognitive measures were not reported, leaving CBZ's effect on cognition and role in therapy of the older bipolar patient unclear.

CBZ kinetics profile is characterized by a peaking of blood concentration approximately 6–10 hours after the oral dose is taken (Evans & Gualtieri, 1985). The late peaking of CBZ has implications for dosing in the morning because of the potential subsequent effects on driving performance later in the afternoon. CBZ's effect on psychomotor performance has chiefly been evaluated in epilepsy patients with the potential resultant confounding of the effects of the illness itself on test results. Several studies have examined normal individuals and found impairment in tests relevant to driving (Kuitunen, Mattila, Aranko, & Mattila, 1990; Mac-Phee, McPhail, Butler, & Bradie, 1986). Other studies of epilepsy patients have also found performance impairments (Brodie, McPhail, MacPhee, Larkin, & Gray, 1987); one study has recently suggested that a significant determinant of performance decline is the presence of high blood concentrations of the active epoxide of CBZ (Gillham et al., 1988). These reports suggest that blood levels should be kept as low as possible to minimize the extent to which psychomotor impairment is produced and that patients be warned of the possible adverse effects of CBZ on driving performance.

Valproate

Valproate is currently being evaluated for its utility in the management of several psychiatric conditions (McElroy, Keck, Pope, & Hudson, 1989). In a study of normal volunteers and patients with epilepsy, valproate produced relatively little consistent evidence of adverse effects on measures of attention, memory, or motor speed. Among the patients it was noted that some manifested adverse cognitive effects in measures of recall and selective attention, and these patients had higher blood levels of the medicine (Trimble & Thompson, 1984). There are at present insufficient data to determine if the effects of valparoate on cognitive function in patients with bipolar disorder or in the elderly are different from those reported for young, normal individuals or those with epilepsy.

REFERENCES

American Psychiatric Association, 1990: *Benzodiazepine dependence, toxicity, and abuse: A task force report of the American Psychiatric Association,* Washington, DC: Author.

Baddeley A, 1986: *Working memory,* Oxford psychological series, no. II. Oxford: Clarendon Press.

Branconnier RJ, DeVitt DR, Cole JO, Spera KF, 1982: Amitriptyline selectively disrupts verbal recall from secondary memory of the normal aged. *Neurobiology of Aging, 3,* 55–59.

Branconnier RJ, Harto NE, Dessain EC, Spera KF, McNiff ME, 1987: Speech blockage, memory impairment and age: A prospective comparison of amitriptyline and maprotiline. *Psychopharmacology Bulletin, 23,* 230–234.

Brodie MJ, McPhail E, MacPhee GJA, Larkin JG, Gray MB, 1987: Psychomotor impairment and anticonvulsant therapy in adult epileptic patients. *European Journal of Clinical Pharmacology, 31,* 655–660.

Brown J, Brown M, Bowes, JB, 1983: Effects of lorazepam on rate of forgetting, on retrieval from semantic memory and on manual dexterity. *Neuropsychologia, 21,* 501–512.

Cassens G, Inglis AK, Appelbaum PS, Gutheil TG, 1990: Neuroleptics: Effects on neuropsychological function in chronic schizophrenic patients. *Schizophrenia Bulletin, 16,* 477–499.

Deptula D, Pomara N, 1990: Effects of antidepressants on human performance: A review. *Journal of Clinical Psychopharmacology, 10,* 105–111.

Dowson J, 1989: Neuronal lipopigment: A marker for cognitive impairment and long-term effects of psychotropic drugs. *British Journal of Psychiatry, 155,* 1–11.

Elwan O, Sonief M, Hassan MA, Allam M, 1976: Psychometric assessment of the therapeutic efficacy of antidepressant agents. *Journal of Internal Medicine Research, 4,* 118–124.

Evans RW, Gualtieri CT, 1985: Carbamazepine: A neuropsychological and psychiatric profile. *Clinical Neuropharmacology, 8,* 221–241.

Franzen MD, 1989: *Reliability and validity in neuropsychological assessment.* New York: Plenum Press.

Ganguli R, Raghu U, 1985: Tardive dyskinesia, impaired recall, and informal consent. *Journal of Clinical Psychiatry, 46,* 434–435.

Ghoneim MM, Hinrichs JV, Mewaldt SP, 1984: Dose response analysis of the behavioral effects of diazepam: Learning and memory. *Psychopharmacology, 82,* 291–295.

Ghoneim MM, Hinrichs JV, Mewaldt SP, 1986: Comparison of two benzodiazepines with differing accumulation: Behavioral changes during and after 3 weeks of dosing. *Journal of Clinical Pharmacology and Therapeutics, 39,* 491–500.

Gillham RA, Williams N, Weidmann K, Butler E, Larkin JG, Brodie MJ, 1988: Concentration—Effect relationships with carbamazepine and its epoxide on psychomotor and cognitive function in epileptic patients. *Journal of Neurology, Neurosurgery and Psychiatry, 51,* 929–933.

Glass RM, Uhlenhuth EH, Hartel FW, Matuzas W, Fischman MW, 1981: Cognitive dysfunction and imipramine in outpatient depressions. *Archives of General Psychiatry, 38,* 1048–1051.

Glue PW, Nutt DJ, Cowen PJ, Broadbent D, 1987: Selective effect of lithium on cognitive performance in man. *Psychopharmacology, 91,* 109–111.

Golombok S, Moodley P, Lader M, 1988; Cognitive impairment in long term benzodiazepine users. *Psychological Medicine, 18,* 365–374.

Greenblatt DJ, Harmatz JS, Engelhardt N, Shader RI, 1989: Pharmacokinetic determinants of dynamic differences among three benzodiazepine hypnotics: Flurazepam, temazepam and triazolam. *Archives of General Psychiatry, 46,* 326–332.

Gur RC, Saykin AJ, Gur RE, 1991: Neuropsychological study of schizophrenia. In: *Advances in neuropsychiatry and psychopharmacology, vol. 1: Schizophrenia research,* edited by CA Tamminga and SC Schulz. New York: Raven Press.

Hatcher S, Sims R, Thompson D, 1990: The effects of chronic lithium treatment on psychomotor performance related to driving. *British Journal of Psychiatry, 157,* 275–278.

Hindmarch I, 1988: A Pharmacological profile of fluoxetine and other antidepressants on aspects of skilled performance and car handling ability. *British Journal of Psychiatry, 153,*(3, suppl.) 99–104.

Hindmarch I, Parrott AC, 1977: Repeated dose comparisons of nomifensine, imipramine and placebo on subjective assessment of sleep and objective measures of psychomotor performance. *British Journal of Clinical Pharmacology, 4,* 167s–173s.

Joffe RT, MacDonald C, Kutcher SP, 1988: Lack of differential cognitive effects of lithium and carbamazepine in bipolar affective disorder. *Journal of Clinical Psychopharmacology, 8,* 425–428.

Johnstone EC, Owens DGC, Firth CD, Calvert LM, 1985: Institutionalization and the outcome of functional psychoses. *British Journal of Psychiatry, 146,* 36–44.

Judd LL, Squire LR, Butters N, Salmon DP, Paller KA, 1987: Effects of psychotropic drugs on cognition and memory in normal humans and animals. In: *Psychopharmacology: The third generation of progress,* edited by HY Meltzer. New York: Raven Press.

Kausler DH, 1990: *Experimental psychology, cognition and human aging,* 2nd edition. New York: Springer-Verlag.

King DJ, 1990: The effect of neuroleptics on cognitive and psychomotor function. *British Journal of Psychiatry, 157,* 799–811.

Kuitunen T, Mattila MJ, Aranko K, Mattila ME, 1990: Actions of zopiclone and carbamazepine, alone and in combination on human skilled performance in laboratory and clinical tests. *British Journal of Clinical Pharmacology, 30,* 453–461.

Lamping DL, Spring B, Gelenberg AJ, 1984: Effects of two antidepressants on memory performance in depressed outpatients: A double blind study. *Psychopharmacology, 84,* 254–261.

Lenzi A, Lazzerini F, Marazziti D, Massimetti G, Lucarelli P, 1988: Prophylaxis of bipolar disorder in elderly: A double blind study with lithium vs. carbamazepine (abstract). *Psychopharmacology, 96*(Suppl. 1), 288.

Levin S, Yurgelin-Todd D, Crafts, 1989: Contributions of clinical neuropsychology to the study of schizophrenia. *Journal of Abnormal Psychology, 98,* 341–356.

Liljequist R, Linnoila M, Mattila MJ, 1978: Effect of diazepam and chlorpromazine on memory functions in man. *European Journal of Clinical Pharmacology, 14,* 339–343.

Liljequist R, Linnoila A, Mattila MJ, Saario I, Seppala T, 1975: Effects of two weeks treatment with thioridazine, chlorpromazine, sulpiride, and bromazepam alone or in combination with alcohol. *Psychopharmacologia* (Berlin), *44,*205–208.

Linnoila M, 1973: Effects of diazepam, chlordiazepoxide, thioridazine, haloperidol, flupenthixol, and alcohol on psychomotor skills related to driving. *Annals Medicinae Experimentacts et Biologiae Fenniae, 51,* 125–132.

Linnoila M, Maki M, 1974: Acute effects of alcohol, diazepam, thioridazine, flupenthixol, and atropine on psychomotor performance profiles. *Arzneim-Forsch, 24* NR4, 565–569.

Lister RG, 1985: The amnestic action of benzodiazepines in man. *Neuroscience and Biobehavioral Reviews, 9,* 87–94.

Lister RG, File SE, 1984: The nature of lorazepam-induced amnesia. *Psychopharmacology, 83,* 183–187.

Loftus EF, 1991: The glitter of everyday memory . . . and the gold. *American Psychologist, 46,* 16–18.

Lucki I, Rickels K, 1988: The effect of anxiolytic drugs on memory in anxious subjects. In: *Benzodiazepine receptor ligands, memory and information processing,* edited by I Hindmarch and H Ott. New York: Springer-Verlag.

MacPhee GJA, McPhail EM, Butler E, Brodie MJ, 1986: Controlled evaluation of a supplementary dose of carbamazepine on psychomotor function in epileptic patients. *European Journal of Clinical Pharmacology, 31,* 195–199.

McElroy SL, Keck PE, Pope HG, Hudson JI, 1989: Valproate in psychiatric disorders: Literature review and clinical guidelines. *Journal of Clinical Psychiatry, 50*(3, suppl), 23–29.

Medalia A, Gold J, Merriam A, 1988: The effects of neuroleptics on neuropsychological test results in schizophrenics: Critical review. *Archives of Clinical Neuropsychology, 3,* 249–271.

Neuchterlein KH, Dawson ME, 1984: Information processing and attentional functioning in the developmental course of schizophrenic disorders. *Schizophrenia Bulletin, 10,* 160–203.

Oxford English Dictionary: The compact edition of the English dictionary: Mind (vol. 1), 1971. New York: Oxford University Press.

Peturson H, Lader MH, 1982: Psychological impairment and low-dose benzodiazepine treatment. *British Medical Journal, 285,* 815–816.

Raskin A, Freedman AS, DiMascio A, 1983: Effects of chlorpromazine, imipramine, diazepam, and phenelzine on psychomotor and cognitive skills of depressed patients. *Psychopharmacology Bulletin, 19,* 649–652.

Roache JO, Griffiths RR, 1985: Comparison on triazolam and pentobarbital: Performance impairment, subjective effects, and abuse liability. *Journal of Pharmacology and Experimental Therapeutics, 234,* 120–133.

Sanders AF, Wauschkuhn CH, 1988: Drugs and information processing in skilled performance. In: *Benzodiazepine receptor ligands, memory and information processing,* edited by I Hindmarch and H Ott. New York: Springer-Verlag.

Seppela T, 1977: Psychomotor skills during acute and two week treatment with mianserine (ORG GB94) and amitriptyline, and their combined effects with alcohol. *Annals of Clinical Research, 9,* 66–72.

Sorokin JE, Giordani B, Mohs RC, Losonczy MF, Davidson M, Siever LJ, Ryan TA, Davis KL, 1988: Memory impairment in schizophrenic patients with tardive dyskinesia. *Biological Psychiatry, 23,* 129–135.

Spiegel R, 1989: *Psychopharmacology: An introduction,* 2nd edition. New York: John Wiley and Sons.

Spohn HE, Coyne L, Lacoursiere R, Mazur D, Hayes K, 1985: Relation of neuroleptic dose and tardive dyskinesia to attention, information-processing, and psychophysiology in medicated schizophrenics. *Archives of General Psychiatry, 42,* 849–859.

Spohn HE, Strauss ME, 1989: Relation of neuroleptic and anticholinergic medication to cognitive functions in schizophrenia. *Journal of Abnormal Psychology, 98,* 367–380.

Sternberg DE, Jarvik ME, 1976: Memory function in depression: *Archives of General Psychiatry, 33,* 219–224.

Struve FA, Willner AE, 1983: Cognitive dysfunction of tardive dyskinesia. *British Journal of Psychiatry, 143,* 597–600.

Takezakl H, Hanaoka M, 1971: The use of carbamazepine in the control of manic-depressive psychosis and other manic depressive states. *Seishin-Igaku, 13,* 173–183.

Taylor JL, Tinklenberg JR, 1987: Cognitive impairment and benzodiazepines. In: *Psychopharmacology: The third generation of progress,* edited by HY Meltzer. New York: Raven Press.

Trimble MR, 1987: Anticonvulsant drugs and cognitive function. *Epilepsia, 28*(3, suppl), S37–S45.

Trimble MR, Thompson PJ, 1983: Anticonvulsant drugs, cognitive function and behavior. *Epilepsia, 24,* S55–S63.

Trimble MR, Thompson PJ, 1984: Sodium valproate and cognitive function. *Epilepsia, 25*(1), S60–S64.

Trimble MR, Thompson PJ, Huppert F, 1980: Anticonvulsant drugs and cognitive abilities. In: *International symposium,* edited by R Canger, F Angeleki, and JK Penry. New York: Raven Press.

Weingartner H, Rudorfer MV, Linnoila M, 1986: Cognitive effects of lithium treatment in normal volunteers. *Psychopharmacology, 86,* 472–474.

Werry JS, 1988: Drugs, learning and cognitive function in children—an update. *Journal of Child Psychology and Psychiatry, 29,* 129–141.

Wittenborn JR, Plante M, Burgess F, Maurer H, 1962: A comparison of imipramine, electroconvulsive therapy and placebo in the treatment of depression. *Journal of Nervous and Mental Disorders, 135,* 131–137.

19

Psychotherapeutic Drug Abuse and Dependence

Shitij Kapur and Matcheri S. Keshavan

A psychoactive substance is one that, when administered, can alter the state of mind. All psychoactive substances are liable to be abused. The revised third edition of the *Diagnostic and Statistical Manual* (*DSM-III-R*; American Psychiatric Association, 1987) divides psychoactive substances disorders into two categories: dependence and abuse. Psychoactive substance dependence is defined by psychological dependence resulting in drug seeking behavior, physical dependence resulting in withdrawal symptoms, and deterioration in physical and mental health as a result of continued substance use. Some symptoms of the disturbance must have persisted for at least a month or have occurred repeatedly over a longer period of time. Psychoactive substance abuse is defined by pathological patterns of use lasting at least a month (occurring either in hazardous situations or despite knowledge of problems related to use).

Prescription drug abuse is a growing public health problem. Among the psychotropic drugs, benzodiazepines (BZDs) are the most ubiquitously prescribed medicines; the widespread recognition of their overprescription, abuse, and dependence has been a source of major concern and is reviewed in this chapter in detail. Some discussion of anticholinergic drug abuse is also presented. Details of stimulant abuse are discussed in Chapter 6. In this chapter, we review the problem of prescription drug abuse in psychiatry. Other prescribed drugs which are abused, such as barbiturates, are not discussed here, since they are not commonly used as psychotherapeutic drugs in current practice.

BENZODIAZEPINE ABUSE AND DEPENDENCE

Chlordiazepoxide, the first BZD, was introduced in the United States in 1957. Since then BZDs have replaced virtually all previous sedative-hypnotics, namely bromides, barbiturates, and meprobamate. BZDs offer a relatively lower addiction potential and a high therapeutic index.

Currently 13 BZDs are approved by the Food and Drug Administration (FDA) for use in the United States. All drugs are classified as class IV (low potential for abuse; use may lead to limited physical or psychological dependence; prescription may be oral or written, 5 refills within 6 months). Chlordiazepoxide, diazepam, oxazepam, lorazepam, clorazepate, prazepam, halazepam, and alprazolam are approved for anxiety disorders. Flurazepam, temazepam, estazolam, triazolam, and quazepam are approved for treatment of insomnia. Diazepam and clonazepam have been approved as anticonvulsants. However, all BZDs have a similar range of action, and their FDA approval and indications might reflect corporate marketing strategy rather than intrinsic differences (Perry, 1988).

Epidemiology

After their introduction in the 1960s the BZDs became the most commonly prescribed drugs for the next two decades. However, this extensive popularity and unrestrained prescribing brought in its wake concern regarding misuse, abuse, and withdrawal. According to a survey, 11.1% of Americans aged 18–79 years reported having used a BZD at least once in the preceding 12 months. These figures vary in different countries, from a low 7.4% in the Netherlands to a high of 17.6% in Belgium. The prevalence in women is twice that of men. The survey also revealed that although greater than two thirds used it for less than a month, between 1% and 2% of the population studied had used it for more than 12 months continuously (Uhlenhuth, DeWit, Balter, Johanson, & Mellinger, 1988). Presently, about 60 million prescriptions of benzodiazepine anxiolytics are dispensed annually by retail pharmacists, with alprazolam being the commonest anxiolytic and triazolam the most common hypnotic agent (American Psychiatric Association, 1990).

Risk Factors for Withdrawal

Studies suggest that there is a relationship between discontinuation symptom severity and dose used; however, there is no identified threshold below which discontinuation symptoms are not observed (American Psychiatric Association, 1990). Studies have suggested that the longer the duration of treatment, the higher the incidence, with all other factors controlled; however, withdrawal has often been observed with as little as 3 weeks of treatment (Noyes, Garvey, Cook, & Perry, 1988). Withdrawal syndromes have been noted with BZDs; however, experience with the newer BZDs such a quazepam and estazolam has been limited. The freqeuency of the withdrawal syndrome as well as the intensity of symptoms is higher after short-acting BZDs (Roy-Byrne & Hommer, 1988). Clinical experience also suggests that a gradual rate of tapering of BZDs should decrease the incidence as compared to abrupt withdrawal.

Discontinuation Syndromes

The understanding of BZD abuse-dependence syndromes is confounded by nosological and methodological issues (Noyes et al., 1988). In any discussion of the discontinuation syndromes in patients with chronic BZD administration, four terms need to be differentiated: withdrawal syndrome, relapse of anxiety, rebound anxiety, and pseudowithdrawal. *Withdrawal syndrome* refers to a set of unique, time-limited, constellation of symptoms that follows discontinuation after a period of continuous administration. However, the symptoms that are attributed to withdrawal from BZDs (e.g., nausea or vomiting, malaise or weakness, autonomic hyperactivity, anxiety, orthostatic hypotension, coarse tremor, marked insomnia, and grand mal seizures; *DSM-III-R* criteria—American Psychiatric Association, 1987) are neither specific nor limited to withdrawal, but may be part of a *relapse* of the initial disorder for which BZDs were being used. Efforts have been made to differentiate between withdrawal and relapse using time course (withdrawal occurs early), outcome (withdrawal is self-limited and gradually improves), and unique symptoms (withdrawal seizures, psychosis, perceptual abnormality are considered by some to be unique to withdrawal). However, none of these approaches have been unequivocally useful. Also described is a concept of *rebound anxiety,* analogous to rebound insomnia described by Kales, Scharf, & Kales (1978). This syndrome is considered to be neither a withdrawal nor a relapse, but a worsening of the underlying process while symptomatic control of anxiety is achieved with BZDs; an even worse than initial symptom picture presents on discontinuing BZDs. *Pseudowithdrawal,* a term based on the concept of conditioned tolerance (King, Bouton, & Musty, 1987), constitutes a kind of placebo response to the perceived discontinuation of the drug without the drug actually being changed (Roy-Byrne & Hommer, 1988). The only systematic study of this concept revealed that 20% of chronic BZD abusers developed symptoms of withdrawal when told that their medication had been switched to a placebo even though their medication continued unchanged (Tyrer, Rutherford, & Huggett, 1983). In an actual clinical situation it is often hard to distinguish between the different discontinuation syndromes.

Pathophysiology

BZDs are understood to exert their effect by enhancing the gamma aminobutyric acid (GABA)-mediated inhibitory effects. BZDs attach to a BZD-GABA receptor complex and enhance transmembrane chloride transport resulting in hyperpolarization of the membrane (American Psychiatric Association, 1990; Cowen & Nutt, 1982). Efforts have been made to explain the clinically observed phenomena of dependence, tolerance, and withdrawal on a neurophysiological basis. The aforementioned phenomena could result from pharmacokinetic changes, or from changes at the level of the BZD-GABA receptor complex or at the level of the chloride channel (Roy-Byrne & Hommer, 1988). Recent animal studies have attempted to address this question. Rats that were chronically administered lorazepam via implanted osmotic pumps were noted to develop behavioral tolerance as measured by a reduction in the induced ataxia. Pharmacokinetic studies revealed that tolerance was not related to enhanced distribution or elimination. However, studies of the BZD receptor suggested that even though receptor affinity remained unchanged, the available receptor number decreased, suggesting downregulation. The functional ability of the BZD-GABA receptor complex to induce chloride ion uptake in membranes in vitro was decreased in parallel with behavioral tolerance (Cowen & Nutt, 1982; Miller, Greenblatt, Barahill, & Shader, 1988a).

The same model was then used to study the effect of abrupt discontinuation of BZDs in rats who displayed behavioral tolerance on chronic administration of BZDs. On discontinuation of BZD, a time-limited behavioral syndrome of increased locomotor activity as measured by open-field activity was observed (Miller et al., 1986). It has been proposed that sudden discontinuation of BZDs exposes the functionally underactive GABA system. And since the GABA system is inhibitory, its underactivity results in excitatory manifestations that range from restlessness and anxiety to seizures (Cowen & Nutt, 1982). Although these studies document neurochemical alterations at a receptor level that accompany tolerance and withdrawal, they do not explain why these alterations should happen. A complementary line of investigation in animals has suggested that production of an endogenous anxiogenic ligand, which increases with BZD administration, may cause the neurochemical changes noted earlier, and could be responsible for the observed clinical and behavioral effects (Baldwin & File, 1988).

As evidence for a neurophysiological basis for tolerance and withdrawal accumulates, separate lines of investigation suggest a strong role for conditioned learning of behavioral tolerance. Experiments using BZDs in rats suggest that tolerance may be partially explained as a "learned behavior" to drug administration (King et al., 1987). Clinical studies suggest the effect of personality factors in development of tolerance-dependence (Johanson & Woods, 1988) and the noted phenomenon of pseudowithdrawal. It is important to note that there is no reason to believe that BZDs or their discontinuation produce any permanent structural or functional brain changes (American Psychiatric Association, 1990).

Clinical Features

Abuse and physical dependence on BZD may be encountered in four settings in clinical practice. The first and most common is the individual, usually an elderly woman with multiple somatic illnesses and depressive symptoms, who is prescribed a BZD for insomnia or anxiety. Noticeable benefit usually exists and she does not take higher than the prescribed dose, but she experiences withdrawal whenever attempts are made to discontinue the drug. Second are individuals with chronic anxiety, dysphoria, and interpersonal problems who first use BZDs as prescribed but may start "self-medicating," increasing the dose or changing the pattern of use. Third is the individual who is primarily dependent on alcohol or some other illicit drug and uses BZDs in an abuse pattern to either alleviate withdrawal or enhance the "rush." Fourth is the relatively rare, exclusively BZD abuser who procures the drug illicitly and abuses it (Jaffe, 1989).

Not every patient who has to discontinue BZD after long-term use develops withdrawal symptoms. Although incidence figures have varied from 0% to a 100% incidence for withdrawal, a figure of 30–50% is more commonly reported (Busto et al., 1986; Noyes et al., 1988; Roy-Byrne & Hommer, 1988). This wide range is accounted for by the different definitions of withdrawal as well as the heterogeneity of the samples in terms of age, sex, duration, dose, personality factors, and other substance abuse patterns (Roy-Byrne & Hommer, 1988). Various approaches have been used to diagnose withdrawal; some authors suggest that the development of new symptoms not experienced at baseline is essential to qualify for withdrawal. Others have used a 50% increase in self-reported subjective symptoms over baseline levels as indicative of withdrawal (Noyes et al., 1988; Tyrer, Owen, & Dawling, 1983). Arbitrary cut-off levels on inventories of symptoms have also been used to diagnose withdrawal (Busto et al., 1986). Thus, even though there is no consensus over what constitutes a withdrawal syndrome to BZDs, the *DSM-III-R* has a distinctly defined category "uncomplicated sedative, hypnotic or anxiolytic withdrawal" (292.00 Code). It is diagnosed when there is a reduction or cessation of BZD use after several weeks or more of moderate to heavy use and is characteristically followed by at least three of eight symptoms:

nausea or vomiting, malaise or weakness, autonomic hyperactivity, anxiety or irritability, orthostatic hypotension; coarse tremor, marked insomnia, and grand mal seizures (American Psychiatric Association, 1987). A recent review of reports of BZD discontinuance symptoms concludes that symptoms seen "very frequently" include anxiety, insomnia, restlessness, agitation, irritability, and muscle tension. Nausea, coryza, diaphoresis, lethargy, blurred vision, hyperacusis, aches and pains, ataxia, depression, and nightmares are "common but less frequent," whereas psychosis, seizures, confusion, delusion, and hallucinations are "uncommon" (American Psychiatric Association, 1990). The usual withdrawal reaction is mild to moderate and of brief duration; severe reactions are seen only in a minority (Noyes et al., 1988). The symptoms may be influenced by coexisting polysubstance abuse.

The temporal profile of these symptoms varies with the specific BZD and the rate of discontinuation. Withdrawal reactions are observed on the first day after abrupt discontinuation in patients on short halflife compounds and around the fifth day in patients on long halflife BZDs. Similarly, peak severity is observed 1 day after abrupt discontinuation of short halflife BZDs and about 10 days after long halflife BZDs. The usual duration of these reactions is 3–4 weeks when no pharmacological adjuncts are used to alleviate symptoms. See Table 1 for details of the important characteristics of available BZDs.

Treatment

Not all patients who are on BZDs need to discontinue them. Even if there is evidence to suggest physical dependence this is not by itself an indication for discontinuation. Anxiety disorders are chronic; therefore, many patients may benefit from continuous BZD administration.

Indications for discontinuation include: reason to believe that the indication for which the BZD was prescribed is in remission, a pattern of abuse (i.e., the patient

Table 1 Pharmacological characteristics of benzodiazepines

	Approx. equiv. (mg)	Metabolites	Absorption	Generic	Available form
Chlordiazepoxide	10	Active	Intermediate	Available	p.o., i.m./i.v.
Diazepam	5	Active	Rapid	Available	p.o., i.m./i.v.
Oxazepam	15	Inactive	Slow	Available	p.o. —
Clorazepate	7.5	Active	Rapid	—	p.o. —
Lorazepam	1	Inactive	Intermediate	Available	p.o., i.m./i.v.
Alprazolam	0.5	Active	Rapid	—	p.o. —
Prazepam	10	Active	Slow	—	p.o. —
Halazepam	20	Active	Intermediate	—	p.o. —
Triazolam	0.25	Active	Rapid	—	p.o. —
Temazepam	15	Inactive	Slow	—	p.o. —
Quazepam	15	Active	Rapid	—	p.o. —
Estazolam	1	Active (minor)	—	—	p.o. —

Table derived from Perry et al. (1988); Gelenberg (1987); Silver and Yudofsky (1988).
Abbreviations: p.o. = per os (by mouth, orally); i.m. = intramuscularly; i.v. = intravenous.

is using more pills than prescribed or using BZD to obtain a "high"); and cognitive side effects or sedations that interfere with social or occupational functioning.

Patients should be involved in the decisionmaking process of evaluating the risk/benefit equation for BZD usage. The patient should understand that despite adequate management of withdrawal, some distressing symptoms are likely to be experienced. The possibility that the patient may experience symptoms similar to those that caused medication to be started should be discussed. Discontinuation can be achieved as an outpatient in many cases and can be scheduled electively at a relatively less stressful time. Patients should be assured of psychological support and of ready clinician availability during BZD discontinuation.

The following patients are thought to be more susceptible to develop withdrawal symptoms: those who have been on a high dose for a long duration and have been using short-acting BZDs (Rickels, Schweizer, Csanalosi, Case, & Chung, 1988; Busto et al., 1986); those patients with a history of other substance abuse particularly alcohol; and those with passive dependent personality traits (Tyrer et al., 1983; Rickels et al., 1988). There is some evidence to suggest that male sex and older age predict a greater likelihood of successful outcome of BZD discontinuation (Schweizer, Case, & Rickels, 1989). Therapeutic strategies are outlined below.

Tapering

Considerable evidence has accumulated that gradual tapering as opposed to an abrupt withdrawal is associated with lesser frequency and severity of the withdrawal syndrome. Abrupt cessation of BZDs has been known to result in seizures. This is a particular problem in the case of short-acting BZDs such as alprazolam (Levy, 1984; Breier, Charney, & Nelson, 1984). Although taper schedules have not been systematically evaluated, recommendations for "gradual" tapering vary from 4 to 16 weeks (Noyes et al., 1988; Busto et al., 1986). Some researchers have cautioned that discontinuation should not proceed faster than the equivalent of 5 mg of diazepam per week, and even slower for shorter half-life agents. It has been observed that as the total dose decreases, successive decrements become more distressing for the patient and the rate of tapering should be slowed toward the end (Noyes et al., 1988).

Substitution

For patients judged to be at a high risk because of a high dose or short half-life BZD use, or those who have been unsuccessful with tapering, "substitution" with a long halflife BZD followed by gradual tapering may be used. The rationale behind this approach is that a higher rate and severity of withdrawal symptoms are observed with short half-life agents and with a fast rate of drop in plasma levels of BZD (Tyrer et al., 1983). As BZDs exhibit cross tolerance it is hoped that substituting an equivalent dose of a long half-life agent provides a favorable withdrawal outcome. Two approaches may be used. If the exact BZD use patterns are known, an equivalent dose of diazepam may be substituted, using the equivalence suggested in Table 1, and then gradual tapering be used as suggested earlier (Perry, Stambaugh, Tsuang, & Smith, 1981). Clonazepam, another long-acting BZD, has also been successfully used as a substitute during alprazolam withdrawal (Patterson, 1988). For patients in whom the nature of BZD use cannot be reliably ascertained, a tolerance test has been suggested. In an inpatient setting, the patient is given 20 mg of diazepam orally every 2 hours until signs of ataxia, coarse nystagmus, dysphasia, or sleep develop. Ten milligrams less than the total amount of diazepam used to reach this end point is considered to be the patient's daily dose. This dose is used to guide further management of tapering (Perry et al., 1981). However, in certain cases a withdrawal syndrome may develop on abrupt switching from a short half-life to a long half-life BZD, even when equivalent doses are used, and therefore a gradual stepwise substitution is recommended before tapering is attempted (Zipursky, Baker, & Zimmer, 1986; Roy-Byrne & Hommer, 1988).

Pharmacological Adjuncts

Several strategies have been suggested to manage the withdrawal symptoms using non-BZD pharmacological adjuncts. The information is largely derived from case reports, and few prospective controlled comparisons are available.

Propranolol. Since tachycardia, hypertension, tremulousness, and sweating are all manifestations of a hypothesized hyperadrenergic state seen in BZD withdrawal, propranolol 10–40 mg every 6–8 hours has been used to ameliorate these symptoms. Although no decrease in incidence of withdrawal was observed, the severity of the aforementioned symptoms was decreased (Tyrer et al., 1981). However, despite control of peripheral manifestations, self-rated dysphoria was noted to have worsened (Abernathy, Greenblatt, & Shader, 1981).

Clonidine. Clonidine has been used with some measure of success in opiate withdrawal, an effect probably related to its ability to reduce central hyperadrenergic state via presynaptic alpha$_2$ agonist activity; it has also been used in BZD withdrawal with some success in an initial case report (Keshavan & Crammer, 1985). However, a subsequent double-blind, placebo-controlled study of 3 patients did not reveal any significant benefit in the intensity, severity, or duration of the syndrome (Goodman, Charney, Bice, Woods, & Heninger, 1986).

Carbamazepine. Lately carbamazepine has been used with some success in alcohol withdrawal, presumably via its "antikindling" properties and its ability to inhibit limbic excitation. It also has been used in BZD withdrawal. Reports to date are anecdotal and uncontrolled; in one study, carbamazepine up to 800 mg a day was able to produce uneventful withdrawal in 9 patients in whom gradual tapering had been unsuccessful (Ries, Roy-Byrne, Ward, Neppe, & Cullison, 1989).

Tricyclic antidepressants. Antidepressants, notably amitriptyline, doxepin, and imipramine, have also been used to attenuate BZD withdrawal. Patients are stabilized on moderate doses of an antidepressant for a few weeks before BZD taper is initiated. Since antidepressants manifest antianxiety and antipanic properties, they may protect against reemergence of primary symptoms; moreover, a specific BZD receptor modulation role has also been suggested (Tyrer, 1985). A concern has been expressed that since antidepressants, such as bupropion, lower the seizure threshold they may increase the propensity for withdrawal seizures, but no systematic studies have addressed this issue (Noyes et al., 1988).

Buspirone. A recent double-blind, randomized, placebo-controlled study revealed no clinical cross-tolerance between buspirone and BZD, and there was no clinical advantage of buspirone over placebo in modifying BZD withdrawal profile. There was some evidence of anxiolytic action, but it did not substantially change overall outcome (Lader & Olazide, 1987).

Psychotherapy

Since it is becoming increasingly clear that psychological factors and behavioral learning may play a significant role in withdrawal reactions, nonpharmacological strategies are being investigated (King et al., 1987; Roy-Byrne & Hommer, 1988). Sanchez-Craig, Ray, and Busto (1986) have used cognitive therapy principles to decrease symptoms associated with abrupt withdrawal. Crouch, Robson, and Hallstrom (1988) employed group therapy using anxiety management techniques in patients who were previously unable to discontinue BZDs and achieved a 50% success rate. Of the six components of the group therapy package, the subjects identified "learning to cope with symptoms" and "sharing problems with others" as being most helpful.

Prevention

Table 2 outlines the guidelines for prescribing BZDs. A careful pretreatment psychiatric evaluation helps to rule out subjects prone to BZD abuse and to identify clear indications of BZD treatment. Routine prescribing of BZDs is to be avoided. There is an increasing trend to limit BZD use to short courses (i.e., less than 6 weeks) whenever possible. It is important to periodically reevaluate the need for continued medications and to attempt discontinuation of BZDs when the patient appears to be in stable remission. Combined treatment with nonpharmacological approaches (i.e., psychotherapy, biofeedback, relaxation training, etc.) will help in preventing BZD dependency.

Some patients require regular long-term use of BZDs in therapeutic doses for symptom control but experience severe difficulties when attempts are made to

Table 2 Guidelines for prevention and management of BZD dependence and withdrawal

	Guidelines
Prevention	Complete a detailed psychiatric, neurologic, and medical evaluation before starting treatment
	Consider nonpharmacological options first
	Use only where clearly indicated
	Use long halflife agents, if abuse is a concern
	Use lowest possible effective dose
	Use for the shortest possible time
	Avoid in patients with substance abuse history
	Avoid in patients with dependent-passive traits
	Caution patient regarding risk of dependence
Management of withdrawal	Inform patient of technique of discontinuation and expected symptoms
	Taper gradually
	If above fails try "substitution"
	If above fails try pharmacological adjuncts
	Provide access to physician or other psychological support during period of discontinuation
	Consider specific nonpharmacological therapy to assist during withdrawal

discontinue them. It is unclear what benefits are derived from persistent or recurrent efforts at discontinuation in such patients.

ANTICHOLINERGIC ABUSE AND WITHDRAWAL

The effect of anticholinergic drugs in causing hallucinations and euphoria is well known; this has led to frequent misuse. In the middle ages, belladonna and related substances were used in witches' brews to conjure up the devil. Patients who are prescribed antiparkinsonian agents for extrapyramidal side effects often refuse discontinuation of these drugs because of "depression" or "feeling unwell" without these drugs.

Epidemiology

About one half of patients treated with antipsychotic drugs are also concurrently treated with anticholinergic agents (Michel & Kolakowska, 1981). Several reports exist of anticholinergic abuse from various countries including Britain, North America, Australia, Israel, and Poland (see Pullen, Best, & Maguire, 1984). Benzhexol (trihexiphenidyl) is by far the most commonly abused drug, but reports of most other anticholinergic drugs exist in the literature. The prevalence of anticholinergic drug abuse is unknown and is likely to be underestimated. Kaminer, Munitz, and Wijsenbeck (1982) have estimated benzhexol abuse prevalence to be in the range of 7%.

Clinical Features

The possibility of anticholinergic abuse should be considered in patients who request additional supplies of these medicines claiming that they have lost their prescriptions or those who develop new unusual symptoms such as excitability, dizziness, euphoria, tachycardia, or visual hallucinations (Pullen et al., 1984). The patients may alternatively present with anticholinergic withdrawal symptoms when they run out of the medication; the withdrawal symptoms typically include nausea, diaphoresis, diarrhea, abdominal pain, dizziness, restlessness, and insomnia. In addition, marked dysphoria and frank depression have also been described (Keshavan, Burton, Murphy, Checkley, & Crammer, 1985). Anticholinergic withdrawal may also lead to worsening of parkinsonian symptoms in patients concurrently treated with antipsychotics.

Treatment

Routinely prescribing anticholinergic agents for all patients on antipsychotic agents, should be avoided. Caution should be exercised in prescribing these agents to patients with a history of substance abuse. Periodic reevaluation of the need for continued treatment with anticholinergic agents is important. For those who continue to need anticholinergic medications, the lowest possible dose should be used and prescriptions of small supplies should be given whenever possible (Pullen et al., 1984). Withdrawing an antiparkinsonian agent should be done gradually to avoid symptoms of withdrawal.

REFERENCES

Abernathy DR, Greenblatt DJ, Shader RI, 1981: Treatment of diazepam withdrawal syndrome with propranolol. *Annals of Internal Medicine, 94*(3), 354–355.

American Psychiatric Association, 1989: *Diagnostic and statistical manual, 3rd edition, revised.* Washington, DC: Author.

American Psychiatric Association Task Force on Benzodiazepine Dependency, 1990: *Benzodiazepine dependence, toxicity and abuse.* Washington, DC: Author.

Baldwin HA, File SA, 1988: Reversal of increased anxiety during benzodiazepine withdrawal: Evidence for an anxiogenic endogenous ligand for the benzodiazepine receptor. *Brain Research Bulletin, 20,* 603–606.

Breier A, Charney DS, Nelson JC, 1984: Seizures induced by abrupt discontinuation of alprazolam. *American Journal of Psychiatry, 141,* 1606–1607.

Busto U, Sellers EM, Narango CA, Cappell H, Sanchez-Craig M, Sykora K, 1986: Withdrawal reaction after long-term therapeutic use of benzodiazepines. *New England Journal of Medicine, 315*(14), 854–859.

Cowen PJ, Nutt DJ, 1982: Abstinence symptoms after withdrawal of tranquilizing drugs: Is there a common neurochemical mechanism? *Lancet, 2,* 360–362.

Crouch G, Robson M, Hallstrom C, 1988: Benzodiazepine dependent patients and their psychological treatment. *Progress in Neuro-Psychopharmacology and Biological Psychiatry, 12,* 503–510.

Gelenberg AJ, 1987: Anxiety. In: *The practitioner's guide to psychoactive drugs,* 2nd edition, edited by E Bassuk, SC Schoonover, and AJ Gelenberg. New York: Plenum.

Goodman WK, Charney DS, Bice LH, Woods SW, Heninger GR, 1986: Ineffectiveness of clonidine in the treatment of benzodiazepine withdrawal syndrome: Report of three cases. *American Journal of Psychiatry, 143*(7), 900–903.

Hallstrom C, Lader M, 1988: Benzodiazepine withdrawal phenomena. *International Pharmacopsychiatry, 16,* 235–244.

Jaffe JH, 1989: Drug dependence: Opiods, nonnarcotics, nicotine, and caffeine. In: *Comprehensive textbook of psychiatry IV,* 5th edition, edited by HI Kaplan and BJ Sadock. Baltimore, MD: Williams and Wilkins.

Johanson CE, Woods JH, 1988: Risk factors in benzodiazepine misuse and dependence. *Psychopharmacology Bulletin, 24*(3), 415–420.

Kales A, Scharf MB, Kales JD, 1978: Rebound insomnia: A new clinical syndrome. *Science, 201,* 1039–1041.

Kaminer Y, Munitz H, Wijsenbeck H, 1982: Trihexiphenidyl abuse: Euphorient and anxiolytic. *British Journal of Psychiatry, 140,* 473–474.

Keshavan MS, Burton S, Murphy M, Checkley SA, Crammer JL, 1985: Benzhexol withdrawal and cholinergic mechanisms in depression. *British Journal of Psychiatry, 147,* 560–564.

Keshavan MS, Crammer JL, 1985: Clonidine in benzodiazepine withdrawal. *Lancet, 1,* 1325–1326.

King DA, Bouton MA, Musty RE, 1987: Associative control of tolerance to the sedative effects of a short-acting benzodiazepine. *Behavioral Neuroscience, 101*(1), 104–114.

Lader M, Olajide D, 1987: A comparison of buspirone and placebo in relieving benzodiazepine withdrawal symptoms. *Journal of Clinical Psychopharmacology, 7*(1), 11–15.

Levy AB, 1984: Delirium and seizures due to abrupt alprazolam withdrawal: Case report. *Journal of Clinical Psychiatry, 45,* 38–39.

Michel K, Kolakowska T, 1981: A survey of prescribing psychotropic drugs in two psychiatric hospitals. *British Journal of Psychiatry, 183,* 217–221.

Miller LG, Greenblatt DJ, Barnhill JG, Shader RI, 1988a: Chronic benzodiazepine administration. I. Tolerance is associated with benzodiazepine receptor downregulation and decreased gamma-aminobutyric acid$_A$ receptor function. *Journal of Pharmacology and Experimental Therapeutics, 246*(1), 170–176.

Miller LG, Greenblatt DJ, Barnhill JG, Shader RI, 1988b: Chronic benzodiazepine administration. II. Discontinuation syndrome is associated with upregulation of gamma-aminobutynic. Acid$_A$ receptor complex binding and function. *Journal of Pharmacology and Experimental Therapeutics, 246-1,* 177–182.

Noyes R, Garvey MJ, Cook BL, Perry PJ, 1988: Benzodiazepine withdrawal: A review of the evidence. *Journal of Clinical Psychiatry, 49*(10), 382–389.

Patterson JF, 1988: Alprazolam dependency: Use of clonazepam for withdrawal. *Southern Medical Journal, 81,* 830–836.

Perry PJ, Alexander B, Liskow BI, 1988: Antianxiety agents. In: *Psychotropic drug handbook,* 5th edition. Cincinnati: Harvey Whitney Books.

Perry PJ, Stambaugh RL, Tsuang MT, Smith RE, 1981: Sedative hypnotic tolerance testing and withdrawal comparing diazepam to barbiturates. *Journal of Clinical Psychopharmacology, 1,* 289–296.

Pullen GP, Best NR, Maguire J, 1984: Anticholinegic drug abuse: A common problem? *British Medical Journal, 289,* 612–613.

Rickels K, Schweizer E, Csanalosi I, Case WG, Chung H, 1988: Long-term treatment of anxiety and risk of withdrawal. *Archives of General Psychiatry, 45,* 444–450.

Ries RK, Roy-Byrne PP, Ward NG, Neppe V, Cullison S, 1989: Carbamazepine treatment for benzodiazepine withdrawal. *American Journal of Psychiatry, 146*(4), 536–537.

Roy-Byrne PP, Hommer D, 1988: Benzodiazepine withdrawal: Overview and implications for the treatment of anxiety. *American Journal of Medicine, 84,* 1041–1052.

Sanchez-Craig M, Kay G, Busto U, 1986: Cognitive behavioral treatment for benzodiazepine dependence. *Lancet, 1,* 388.

Schweizer E, Case WG, Rickels K, 1989: Benzodiazepine dependence and withdrawal in elderly patients. *American Journal of Psychiatry, 146*(4), 529–531.

Silver JM, Yudofsky SC, 1988: Psychopharmacology and electronconvulsive therapy. In: *Textbook of psychiatry,* edited by JA Talbott, RE Hales, and SC Yudofsky. Washington, DC: American Psychiatric Press.

Tyrer P, 1985: Clinical management of benzodiazepine dependence (letter). *British Medical Journal, 291,* 1507.

Tyrer P, Owen R, Dawling S, 1983: Gradual withdrawal of diazepam after long-term therapy. *Lancet, 1,* 1402–1406.

Tyrer P, Rutherford D, Huggett D, 1981: Benzodiazepine withdrawal symptoms and propranolol. *Lancet, 1,* 520–522.

Uhlenhuth EH, DeWit H, Balter MB, Johanson CE, Mellinger GD, 1988: Risks and benefits of long term benzodiazepine use. *Journal of Clinical Psychopharmacology, 8*(3), 161–167.

Zipursky RS, Baker RB, Zimmer B, 1985: Alprazolam withdrawal delirium unresponsive to diazepam: Case report. *Journal of Clinical Psychiatry, 46,* 344–345.

Concluding Remarks

Neurological Syndromes

Extrapyramidal symptoms are well-known effects of antipsychotic medications. They can be classified into two arbitrary categories, acute and tardive types. The acute syndromes include acute dystonia and drug-induced parkinsonism; delayed-onset (tardive) syndromes include tardive dyskinesia and tardive dystonia. Extrapyramidal syndromes that are not so easily classified include akathisia and neuroleptic malignant syndrome.

Dystonias are characterized by slow, sustained muscular contractions occurring early in treatment. These can be painful, alarming, and potentially fatal and often result in noncompliance with treatment. The parkinsonian syndrome, which occurs somewhat later during treatment, includes muscle stiffness, cogwheel rigidity, tremors, shuffling gait, and drooling. Akathisia, which refers to a subjective experience of restlessness, can cause the patient to appear agitated and feel dysphoric. This can present at any time during treatment. A similar syndrome with a like subjective experience of jitteriness has also been described during treatment with tricyclic antidepressants. Neuroleptic malignant syndrome is a potentially fatal disorder characterized by extrapyramidal symptoms, elevated temperature, and often distinct autonomic dysfunction and laboratory test changes.

The current thinking is that the aforementioned extrapyramidal symptoms are related to the dopaminergic blockade caused by antipsychotic drugs. A variety of drugs may be used to prevent and manage such adverse effects. Acute dystonias and drug-induced parkinsonism are effectively treated with anticholinergic, antiparkinsonian agents. Akathisia may also benefit from such treatment in some cases. Amantadine, a dopaminergic agonist, is beneficial in some patients with drug-induced parkinsonism. Propranolol may be especially helpful in akathisia. The management of neuroleptic malignant syndrome initially involves antipsychotic medication discontinuation, supportive therapies to maintain vital functions, and use of dopaminergic agonists such as bromocriptine; other treatments may be of assistance.

Tardive dyskinesia is a delayed sequel of antipsychotic treatment and is characterized by abnormal involuntary choreoathetoid movements of head, limb, and trunk muscles. All neuroleptics have been associated with causing these complications; although, there is some evidence that clozapine may be less prone to result in this condition. Tardive dyskinesia is considered to be caused by dopaminergic supersensitivity resulting from chronic dopaminergic blockade. This complication is best prevented by using antipsychotic drugs only when necessary—and in the minimum effective doses. Tardive dyskinesias may be reversible in some cases, particularly if recognized early. Once a diagnosis is made, an attempt should be made to decrease or stop the antipsychotic—

particularly if the movement disorder is severe. There is no single satisfactory treatment for tardive dyskinesia.

Another neurological adverse effect, sometimes seen with psychotropic drugs, is epilepsy. In view of its rarity, this problem has not been discussed as a separate chapter in this book; however, it is important to note that some antipsychotics, notably chlorpromazine, loxapine, and other low-potency antipsychotics, are more epileptogenic than high-potency drugs. Clozapine is especially prone to reduce the seizure threshold. Among antidepressants, amoxapine maprotiline, and bupropion may be more epileptogenic than the others. These issues need to be kept in mind when treating patients with seizure disorders or organic brain lesions with psychotropic drugs. The interested reader may refer to a recent comprehensive review for reference (Lipka & Lathers, 1987).

Psychiatric Syndromes

Drugs used to treat extrapyramidal syndromes (i.e., anticholinergic drugs) themselves have significant neuropsychiatric complications. The anticholinergic syndrome is characterized by peripheral and central anticholinergic effects such as dry mouth, blurred vision, constipation, confusion, and impaired memory. Older adults and those with preexisting organic mental syndromes are particularly prone to developing this syndrome. Antipsychotic and antidepressant drugs with anticholinergic properties are also capable of contributing to this syndrome.

A wide variety of prescribed drugs can cause depression and mania. It has been generally believed that antidepressant treatments can cause a switch into mania and that antipsychotic agents can cause depression. However, a careful review of the literature in regard to both these contentions raises questions about the validity of these assumptions.

Certain psychotropic drugs can cause psychotic reactions and/or provoke exacerbation of preexisting psychotic disorders. In particular, stimulants such as amphetamines and methylphenidate can cause characteristic schizophreniform syndromes. Discontinuation of antipsychotics is known to be associated with psychotic relapse; this is sometimes called "supersensitivity psychosis" and is a controversial topic. Abrupt benzodiazepine withdrawal is known to be associated with a wide range of psychotic reactions.

Cognitive impairments are often seen with psychotherapeutic drug treatments, notably anticholinergic agents and benzodiazepines. The literature in regard to the cognitive side effects of antidepressants and antipsychotic drugs is less clear. Cognitive impairments are also seen during treatment with antiepileptic drugs; however, it is frequently difficult to disentangle the cognitive impairments associated with the primary conditions being treated with these drugs. The use of electroconvulsive treatment is also associated with significant, albeit controversial, cognitive dysfunction.

Abuse of prescription drugs is a health problem of increasing magnitude. Benzodiazepines are among the most commonly prescribed psychotropic medications. The problems of their abuse and dependence have been widely recognized. Discontinuation of benzodiazepines in a patient dependent on these drugs is a particularly difficult clinical problem. Several approaches have been suggested, none of which are entirely satisfactory. Anticholinergic drugs are also frequently abused.

REFERENCE

Lipka LJ, Lathers CN, 1987: Therapeutic review: Psychoactive agents, seizure, product and sudden death in epilepsy. *Journal of Clinical Psychopharmacology Pharmacology and Therapeutics, 27,* 169–183.

III

DRUG-INDUCED SYSTEMIC SYNDROMES

Psychotropic drugs have effects on the diverse systems of the body. The physician needs to conduct a careful systems review of the patient receiving these drugs to ascertain the presence and severity of such adverse effects. This section reviews the systemic adverse effects and is organized in a manner similar to the way a physician approaches a review of the patient's systems: skin; special sense organs; liver; cardiovascular system; reproductive system; and, finally, the hematologic, endocrine, and immune systems. Each chapter reviews the significant drug reactions and discusses the frequency, clinical presentations, diagnosis, management, and prevention of these dysfunctions.

20

Adverse Cutaneous Reactions

Matcheri S. Keshavan

Some of the more conspicuous and distressing side effects of psychotherapeutic drugs involve skin. Dermatological side effects are common and can pose problems in diagnosis and management. Establishing cause-effect relationship in drug-induced skin reaction in a given patient is also problematic, since the patient may be simultaneously receiving more than one drug and or other agents (e.g., cosmetics) that could cause similar reactions. Furthermore, skin reactions have been seen during placebo treatment also. In a given case, the diagnosis of drug-induced cutaneous reaction is made by the temporal relation between drug ingestion and emergence of the reaction, and disappearance of the reaction on drug discontinuation. In difficult cases, drug rechallenge may be needed for a firm diagnosis.

PATHOPHYSIOLOGY

Adverse cutaneous reactions could result from several mechanisms. Immunological mechanisms may be mediated by immune complex dependent reactions (e.g., serum sickness), IgE dependent hypersensitivity reactions (e.g., urticaria), and cell-mediated cytotoxic reactions (e.g., contact dermatitis). Nonimmunological mechanisms are exemplified by phototoxicity (e.g., phenothiazine-induced light sensitivity), metabolic effects (e.g., phenothiazine-induced pigmentation), or worsening of preexisting disease (e.g., lithium-worsening psoriasis). In many cases, the precise pathophysiological mechanism(s) remain unclear.

This chapter reviews common dermatological problems with psychotherapeutic medications (Table 1). Rarer and secondary cutaneous manifestations such as drug-induced lupus are discussed elsewhere in this book (Chapter 28). This topic has been well reviewed by Appleton, Shader, and Dimascio (1971), Bruinsma (1973), and Warnock and Knesevich (1988).

ANTIPSYCHOTIC AGENTS

Antipsychotic agents frequently cause uncomfortable skin reactions both acutely and long-term. These maybe of three types: allergic skin reactions, photosensitivity reactions, and pigmentary changes.

Allergic Reactions

Like most other drugs, antipsychotic drugs can cause maculopapular rashes. These are erythematous and itchy and appear on the face, neck, chest, and limbs

Table 1 Dermatological side effects of psychotherapeutic drugs

Side effects	Drugs
Pruritus	Amoxapine, maprotiline, TCAs, antipsychotics, MAOIs
Urticaria	Antipsychotics, carbamazepine, trazodone, TCAs, Maprotiline, disulfiram, amantadine, amphetamines, MAOIs
Exanthematous eruptions	Carbamazepine, maprotiline, TCAs, trazodone, fluoxetine, alprazolam, disulfiram, amphetamines, lithium
Exfoliative dermatitis	Crbamazepine, TCAs, antipsychotics, lithium
Erythema multiform	Carbamazepine, mianserin, fluoxetine
Stevens-Johnson syndrome	Carbamazepine
Fixed-drug eruptions	Carbamazepine, chloral hydrate, chlordiazepoxide, disulfiram
Purpuric eruptions	Crbamazepine
Photosensitivity	Carbamazepine, TCAs, mianserin, chlordazepoxide
Vestibulobullous eruptions	Carbamazepine
Toxic epidermal necrolysis	Amoxapine, carbamazepine, mianserin
Lichen planus-like eruptions	Carbamazepine
Acneiform eruptions	TCAs, maprotiline, lithium
Pigmentary changes	Amitriptyline, imipramine, antipsychotics
Alopecia	Carbamazepine, trazodone, lithium
Increased sweating	TCAs, CNS stimulants
Pretibial edema	Lithium

typically between 2–10 weeks after beginning treatment. The reactions occasionally may be severe and manifest with exfoliative dermatitis, localized or generalized urticaria, and erythema multiforme; angioneurotic edema, which can be life-threatening, has also been described. The signs and symptoms promptly subside with discontinuation of the drug (Simpson, Pi, & Sramek, 1981). However, since phenothiazines are slowly excreted, the rashes may persist, or even appear to get worse for some time after the drug is discontinued. For this reason, a treatment-free interval of about a week should be allowed before beginning another antipsychotic drug. The possibility of a "cross allergy" to the newly started drug should also be kept in mind (Appleton, Shader, & Dimascio, 1971). Treatment of the skin reactions with antihistamines and topical steroids may be required. Alternative treatments of the psychotic illness, perhaps with nonantipsychotic drugs or electroconvulsive therapy, may also have to be considered.

Photosensitivity Reactions

Photosensitivity reactions are thought to result from interactions between certain drugs and light energy resulting in the formation of free radicals with adverse biological effects. Low-potency antipsychotic agents, most commonly chlorpromazine, result in increased sensitivity to sunlight in about 3% of patients (Winkelman, 1957). The reactions are commonly seen in areas of the body exposed to sunlight and resemble sunburns in appearance. The patients should be advised to limit exposure to the sun; the use of a sunscreen (usually containing paramino benzoic acid, or PABA) and protective clothing are also helpful. The patients should be educated about the side effects, especially during the summer months. Switching to a high-potency antipsychotic drug may be necessary.

Cutaneous Pigmentation

Chronic treatment with antipsychotic drugs, especially low-potency drugs such as chlorpromazine, often result in discoloration of the skin, particularly in areas of skin exposed to the sun. Alteration in melanin metabolism by phenothiazines has been postulated as a causative mechanism (Ban & Lehmann, 1965). The skin changes may range from a tan color to a purple; pigmentary changes in the eye are frequently associated. The frequency of this reaction is about 1% (Ban & Lehmann, 1965) and may be dose-related; long-term treatment with high-dose antipsychotics should therefore be avoided. Avoidance of excessive exposure to direct sunlight is important. The pigmentary skin changes cause a good deal of cosmetic embarrassment; reducing the antipsychotic drug dose and switching to high-potency agents are helpful measures. Haloperidol and other high-potency antipsychotic drugs are less prone to cause this side effect (Shader & Dimascio, 1970).

ANTIDEPRESSANTS

Urticarial Rashes

Urticarial rashes are erythematous, itchy wheals. When the dermal and subcutaneous tissues are swollen, this reaction is termed angioedema, which could be life-threatening. These reactions are seen rarely after treatment with tricyclic antidepressants (TCAs) and occur within hours or days of the drug administration.

Maculopapular or Exanthematous Rashes and Petechiae

These are occasionally seen and respond well to discontinuation of the drug and may occasionally disappear with continued therapy. Symptomatic treatment with antihistamines and topical steroids is helpful. The skin reactions are typically seen during the first 2 months after starting treatment. Allergic reactions are more often seen with amitriptyline than imipramine. Among the second generation of antidepressants, fluoxetine has been reported to be associated with cutaneous rashes in 48 of 1,378 patients studied (Wernicke, 1985); maprotiline has been reported to cause cutaneous rashes twice as frequently as imipramine and amitriptyline (Wells & Gelenberg, 1981).

Other Antidepressant-Related Reactions

Acneiform eruptions have been noted with maprotiline therapy (Ponte, 1982). Exfoliative dermatitis has rarely been described during imipramine and desipramine treatment (Powell, Koch-Weser, & Williams, 1968). Erythema multiform is an acute, self-limited inflammatory disorder of the skin often associated with constitutional symptoms and has been seen during treatment with mianserin (Cox,

1985) and fluoxetine (Wernicke, 1985). Photosensitivity reactions have been described with most TCAs (Medical Economics Company, 1989). These reactions are caused by the drug interacting with light energy and are seen in light exposed body parts such as face, neck, hands, and arms. Usually, photosensitivity reactions are benign and disappear on drug discontinuation. Toxic epidermal necrolysis, characterized by a rapidly developing generalized erythematous rash with epidermal necrosis that is potentially life-threatening, has been reported in association with mianserin (Camisa & Grines, 1983).

ANTIMANIC AGENTS

Lithium

A wide range of skin reactions have been associated with lithium treatment (Deandrea, Walker, Menmauer, & White, 1982). Maculopapular rashes, typically pruritic and erythematous, may appear during the first month of therapy. This reaction can sometimes progress to severe dermatitis. Acneiform eruptions may also appear or worsen during lithium treatment. Follicular eruptions are also common, occurring in up to one third of the patients. They may be a symptomatic and transient. Psoriasis may be induced or exacerbated by lithium. Other potential cutaneous effects of lithium include exfoliative dermatitis, hyperkeratotic papules, xerosis cutis, cutaneous anesthesia, and alopecial of the scalp.

Many of the above skin reactions respond to symptomatic treatment, including dosage reduction, In severe and persistent cases, discontinuation of lithium and institution of alternative treatment such as cabamazepine may be warranted. If tetracycline is used for treatment of acne, lithium levels should be monitored closely since the former drug may lead to retention of lithium.

Carbamazepine

About 3–17% of patients treated with carbamazepine report exanthematous skin reactions (Warnock & Knesevich, 1988). Typically, skin reactions begin within 2–20 weeks after beginning treatment. The rash responds promptly to stopping the drug (Harman, 1967). Skin rashes have been thought to be often associated with concomitant bone marrow suppression; blood counts should therefore be closely monitored in such patients (Killian & Fromm, 1968).

Stevens-Johnson syndrome, a severe, bullous form of erythema multiform involving the eyes, mouth, and genital tract, has been described during carbamazepine treatment (Bottinger, Strandberg, & Westerholm, 1975; Coombes, 1965).

Exfoliative dermatitis is characterized by a generalized erythematous reaction with scaling, usually accompanied by constitutional symptoms such as fever, and can often be diagnosed by a patch test (Camarasa, 1985). The drug should be immediately discontinued.

Fixed drug eruptions have been described with carbamazepine (Shuttleworth & Graham-Brown, 1984). These are sharply defined circular, pruritic lesions usually measuring 2–3 inches, which recur at the same site each time the drug is administered. The eruptions slowly disappear after the drug is discontinued and may leave residual hyperpigmentation.

ANXIOLYTIC AGENTS

Use of benzodiazepines has been associated with allergic cutaneous rashes, although this is rare. Allergic skin reactions were observed in 21 of 236 depressive patients receiving alprazolam (Feighner et al., 1983). In contrast, 26 of 243 patients receiving a placebo in this study also developed allergic skin reactions. This illustrates the difficulty in drawing conclusions about cause-effect relationships in studies of drug-related reactions. Photosensitivity reactions have been rarely described during treatment with chlordiazepoxide (Luton & Finchum, 1965). Erythematous rashes, maculopapular rashes, and erythema multiform also have been reported during propranolol administration (Robinson, 1975).

DISULFIRAM

Allergic cutaneous rashes occur in 1–5% of patients on disulfiram. Typically, this consists of pruritic, vesicular erythematous eruptions over the face and extremities. Usually the reaction is transient and is helped by giving the daily dose at bedtime (Gerrein, Roseberg, & Monohan 1973). Acneiform reactions, fixed drug eruptions, and flushing are also seen.

REFERENCES

Appleton WS, Shader RI, Dimascio A, 1970: Dermatological effects. In: *Psychotropic drug side effects*, edited by RI Shader and A Dimascio. Baltimore: Williams and Wilkins.

Ban TA, Lehmann H E., 1965: Skin pigmentation, a rare side effect of chlorpromazine. *Canadian Psychiatric Association Journal, 10,* 112–124.

Bottinger LE, Strandberg I, Westerholm B, 1975: Drug-induced febrile mucocutaneous syndrome: With a survey of the literature. *Acta Medica Scandinavica, 198,* 229–233.

Bruinsma W, 1973: A guide to drug eruptions. *Excerpta Medica.*

Camarasa JG, 1985: Patch test diagnosis of exfoliative dermatitis due to carbamazepine. *Contact Dermatitis, 12,* 49.

Camisa C, Grines C, 1983: Amoxapine: A cause of toxic epidermal necrolysis (letter). *Archives of Dermatology, 119,* 709–710.

Coombes BW, 1965: Stevens-Johnson syndrome associated with carbamazepine (Tegretol). *Medical Journal of Australia, 1,* 895–896.

Deandrea D, Walker N, Menmauer M, White K, 1982: Dermatological reactions to lithium: Critical review. *Journal of Clinical Psychopharmacology, 2,* 199–204.

Feighner JP, Aden GC, Fabre LF, Rickels K, Smith WT, 1983: Comparison of alprazolam, imipramine, and placebo in the treatment of depression. *Journal of the American Medical Association, 249,* 3057–3064.

Gerrein J, Roseberg CM, Monohan V, 1973: Disulfiram maintenance in outpatient treatment of alcoholism. *Archives of General Psychiatry, 28,* 793–802.

Harman RRM, 1967: Carbamazepine drug eruptions. *British Journal of Dermatology, 79,* 100–101.

Killian FM, Fromm GH, 1968: Carbamazepine in the treatment of neuralgia. *Archives of Neurology, 19,* 129–136.

Luton EF, Finchum RN, 1965: Photosensitivity reaction to chlordiazepoxide. *Archives of Dermatology, 91,* 362.

Medical Economic Company, 1989: *Physician's Desk Reference, 43rd Edition.* Oradell, New Jersey: Author.

Ponte CD, 1982: Maprotiline-induced acne (letter). *American Journal of Psychiatry, 139,* 141.

Powell WJ, Koch-Weser J, Williams RA, 1968: Lethal hepatic necrosis after therapy with imipramine and desipramine. *Journal of the American Medical Association, 206,* 642–645.

Robinson BF, 1975: Drugs acting on the cardiovascular system. In: *Meyler's side effects of drugs, Volume 8,* edited by MNG Dukes (pp. 442–445). New York: Excerpta Medica.

Shader RI, Dimascio A, 1970: *Psychotropic drug side effects, clinical and theoretical perspectives.* Baltimore: Williams and Wilkins.

Shuttleworth D, Graham-Brown RAC, 1984: Fixed drug eruption due to carbamazepine. *Clinical and Experimental Dermatology, 9,* 424–426.

Simpson GM, Pi EH, Sramek JJ, 1981: Adverse effects of antipsychotic agents. *Drugs, 21,* 138–151.

Wells BG, Gelenberg AJ, 1981: Chemistry, pharmacology, pharmacokinetics, adverse effects and efficacy of the antidepressant maprotiline hydrochloride. *Pharmacotherapy, 2,* 255–265.

Wernicke JF, 1985: The side effect profile and safety of fluoxetine. *Journal of Clinical Psychiatry, 46*(3, section 2), 59–67.

Warnock JK, Knesevich J, 1988: Adverse cutaneous reactions to antidepressants. *American Journal of Psychiatry, 145,* 425–430.

Winkelman NW, 1957: An appraisal of chlorpromazine. *American Journal of Psychiatry, 113,* 961–971.

21

Otologic and Ophthalmologic Side Effects

John R. DeQuardo and Rajiv Tandon

Side effects associated with psychotropic medications are commonplace and can occupy significant amounts of a clinician's time. Complications involving the eye and ear tend to be relatively innocuous when compared with those involving other organ systems. In this chapter, we discuss side effects of psychotropic medications that involve the eye and ear, their cause (if known), and a plan of management to minimize or eliminate them. Side effects that result from interactions of psychotropic medications with other types of medication are beyond the scope of this chapter and are not discussed.

OTOLOGIC SIDE EFFECTS

Complications involving the ear are considerably less common, less severe than those affecting the eye, and by and large are wholly reversible. As a result, patient discomfort and noncompliance are relatively insignificant. This section details the medications associated with otologic side effects on a class by class basis, and where possible individual "offenders" will be identified.

Antidepressants

The most commonly reported otologic side effect associated with antidepressants is tinnitus. It has been seen with the tricyclics amitriptyline (Miles, 1980), imipramine (Racy & Ward-Racy, 1980), protriptyline (Evans & Golden, 1981), and doxepin (Golden, Evans, & Nau, 1983); with the monoamine oxidase inhibitors (MAOIs) tranylcypromine (*Physician's Desk Reference*, 1989) and phenelzine (Glass, 1981); and with the atypical agents fluoxetine (Feighner, 1985) and trazodone (Golden & Evans, 1987). It can occur at therapeutic and subtherapeutic doses, with a frequency of up to 1% (Tandon, Grunhaus, & Greden, 1987). A number of causes for this complication have been proposed, including aminergic overstimulation (Miles, 1980); adrenergic/cholinergic system alteration causing changes in blood flow or autonomic imbalance leading to vasospasm and subsequent end-organ ischemia (Evans & Golden, 1981); endolymphatic hydrops (Gordon, 1987); and direct neurotoxicity to the auditory, tympanic, and/or chorda tympani nerves (Golden et al., 1983). Management begins with the determination of antidepressant serum level, followed by observation for 2 or 3 weeks; most cases will resolve or diminish considerably over this time (Tandon et al., 1987). Should tinnitus persist, reduction in dose or a change to an agent of a different class is advised (Laird & Lydiard, 1989). Although tinnitus is bothersome, few patients discontinue therapy as a direct result of it.

Diminished auditory acuity, including transient deafness (Barker, Ashcroft, & Binns, 1960), impaired tone discrimination (Smith, Reece, & Kaufmann, 1972), and hypacusis (Fleischhauer, 1982) have been reported in association with imipramine, nortriptyline, and amitriptyline, respectively. These symptoms may occur at subtherapeutic doses. Proposed mechanisms include direct neurotoxicity and capillary microcirculation dysregulation resulting in cochlear circulatory disturbance. Discontinuing the drug and changing to another antidepressant were associated with resolution of these side effects.

Bupropion, a new nontricyclic antidepressant, has "auditory disturbance" listed as a possible side effect on the package insert. No information is given regarding the relationship to dose or a possible mechanism of action. Its occurrence appears to be uncommon. Should problems arise, another agent should be substituted.

Anticonvulsants

Carbamazepine has been associated with tinnitus (package insert); it is benign and reversible. No data exist on its relationship to dose or serum level; etiology is unclear. Given its structural similarity to the tricyclic agents, possible etiological mechanisms for tinnitus proposed for them may apply in the case of carbamazepine. Should tinnitus pose a significant problem, carbamazepine serum level should be checked. Appropriate courses of action include reducing the dose to achieve a lower (yet therapeutic) level and observing the response—or changing to another agent such as valproate.

The package insert also lists hyperacusis as a side effect associated with the use of carbamazepine. No mention is made of a possible mechanism, time course, or relationship to serum level. If hyperacusis is troubling to patients despite therapeutic levels, one should consider using another medication.

Dizziness and/or vertigo have been attributed to the anticonvulsants with psychiatric indications (e.g., carbamazepine and valproic acid). These may be more likely to occur at higher serum levels. The etiological mechanism is unknown. If a patient experiences significant problems with dizziness or vertigo, it would seem prudent to determine the serum level of the medication and, if possible, reduce it or switch to another agent.

Benzodiazepines

Triazolam has been reported to be associated with hyperacusis and "pressure on the ears" (van der Kroef, 1979); the relationship to dosage was not given. The symptoms subsided within several days of discontinuation of the drug. No mention was made of a possible mechanism of action. Discontinuation of the medication is indicated should patients be severely troubled by these symptoms. Tinnitus has also been reported as a rare side effect (frequency less than 5%) of triazolam, according to the package insert. No speculation as to mechanism or relationship to dose is offered. Should this problem be extremely troubling, the drug should be withdrawn or replaced if needed.

Virtually all of the benzodiazepines have been associated with dizziness and/or vertigo; the mechanism and relationship to dosage are unclear. If severe, the drug involved should be withdrawn or replaced.

Lithium

Brown (1976) lists dizziness and vertigo as side effects associated with the use of lithium; a relationship to serum level is suggested. Dizziness is regarded as "innocuous," occurring at therapeutic levels. On the other hand, vertigo is associated with toxic levels. Brown does not speculate about a possible mechanism underlying these problems. They may be related to neurotoxic effects or hypotension secondary to lithium-induced polyuria, or they may be idiopathic. If these problems develop, one should immediately check a lithium level and, if high, reduce the patient's dose. Should these difficulties persist at therapeutic serum levels, a change to another medication must be considered.

Others

Dizziness/vertigo has been associated with a number of medications used in psychiatric practice, including antipsychotics, psychostimulants, anticholinergics, amantadine, calcium channel blockers, beta-blockers, disulfiram (when combined with alcohol), opioid antagonists, and clonidine. In some cases (e.g., beta-blockers), it is likely that this complication results from hemodynamic effects of the medications; in others, the precise mechanism is unknown. When this problem is disabling, it is best to adjust the dose downward and optimize blood pressure; when adjustment is not possible or unsuccessful, a change in medication is indicated.

Antihistamines have been associated with a number of minor otologic side effects (*Physician's Desk Reference*, 1989), including acute labyrinthitis, dizziness/vertigo, and tinnitus, which resolve on discontinuation. No mention is made of etiology or relationship to dose. If these complications occur and interfere with patient function, the drug should be discontinued.

Tinnitus and ear aching and congestion have been reported as side effects of naltrexone, an oral opioid antagonist, with a frequency of less than 1% (McEvoy, 1988). No speculation as to mechanism or relationship to dose is offered. Should these effects be extremely troubling to a patient, naltrexone should be withdrawn.

The *Physician's Desk Reference* (1989) lists tinnitus as a possible side effect of the calcium channel blocker diltiazem, occurring in less than 1% of patients. The relationship to dose and cause are not stated, although alteration of inner-ear hemodynamics is a possibility. Given that tinnitus is reversible, the drug should be withdrawn, and replaced if necessary, should the problem persist.

Beta-adrenergic blocking agents (e.g., propranolol) have been associated with oculomucocutaneous syndrome, an idiosyncratic immune reaction that affects skin, ears, eyes, and mucous and serous membranes; it is often seen with a positive antinuclear antibody (Frishmann, Silverman, Strom, Elkayam, & Sonnenblick, 1979). This syndrome is most commonly seen with practolol. Otologic involvement can result in deafness secondary to serous otitis media. The authors recommend immediate drug withdrawal and substitution of another beta-blocker, if needed.

OPHTHALMOLOGIC SIDE EFFECTS

Psychotropic drug side effects that involve the eye are far more common, and carry a significantly higher morbidity, than those affecting the ear. This section will detail, on a class-by-class basis, the ocular complications associated with psychotropic drug use. As in the previous section, information on relationship to dose, mechanism, time course, and management options is presented.

Antidepressants

Virtually all antidepressant medications of all classes are associated with some degree of antimuscarinic (anticholinergic) activity; notable exceptions are bupropion and fluoxetine. The tricyclic agents are the most likely to produce this effect, with amitriptyline most potent and desipramine least potent in this respect (Snyder & Yamamura, 1977). As a result, they have the potential to cause blurred vision, mydriasis, and restricted accommodation. These side effects are related to dose, but there is a ceiling effect in that they do not worsen as the dose is increased above the lower end of the therapeutic range. There tends to be an adaptation that occurs as a patient is maintained on the medication for several weeks. Corrective lenses, however, may be necessary for improving near vision in some patients. If the visual disturbance is intolerable or interferes with a patient's livelihood, a switch to a less anticholinergic drug (e.g., desipramine) or one without this property (e.g., fluoxetine) should improve the situation. An associated complication, related to the anticholinergic potential of antidepressants, is precipitation of acute narrow-angle glaucoma. Because of pupillary dilatation in susceptible patients, aqueous humor drainage from the anterior chamber is impeded with a resultant increase in intraocular pressure and subsequent pain and visual impairment; this situation constitutes a medical emergency. Glaucoma patients may be treated with these agents if their condition is under adequate medical control, and they have close ophthalmologic follow-up. In tenuously controlled patients, the physician should consider a nonanticholinergic drug.

Fraunfelder and Meyer (1982) mention that diminished lacrimation has been associated with tricyclic antidepressants (although amoxapine has been related to increase lacrimation); in severe cases this diminution can result in keratoconjunctivitis. The phenomenon is thought to be more common in patients with a preexistent deficiency in tear production. Given that tear production is partially under cholinergic control, the anticholinergic activity of these agents is a likely etiology. Relationship to dose is not specified. Switching to a less anticholinergic or nonanticholinergic medication will likely improve this symptom and prevent possible corneal damage.

Tricyclic antidepressants have been noted to cause transient paresis/paralysis of the extraocular muscles, with subsequent gaze impairment and/or diplopia. This side effect is especially likely with amitriptyline at toxic doses (Mladinich & Carlow, 1977; Smith, 1979). Physostigmine treatment may reverse this, which suggests that impaired cholinergic transmission may be the cause. In less severe cases, dosage adjustment or withdrawal of the medication should result in return to a normal function. Bupropion has also been rarely associated with diplopia, according to the package insert; no relationship to dose or mechanism is specified.

Other antidepressant-related ocular side effects (associated with either tricyclic antidepressants or MAOIs) include decreased corneal reflex, dyschromatopsia, toxic amblyopia, blepharospasm, oculogyric crisis, photophobia, and nystagmus. The latter has been mentioned in association with hypertensive crises with MAOIs (*Physician's Desk Reference,* 1989) and bupropion (package insert). Although no specific references were made to dose or mechanism, return to normal function is likely after the offending drug is withdrawn or replaced (Fraunfelder & Meyer, 1982).

Antipsychotics

Chlorpromazine has long been associated with ocular changes, with the first reports surfacing in 1963 (Greiner & Berry). Since that time, many authors (e.g., Prien, DeLong, Cole, & Levine, 1970; Siddall, 1965, 1968) have elaborated on these changes, generally seen in patients treated with high doses over long periods of time (i.e., several years). The structures involved include the lens, cornea, and possibly the retina. Changes in the lens include anterior capsule granular deposits of white to yellow-brown color; when mild they are disc-shaped and when advanced, stellate. Corneal alterations include granular deposits on the posterior surface when mild, which spread to the stroma when more severe. Changes involving the anterior cornea have also been reported, consisting of clouding in the area of the palpebral fissure (epithelial keratopathy). From 15–79% of patients taking chlorpromazine demonstrate corneal and/or lens involvement, probably depending on dose and duration of therapy. Retinal involvement consists of pigment deposits that range from fine granules to clumps; approximately 20% of patients are affected. Patients who develop skin pigmentation are at increased risk of developing ocular changes. Whether or not these changes produce impairment of visual acuity is controversial. It appears that with the accumulation of multiple structural abnormalities vision can be impaired, but this outcome tends to be the exception rather than the rule. Some authors suggest that there is a relationship between dose and time on the medication; for example, Siddall (1965) proposes that a dose of 800 mg for more than 20 months is toxic. The composition and mechanism of these pigmentary changes are complex. It is hypothesized that melanin forms complexes with phenothiazine derivatives (chlorpromazine and possibly perphenazine), possibly facilitated by light exposure (McClanahan et al., 1966). The involvement of light is by no means certain, in that pigment deposits are observed to involve the skin, gastrointestinal tract, and conjunctiva. These changes appear to be either very slowly reversible or nonreversible. The best management thus involves prevention (i.e., using the lowest possible dose for the shortest possible time); if long-term therapy is envisioned, use of a nonaliphatic phenothiazine antipsychotic is advised.

Perphenazine has been shown to produce corneal opacities in dogs, similar to but less frequently than those seen with chlorpromazine (Barron et al., 1972). Cornea and lens deposits/pigmentation were mentioned by Fraunfelder and Meyer (1982) in association with long-term thioxanthene derivative use; rare retinal pigmentation was also noted. Prien et al. (1970) examined the long-term ocular effects of trifluoperazine (80 mg per day) and found the incidence to be quite low (less than 3%). When phenothiazines are taken during pregnancy, ocular pigmentary changes have been reported to occur in the infant. Ulberg, Linquist, & Sjostrand (1970) reported on these melanin-like deposits; their occurrence is considered rare.

Thioridazine is also associated with pigmentary changes involving the lens and cornea; however, its most frequent site of toxicity is the retina. Siddall (1968) reported that this medication, in doses over 800 mg per day for 3 to 5 years, resulted in granular pigment deposits in the cornea (stroma, especially Descmet's membrane) and lens. These changes were similar to those involving other organs and believed to be reversible. By far the most common and troubling pigmentary changes associated with thioridazine involve the retina (Cameron, Lawrence, & Olrich, 1972; Weekley, Potts, Reboton, & May, 1960). Fine granular deposits that coalesce into clumps over time can be seen via ophthalmoscopy. There is pigmentary epithelium and choreocapillaris damage that accompany the deposits. In addition, these changes result in abnormal fluorescein angiography and electroretinography; the latter, elaborated on by Miyata, Imai, Ishikawa, and Nakajima (1980), can be seen in the absence of pigmentary changes in patients on relatively low doses (e.g., 400 mg per day). Clinical correlates include diminished visual acuity, peripheral vision, and scotoma (predominantly central annular type). The clinical and anatomic changes are (generally) irreversible and may progress even after the drug is stopped. Dosages resulting in these deficits are usually greater than 800 mg per day for periods of months to years; there have been reports of pigmentary changes on lower doses for longer exposure times (Heshe, Engelstoft, & Kirk, 1961). Thus, cumulative dose may be an important variable. The percentage of all patients exposed to this medication who develop ocular complications is unknown.

Davidorf (1973) suggested a possible mechanism behind the retinal damage. Phenothiazines, including thioridazine, are selectively absorbed by uveal tract melanin; this absorption is associated with alterations in enzymes in Müller cells and photoreceptors, possibly including succinic dehydrogenase (a cellular phosphorylating enzyme). Changes in the activity of this enzyme could result in impaired amino acid incorporation and rhodopsin formation with subsequent cellular destruction; rods would be affected more than cones. Other hypotheses (Giannini & Mahar, 1980) include increased free-radical destruction of rods resulting from decreased ability of melanin to protect them secondary to complexing with thioridazine and direct receptor toxicity by the drug. Given the high potential for substantial impairment with the use of high-dose thioridazine, the manufacturer's recommended maximum dose of 800 mg per day must be adhered to strictly. In addition, patients should have, when possible, pretreatment and yearly follow-up ophthalmological exams so that retinal changes can be detected early and the drug discontinued or replaced where indicated.

Thioridazine has also been associated with chromatopsia. Davidorf (1973) presented a case in which a patient on relatively high doses (450–1800 mg per day) complained of "red vision"; she also suffered from classic thioridazine retinopathy. In another case (Giannini & Mahar, 1980) "yellow vision" occurred on low doses (75 mg per day) and was unrelated to retinal changes; fundoscopic exam was normal. Before this report, chromatopsia had only been observed in association with retinopathy, and indeed was considered a prodromal symptom. These authors suggest that the mechanism behind this side effect may be interference with retinal integrity by the processes mentioned earlier. Because this symptom may accompany or predict retinopathy, medication should be discontinued in patients complaining of chromatopsia.

Antipsychotics, like antidepressants, are associated with anicholinergic effects—low-potency agents (e.g., thioridazine, clozapine) more so than high-potency agents (e.g., haloperidol). The symptoms associated with cholinergic blockade include blurred vision, decreased lacrimation, restricted accommodation, and mydriasis. Indeed, complete reversible pupillary paralysis has been associated with pimozide (Crawford, 1971). The incidence of iridocycloplegia with thioridazine has been estimated to be less than 1% (Reboton, Weekley, Bylegna, & May, 1962). Here too there appears to be a ceiling effect, and above a certain dosage (usually the lower end of the therapeutic range) these symptoms do not worsen significantly and in fact seem to diminish with time if patients are maintained on a static dose. Management techniques in this instance are the same as those recommended for antidepressants.

Acute narrow-angle glaucoma can also be precipitated by antipsychotic medications; this complication is more likely to occur with the low-potency agents. Mechanism and management are the same as those delineated in the section on antidepressants.

Antipsychotic agents have been associated with oculomotor palsies, subsequent gaze impairment, and diplopia (Simpson, Pi, & Sramek, 1981). Although a specific mechanism was not suggested, it is possible that, as with the antidepressants, impaired cholinergic transmission may underlie this problem. These symptoms are reversed by drug withdrawal.

An additional oculomotor difficulty found with the use of antipsychotic agents is oculogyric crisis, most commonly associated with acute dystonia; this difficulty is more common early in treatment or after an increase in dosage, and in young male patients. It also tends to be more common with high-potency agents (e.g., haloperidol) than with low-potency agents (e.g., chlorpromazine). The mechanism underlying this problem is thought to involve dopamine-acetylcholine imbalance in the nigrostriatal system brought about by antipsychotic-induced postsynaptic dopamine receptor blockade. Low-potency drugs are less likely to cause problems in this regard because low affinity for dopamine receptors, coupled with high anticholinergic activity, results in less neurotransmitter imbalance; the high-potency drugs are more likely to cause this problem because they possess the opposite receptor properties. Treatment with intravenous anticholinergic drugs (e.g., benztropine, diphenhydramine) is rapidly effective in most cases; if the crisis proves refractory, intravenous diazepam is often an effective alternative. Oculogyric crisis can be avoided by starting with low doses and by providing oral antiparkinson medications as outlined in Chapter 8.

Other ocular side effects associated with antipsychotic medications include corneal edema, night blindness, toxic amblyopia, haloes around objects, photosensitivity, papilledema, Stevens-Johnson syndrome (which can leave permanent corneal scarring), and optic atrophy (Fraunfelder & Meyer, 1982). No specific mechanisms are proposed. One can expect resolution of these problems, in most cases, after the drug is withdrawn. Stevens-Johnson syndrome can rarely be fatal.

Anticonvulsants

Carbamazepine has been associated with oculomotor disturbances including transient ophthalmoplegia (Mullally, 1982; Noda & Umezaki, 1982) oculogyric crisis (Berchou, 1979), nystagmus (Sullivan, Rumack, & Peterson, 1981), downbeat nystagmus and oscilopsia (Chrousos et al., 1987), and diplopia. These problems are usually (although not always) seen when carbamazepine is given in toxic doses or in combination with other anticonvulsants. Chrousos et al. (1987) reported two cases of downbeat nystagmus (primary position vertical jerk nystagmus, fast phase downward, usually exacerbated by lateral or downward gaze) associated with high-normal serum carbamazepine levels. Patients complained of rhythmic jumping of their visual field. These authors proposed several possible mechanisms, including (1) imbalance of vestibulocerebellar connections resulting in inappropriate tonic vertical vestibuloocular signals that generate slow upward eye drift and corrective downward saccades; (2) pursuit system deficits; and (3) loss of vestibulocerebellar inhibition of upward otolith-ocular reflexes. The authors suggest that when a patient develops downbeat nystagmus, serum level must be determined and the dose lowered. If the problem persists, further work-up should be carried out (i.e., magnetic resonance imaging, [MRI] scan), since this symptom is common in structural lesions at the craniocervical junction. In the majority of cases these side effects will disappear with discontinuation of the drug; an appropriate alternative should be instituted where needed.

Diplopia and nystagmus have also been reported in association with valproic acid use. These complications are rare and are likely to disappear with discontinuation; the mechanism is unknown. It seems prudent to check serum levels and, if high, lower the dose; if side effects persist, the physician should stop the drug and, if needed, switch to a different medication.

Visual disturbances (i.e., blurred vision, "spots before eyes") have been reported in association with both carbamazepine (Pellock, 1987) and valproic acid (McEvoy, 1988). These disturbances can occur at both therapeutic and toxic doses. In neither case is the mechanism clear, although, with carbamazepine (as mentioned later), retinotoxicity may underlie these complications. Again, the physician needs to determine the serum level of these agents, consider lowering the dose, or discontinue and replace it when this strategy is ineffective.

Nielsen and Syversen (1986) reported two cases of retinotoxicity associated with carbamazepine that manifested with diminished visual acuity and scotomata. These symptoms were accompanied by retinal pigment epithelium degeneration (observable via ophthalmoscopy) and abnormal fluorescein angiography. The dosages ranged from 600 mg to 1,000 mg per day, producing supratherapeutic serum levels in one case. Visual disturbances and retinal abnormalities improved after the drug was discontinued; visual-evoked potentials and electroretinography were essentially normal. The authors suggested that carbamazepine-induced impairment of the barrier function of pigment epithelium may have caused the observed changes. They mention that given the structural similarities of carbamazepine to thioridazine, it may have similar toxic effects on pigment epithelium in some patients. In individuals who develop visual symptoms while taking this medication, serum level must be determined and ophthalmologic consultation should be considered, if indicated the dosage should be lowered or the drug discontinued.

Additional complications of carbamazepine use include conjunctivitis, cataracts, ocular teratogenic effects, and papilledema (Fraunfelder & Meyer, 1982). These complications are all considered rare; the latter is mentioned only in the context of overdose. No etiological mechanism is specified. Response to drug withdrawal is unknown. In light of the possibility of teratogenicity, its use in pregnancy should be carefully considered (see Chapter 5).

Lithium

Exophthalmos, both unilateral and bilateral, has been linked to the use of lithium in maintenance treatment of bipolar affective disorder (Segal, Rosenblatt, & Eliasoph, 1973). This complication was seen in patients with and without thyroid abnormalities. It tended to improve with cessation of the medication. Lithium levels ranged between 0.7 and 1.2 mEq/L. Other related ocular abnormalities included chemosis and episcleral edema; there was no evidence of "malignant" exophthalmos. Mechanisms cited by the authors as possible causes of exophthalmos included direct lithium effects on retroorbital tissue; lithium-related effects on the hypothalamus, pituitary, or thyroid gland resulting in excess thyroid hormone activity/availability; production of altered thyrotropin molecules by lithium-treated patients; lithium acting as a trigger or cofactor in susceptible patients; and lithium-mediated interference with an endogenous enophthalmic agent. Patients in whom exophthalmos occurs need ophthalmologic evaluation and follow-up. Should it be severe or associated with other severe side effects (despite therapeutic blood levels), lithium should be discontinued and replaced when indicated.

Lithium has been associated with papilledema, usually in the context of pseudotumor cerebri. Lobo, Pilek, and Stokes (1979) reported a case in which lithium used to treat bipolar affective disorder produced this syndrome after 11 months of therapy. Lithium levels ranged from 0.7 to 1.2 mEq/L; there were no symptoms of toxicity. Subjective difficulty was limited to blurred vision; however, plotted visual fields indicated bilaterally enlarged blind spots. Work-up, including skull x rays, brain scan, CT scan, physical and neurological exams, EEG, and lumbar puncture (without record of opening pressure), was unremarkable. The patient's visual symptoms and fundoscopic abnormalities improved with discontinuation of lithium and treatment with dexamethasone, but recurred when lithium was reinstituted. No etiological mechanism was proposed; however, pseudotumor cerebri has been ascribed to a disturbance in cerebrospinal fluid dynamics (production, circulation, and/or absorption) that is currently not well understood. It is prudent to perform fundoscopic exams before starting lithium and yearly thereafter, as well as whenever patients complain of visual disturbance. Any evidence of papilledema requires discontinuation of lithium pending the outcome of neurological consultation.

Blurred vision and transitory blindness have been seen in patients receiving lithium (Fraunfelder & Meyer, 1982), usually at toxic levels (i.e., 2.0 mEq/L or greater). These authors suggest that the blindness probably results from problems at the cortical level; no cause for blurred vision is mentioned. Should these symptoms occur, an immediate blood level determination is indicated. If high, the dose should be adjusted accordingly; if there is no improvement, the drug should be stopped. These problems will, in most cases, resolve after discontinuation of lithium.

Downbeat nystagmus has been noted in association with lithium administration (Rosenberg, 1989; Williams, Troost, & Rogers, 1988) in the absence of other demonstrable pathology. It begins from months to years after initiation, with dosages in the therapeutic range (900 mg per day; no blood levels reported). No speculation about mechanisms underlying this complication was offered by either author. This troubling side effect may gradually resolve after the drug is discontinued; in some cases, however, it may persist for years. If stopping the medication is unsuccessful, and the visual disturbance disabling, valproic acid may be effective in reducing nystagmus. This complication may be minimized or avoided by early detection through clinical examination of extraocular movements (downbeat nystagmus is often worsened by having the patient look down and out) before treatment and yearly thereafter. When patients treated with lithium complain of visual instability ("jiggling" of the eyes), lithium level should be determined and a neuroophthalmological consultation considered.

A number of other side effects have also been associated with the use of lithium, including nystagmus (horizontal and vertical), scotoma, oculogyric crises, photophobia (Fraunfelder & Meyer, 1982), impaired accommodation in up to 10% of patients (McEvoy, 1988), and chemosis and episcleral edema (Segal et al., 1973). These complications may occur at therapeutic blood levels. No etiologic mechanisms are specified. If any of these problems should arise, a lithium level should be determined and the dose adjusted accordingly. If this action is unsuccessful in relieving the symptom, lithium should be withdrawn or, if possible, replaced.

Benzodiazepines

Lutz (1975) reported conjunctival hypersensitivity in association with the use of diazepam. In doses of 5 to 10 mg patients experienced burning and light sensitivity that began within 30 minutes, lasted approximately 4 hours, and subsided within 24 hours. The symptoms resolved completely after discontinuation of the drug and were improved with tetrahydrozoline eye drops. No speculation about mechanisms was made. If this problem arises, discontinuation of diazepam or change to another medication is suggested; however, it should be noted that cross sensitivity with other benzodiazepines is possible.

Benzodiazepines have been associated with many adverse effects, probably reflecting the high frequency and diverse uses for which they are prescribed. These included decreased (blurred) vision, photosensitivity, decreased corneal reflexes, impaired accommodation, dyschromatopsia, diplopia, abnormal electrooculograms, precipitation of narrow-angle glaucoma, and lens deposits (Fraunfelder & Meyer, 1982). These side effects can occur at therapeutic doses. Diazepam is the medication most frequently implicated; however, it is likely that any drug in this class has the potential to produce these difficulties. Van der Kroef (1979) mentioned hyper- and hypoaesthesia for light associated with triazolam; no mention is made of dosage or time course. In these cases the etiology is unknown. If any of these symptoms occur and cause significant patient discomfort, the dosage should be decreased. If decreasing dosage does not alleviate the problem, the medication should be withdrawn or replaced.

Disulfiram

Rainey (1977), in a review of disulfiram toxicity, cited two potential ocular complications: optic neuritis and nystagmus. The former occurs after months of therapy at doses of 250 to 500 mg per day. It can manifest with visual disturbance and enlargement of the blind spot; fundoscopic exam reveals hyperemia and edema of the disk. Symptoms resolve 1–3 weeks after discontinuation. The author suggests periodic evaluation of blind spot size, especially in workers exposed to carbon disulfide. In addition, it would be prudent to perform pretreatment fundoscopic examinations on all patients, and yearly examinations thereafter. Should visual disturbances occur during therapy, in the absence of alcohol exposure (a disulfiram-alcohol reaction is associated with blurred vision), withdrawal of the medication is suggested.

Psychostimulants

The psychostimulant drugs in current psychiatric use—pemoline, d-amphetamine, and methylphenidate—have all been associated with ocular difficulties (Fraunfelder & Meyer, 1982; McEvoy, 1988). Pemoline has been associated with oculomotor disturbances, including oculogyric crisis, nystagmus, and decreased vision. d-Amphetamine has been linked to narrow-angle glaucoma because of drug-induced mydriasis, blurred vision, impaired accommodation and convergence, and chromatopsia. Administration of methylphenidate has resulted in impaired visual acuity, Stevens-Johnson syndrome, and mydriasis leading to narrow-angle glaucoma. Mechanisms of action are not suggested by the authors; however, increased sympathetic activity leading to pupillary dilatation probably underlies the exacerbation of glaucoma. All of these side effects can occur at therapeutic doses and resolve with discontinuation of the offending agent. The use of these medications in patients known to have narrow-angle glaucoma is contraindicated.

Antiparkinsonian Drugs

The antiparkinsonian drugs in common use in psychiatry fall into two categories: anticholinergic and presynaptic dopamine-releasing drugs. The former includes trihexyphenidyl, biperiden, procyclidine, and benztropine, and the latter is limited to amantadine; each class is considered separately.

The most prominent difficulties seen with anticholinergic agents are a result of antimuscarinic effects (blurred vision, impaired accommodation, and mydriasis precipitating narrow-angle glaucoma). These effects occur at therapeutic doses, can be additive with the antimuscarine effects of other medications, and are eliminated by drug withdrawal. Accommodation problems may be treated with a long-acting, topical, ocular anticholinesterase (e.g., echothiophate iodide). Use of these agents in patients with glaucoma is appropriate if the condition is under good medical control. An additional complication of anticholinergic drug use is possible retinal pigmentary changes (Fraunfelder & Meyer, 1982); this association is questionable.

The incidence of ocular complications with amantadine is about 1% (McEvoy, 1988), including decreased acuity, oculogyric crisis, photosensitivity, keratitis, and mydriasis, which may precipitate narrow-angle glaucoma. These complications are dose-related and disappear on drug withdrawal; the mechanism of action is unclear.

The greatest difficulty in managing side effects related to the antiparkinsonian drugs as used in psychiatry may be determining which agent is responsible. The medications with which they are most often used (antipsychotics) can cause the same ocular complications, and in most cases the effects are additive. Systematic single-drug dosage adjustment and/or withdrawal is recommended in this situation to ferret out the offending agent.

Other Drugs

Several cardiovascular medications have found their way into psychiatric practice, including beta-blockers, calcium channel blockers, and clonidine, (an alpha-2 adrenergic receptor agonist). Beta-adrenergic blocking agents, as mentioned earlier, have been associated with oculomucocutaneous syndrome (Frishman et al., 1979), an immune-mediated disorder that can manifest with conjunctivitis and keratitis and result in blindness; eye changes can take, on average, 2 years to arise. These authors recommend immediate drug withdrawal at the earliest sign of the disorder (e.g., rash, conjunctivitis) and change to another beta-blocker. This class of medication has also been related to numerous other side effects, including impaired vision, teichopsia, Stevens-Johnson syndrome, decreased tear production with resultant dryness and eye pain, diplopia, exophthalmos (in withdrawal), and extraocular muscle paralysis and ptosis resulting from myasthenic neuromuscular blockade (Fraunfelder & Meyer, 1982; McEvoy, 1988). In most cases these problems resolve with drug withdrawal; the exact relationship to dose and timing and the etiological mechanism(s) are unknown.

Calcium channel blockers (e.g., verapamil) have been shown to produce ocular side effects in less than 1% of patients. Verapamil produces blurred vision and rotary nystagmus when used i.v. (McEvoy, 1988). Diltiazem is associated with amblyopia (*Physician's Desk Reference, 1989*). Nifedipine use has been accompanied by eye pain (Coulter, 1988) and dose-dependent periorbital edema—thought to be secondary to arteriolar dilatation and subsequent increased capillary hydrostatic pressure (Tordjman, Rosenthal, & Bursztyn, 1985). Other than as stated, the cause and relationship to dose and timing of these difficulties are unknown; in the majority of cases they are reversible. Should these side effects develop, discontinuation or substitution for another agent is suggested.

Lastly, clonidine has been associated with decreased vision, diplopia, miosis, keratoconjunctivitis, dry eyes, exacerbation of glaucoma, and retinal degeneration and pigmentary changes (Fraunfelder & Meyer, 1982). In addition, electrooculographic abnormalities that may reflect retinal changes caused by the drug have been demonstrated in some patients (Turacli, 1974). Retinal abnormalities have been seen in animal studies and may be related to the concentration of clonidine in the choroid; the changes are correlated with dose and amount of light exposure. The ocular complications of clonidine use, with the possible exception of retinal changes, are reversible; the relationship to dose and timing is unclear. Caution is recommended when using clonidine in patients with glaucoma; McEvoy (1988) recommends periodic ophthalmological evaluation in clonidine-treated individuals.

Three additional classes of medication have found their way into psychiatric practice: antihistamines, opioid antagonists, and thyroid hormones. The antihistamines in most frequent use are hydroxyzine, diphenhydramine, and cyproheptadine. They are used for anxiolysis, treatment of antipsychotic-related parkinsonism, and appetite enhancement, respectively. Fraunfelder and Meyer (1982) list numerous reversible ocular side effects, including decreased visual acuity, impaired accommodation, diplopia, photosensitivity, anisocoria, nystagmus, decreased lacrimation, and mydriasis. The relationship to dose is not stated. Most of these difficulties are the result of antimuscarinic effects. The drug involved should be withdrawn if any of these problems cause severe discomfort; caution is advised when used in patients known to have glaucoma.

The most commonly used opioid antagonist is the orally active agent naltrexone. Ocular side effects are limited to blurred vision, photosensitivity, and eye pain, occurring with a frequency of less than 1% (McEvoy, 1988). The relationship to dose and etiologic mechanism is unknown. These difficulties are reversible, and drug discontinuation is recommended if they persist.

Thyroid hormones have found a place in the treatment of affective disorders. Their ocular complications are decreased vision, diplopia, extrocular muscle dysfunction, exophthalmos, and optic neuritis/atrophy (Fraunfelder & Meyer, 1982). The majority of these problems have not been reported in several years and may have been related to the preparation rather than the hormone itself. If any of these complications develop, the drug should be withdrawn and replaced with an equivalent alternative preparation.

REFERENCES

Barker PA, Ashcroft GW, Binns JK, 1960: Imipramine in chronic depression. *Journal of Mental Science, 106,* 1447–1449.

Barron CN, Murchison TE, Rubin ML, Herron W, Muscarella M, Birkhead H, 1972: Chlorpromazine and the eye of the dog VI. A comparison of phenothiazine tranquilizers. *Experimental and Molecular Pathology, 16,* 172–179.

Berchou RC, 1979: Carbamazepine-induced oculogyric crisis. *Archives of Neurology, 36,* 522.

Brown WT, 1976: Side effects of lithium therapy and their treatment. *Canadian Psychiatric Association Journal, 21,* 13–21.

Cameron ME, Lawrence JM, Olrich JG, 1972: Thioridazine (Melleril) retinopathy. *British Journal of Ophthalmology, 56,* 131–134.

Chrousos GA, Cowdry R. Schuelein M, Abdul-Rahim S, Matuso V, Currie JN, 1987: Two cases of downbeat nystagmus and oscillopsia associated with carbamazepine. *American Journal of Ophthalmology, 103,* 221–224.

Crawford R, 1971: Pupillary paralysis after tranquilizer. *British Medical Journal, 3,* 530–531.

Coulter DM, 1988: Eye pain with nifedipine and disturbance of taste with captopril: A mutually controlled study showing a method of postmarketing surveillance. *British Medical Journal, 296,* 1086–1988.

Davidorf FH, 1973: Thioridazine pigmentary retinopathy. *Archives of Ophthalmology, 90,* 251–255.

Evans DL, Golden RN, 1981: Protriptyline and tinnitus. *Journal of Clinical Psychopharmacology, 1,* 404–406.

Feighner JP, 1985: A comparative trial of fluoxetine and amitriptyline in patients with major depressive disorder. *Journal of Clinical Psychiatry, 46,* 369–372.

Fleischhauer J, 1982: Acute hypacusic of the inner ear as a result of reduced blood pressure by amitriptyline. *International Pharmacopsychiatry, 17,* 123–128.

Fraunfelder FT, Meyer SM, 1982: *Drug-induced ocular side effects and drug interactions,* 2nd edition. Philadelphia: Lea and Febiger.

Frishman W, Silverman R, Strom J, Elkayam U, Sonnenblick E, 1979: Clinical pharmacology of the new beta-adrenergic blocking drugs. Part 4. adverse effects. Choosing an adrenoreceptor blocker. *American Heart Journal, 98,* 256–262.

Giannini AJ, Mahar PJ, 1980: An unusual ocular complication of thioridazine. *International Journal of Psychiatry in Medicine, 10*, 217–220.

Glass, RM, 1981: Ejaculatory impairment from phenelzine and imipramine, with tinnitus from phenelzine. *Journal of Clinical Psychopharmacology, 1*, 152–154.

Golden, RN, Evans DL, 1987: Imipramine and tinnitus. *Journal of Clinical Psychiatry, 48*, 496.

Golden, RN, Evans DL, Nau CH, 1983: Doxepin and tinnitus. *Southern Medical Journal, 76*, 1204–1205.

Gordon AG, 1987: Imipramine and tinnitus. *Journal of Clinical Psychiatry, 48*, 496.

Greiner AC, Berry K, 1963: Skin pigmentation and corneal and lens opacities with prolonged chlorpromazine therapy. *Canadian Medical Association Journal, 90*, 663–665.

Heshe J, Engelstoft FH, Kirk L, 1961: Retinal injury developing under thioridazine treatment *Nordisk Psykiatrisk Tidsskrift, 15*, 442–447.

Laird LK, Lydiard RB, 1989: Imipramine-related tinnitus. *Journal of Clinical Psychiatry, 50*, 146.

Lobo A, Pilek E, Stokes PE, 1979: Papilledema following therapeutic dosages of lithium carbonate. *Journal of Nervous and Mental Disease, 166*, 526–529.

Lutz EG, 1975: Allergic conjunctivitis due to diazepam. *American Journal of Psychiatry, 132*, 548.

McClanahan WS, Harris JE, Knobloch WH, Tredici LM, Udasco RL, 1966: Ocular manifestations of chronic phenothiazine derivative administration. *Archives of Ophthalmology, 74*, 319–325.

McEvoy GK, 1988: *American hospital formulary service drug information guide*, 30th edition. Bethesda: American Society of Hospital Pharmacists.

Medical Economics, 1989: *Physician's desk reference*, 43rd edition. Oradell: Author.

Miyata M, Imai H, Ishikawa S, Nakajima S, 1980: Change in human electroretinography associated with thioroidazine administration. *Ophthalmologica, 181*, 175–180.

Miles SW, 1980: Amitriptyline side effect. *New Zealand Medical Journal, 92*, 66–67.

Mladinich EK, Carlow TJ, 1977: Total gaze paresis in amitriptyline overdose. *Neurology, 27*, 695.

Mullally WJ, 1982: Carbamazepine-induced ophthalmoplegia. *Archives of Neurology, 39*, 64.

Nielsen NV, Syversen K, 1986: Possible retinotoxic effect of carbamazepine. *Acta Ophthalmologica, 64*, 287–290.

Noda S, Umezaki H, 1982: Carbamazepine-induced ophthalmoplegia. *Neurology, 32*, 1320.

Pellock JM, 1987: Carbamazepine side effects in children and adults. *Epilepsia, 28*(3, supp.), 64–70.

Prien RF, DeLong SL, Cole JO, Levine J, 1970: Ocular changes occurring with prolonged high dose chlorpromazine therapy. *Archives of General Psychiatry, 23*, 464–468.

Racy J, Ward-Racy EA, 1980: Tinnitus and imipramine therapy. *American Journal of Psychiatry, 137*, 371–378.

Rainey JM, 1977: Disulfiram toxicity and carbon disulfide poisoning. *American Journal of Psychiatry, 134*, 371–378.

Reboton J, Weekley RD, Bylegna ND, May RH, 1962: Pigmentary retinopathy and iridocycloplegia in psychiatric patients. *Journal of Neuropsychiatry, 3*, 311.

Rosenberg ML, 1989: Permanent lithium-induced downbeating nystagmus. *Archives of Neurology, 46*, 839.

Segal RL, Rosenblatt S, Eliasoph I, 1973: Endocrine exophthalmos during lithium therapy of manic-depressive disease. *New England Journal of Medicine, 289*, 136–138.

Siddall JR, 1965: The ocular toxic findings with prolonged and high dosage chlorpromazine intake. *Archives of Ophthalmology, 74*, 460–464.

Siddall JR, 1968: Ocular complications related to phenothiazines. *Diseases of the Nervous System, (29,* supp.) 10–13.

Simpson GM, Pi EH, Sramek JJ, 1981: Adverse effects of antipsychotic agents. *Drugs, 21*, 138–151.

Smith KE, Reece CA, Kauffman R, 1972: Ototoxic reaction associated with use of nortriptyline hydrochloride: Case report. *Journal of Pediatrics, 6*, 1046–1048.

Smith MS, 1979: Amitriptyline ophthalmoplegia. *Annals of Internal Medicine, 91*, 793.

Snyder SH, Yamamura HI, 1977: Antidepressants and the muscarine acetylcholine receptor. *Archives of General Psychiatry, 34*, 236–239.

Sullivan JB, Rumack BH, Peterson RG, 1981: Acute carbamazepine toxicity resulting from overdose. *Neurology, 31*, 621–624.

Tandon R, Grunhaus L, Greden JF, 1987: Imipramine and tinnitus. *Journal of Clinical Psychiatry, 48*, 109–111.

Tordjman K, Rosenthal T, Bursztyn M, 1985: Nifedipine-induced periorbital edema. *American Journal of Cardiology, 55*, 1445.

Turacli ME, 1974: The clonidine side effect in the human eye. *Annals of Ophthalmology, 6*, 699–710.

Ulberg S, Linquist N, Sjostrand S, 1970: Accumulation of chorio-retinotoxic drugs in the foetal eye. *Nature, 225,* 1257.

Van der Kroef C, 1979: Reactions to triazolam. *Lancet, 2,* 526.

Weekley RD, Potts AM, Reboton J, May RH, 1960: Pigmentary retinopathy in patients receiving high doses of a new phenothiazine. *Archives of Ophthalmology, 64,* 65–76.

Williams DP, Troost BT, Rogers J. 1988: Lithium-induced downbeat nystagmus. *Archives of Neurology, 45,* 1022–1023.

22

Adverse Hepatic Effects

Matcheri S. Keshavan and K. N. Roy Chengappa

Drugs are an important cause of liver dysfunction, and psychotropic drugs are commonly involved. Drug-induced liver disease accounts for up to 4–7% of all adverse drug reactions reported to central registries (Jones, 1981). In a study of drug-induced hepatotoxicity between 1968 and 1978, psychotropic drugs were second only to halothane as causative agents (Dossing & Andreasen, 1982). Some drugs used in psychiatric practice also induce hepatic enzymes, thus stimulating their own catabolism. This effect is usually nonspecific; thus, the metabolism of other drugs could be enhanced with significant clinical consequences (see Chapter 3).

The liver is the major site of biotransformation of many psychotropic drugs. It is therefore not surprising that hepatic dysfunction could cause the drugs to accumulate and could alter their effect (Sellers & Bendayan, 1987). Liver disease also alters cerebral sensitivity to sedatives and other psychotropic drugs; this accounts for the increased risk of hepatic encephalopathy by sedatives in patients with liver disease.

In this chapter, we focus on the hepatotoxic effects of psychotropic drugs. Phenothiazines and the monoamine oxidase inhibitors are among the most commonly blamed agents. On the other hand, newer antidepressants and benzodiazepines are relatively safe.

PATHOPHYSIOLOGY

Hepatotoxic reactions can be a result of direct toxic effect (e.g., carbon tetrachloride and acetaminophen), or they can be unpredictable and idiosyncratic (e.g., chlorpromazine). The former tend to be dose-dependent, and the latter are not. Idiosyncratic reactions may occur at any time during or shortly following ingestion of the drug. Extrahepatic manifestation such as fever and leucocytosis are sometimes associated with idiosyncratic drug reactions, suggesting immunological mechanisms. However, there is some evidence that even some of the so-called idiosyncratic reactions may be caused by toxicity related to intermediary metabolites (Deanstag, Wands, & Isselbacher, 1991).

DIAGNOSIS

Drug-induced hepatic disease may be clinically asymptomatic, being manifest only by laboratory test results. Therefore, a high index of suspicion is warranted, and liver function tests should be routinely carried out before and periodically during treatment with psychotropic drugs. Furthermore, the clinical picture of drug-induced liver disease is nonspecific, and it is not always easy to rule out non-drug-related causes of hepatic disease (e.g., viral or bacterial hepatitis, choledocholithiasis, or deterioration of preexisting chronic hepatic disease). The temporal relation behind drug initiation and hepatic dysfunction—and the improvement following drug discontinuation—are helpful diagnostic clues. In doubtful cases, rechallenge with the suspected agent may be useful, but it is potentially risky and should be avoided.

ANTIPSYCHOTIC DRUGS

Jaundice and liver function alterations were described during chlorpromazine therapy soon after introduction of this drug (Ebert & Shader, 1970). Transient increases in hepatic enzymes are seen following initiation of treatment with most antipsychotics; these are usually benign and do not necessitate stopping the antipsychotic.

Chlorpromazine is most frequently implicated in hepatotoxicity, since it has been the most widely prescribed antipsychotic and also has been available longer than most other antipsychotic drugs.

Epidemiology

Ishak and Irey (1972) reviewed eight large series involving a total of 12,210 treated patients. Clinical jaundice developed in 149 (1.2%) patients. Elevated liver enzymes were noted in a larger number of patients (22–50%). Jaundice has also been reported in patients treated with thioridazine, fluphenazine, perphenazine, promazine, mepazine, and all the phenothiazine subclasses. Haloperidol has also been implicated in hepatotoxicity. There are no published reports of jaundice caused by thiothixene or other thioxanthene derivatives (*Physcian's Desk Reference,* 1989).

Pathology

Histopathological examination reveals evidence of cholestasis in the canaliculi, hepatocytes, and Kupffer cells. The patterns of cholestasis are centrilobular or central and midzonal. In addition, some degree of inflammation, sinusoidal eosinophilia, and focal necrosis may be seen (Ishak & Irey, 1972). The time course, eosinophilia, and rare occurrence after a single dose point to an immunogenic hypersensitivity reaction. However, it has been suggested that the higher incidence of liver enzyme elevations and necrosis may point to a cytotoxicity mechanism. Both mechanisms may be operative in clinically significant cholestasis independently or acting in concert. Chlorpromazine may form free radicals that inhibit transport systems (Na^+/ K^+-ATPase activity), which in turn may impair biliary flow (Sherlock, 1979). These cytotoxic effects may possibly lead to membrane alterations that then trigger a hypersensitivity response. It has been suggested that the pathology and mechanisms may be the same in haloperidol-induced liver disease.

Clinical Features and Outcome

Typically, jaundice or other evidence of hepatotoxicity appears during the first month after beginning antipsychotic treatment. Phenothiazines are more commonly implicated. Ishak and Irey (1972) confirmed that 36 of the 96 alleged cases of liver disease were chlorpromazine induced. On average, these patients had received 2.78 g of chlorpromazine over a mean of 15 days before treatment. Two thirds of these patients had a prodromal illness for 2–14 days before jaundice, manifest by fever, chills, malaise, fatigue, muscle aches, nausea, vomiting, and bowel alterations. Liver enzymes [aspartate transaminase (AST, formerly SGOT) and alanine transfererase (ALT, formerly SGPT)] were between 50 and 300 Karmen units and most had peripheral eosinophilia. Most patients recovered in 8 weeks, although laboratory values took longer to recover (3–18 months). Rarely, a patient may develop chronic biliary cirrhosis (Ishak & Irey, 1972; Dossing & Andreasen, 1982). The laboratory picture is usually similar to that of obstructive jaundice with elevations in conjugated bilirubin and alkaline phosphatase levels. The hepatotoxic reaction is idiosyncratic and unrelated to age, sex, dosage, or prior hepatic disease.

Treatment

Although some patients may recover despite continuation of the treatment, it is prudent to stop the antipsychotic drug. A nonphenothiazine antipsychotic, such as thiothixene, provides an effective alternative, but treatment resumption should await normalization of liver parameters. Liver function should also be closely monitored after institution of such treatment. The drugs should be used cautiously in patients with already existing liver disease. Patients on antipsychotics who develop fever, jaundice, or flu-like symptoms should have appropriate liver function tests and a complete blood count and differential count (Chapter 28) done promptly.

ANTIDEPRESSANTS

Transient elevations of hepatic enzymes and alkaline phosphatase without jaundice are not uncommon during treatment with tricyclic antidepressants (TCAs). Cross-sensitization between TCAs may occur. Cholestatic jaundice also has been rarely observed (less than 0.5–1% of patients treated). This reaction is similar to that seen with antipsychotic drugs. Except for a few reports of mild hepatic reactions, the newer tetracyclic antidepressants have not been reported to be associated with hepatotoxicity (Bass & Ockner, 1990); this may change as the use of these agents increases.

Hepatotoxicity has been reported with monoamine oxidase inhibitors (MAOIs) as well, and this led to the withdrawal of Iproniazid from the market. Among the currently used MAOIs, phenelzine and isocarboxazid have a higher incidence (5%) of hepatotoxicity as compared to tranylcypromine (1%) (Sheehan, Claycomb, & Kauretas, 1980–1981). Biochemically and histopathologically, MAOI-induced jaundice results in changes very similar to viral hepatitis.

CARBAMAZEPINE

Carbamazepine use has been reported to be associated with cholestatic and hepatocellular jaundice. The usual pattern is one of a granulomatous reaction, and this may be very slow to resolve (Levy, Goodman, Van Dyne, & Summer, 1981).

Both allergic and direct toxic effects caused by carbamazepine and its metabolites have been implicated. Concurrent administration of enzyme-inducing agents such as phenobarbital and phenytoin is likely to enhance the risk of hepatotoxicity. Management of carbamazepine-induced hepatitis is essentially supportive. Periodic monitoring of ALT, AST, alkaline phosphatase, and bilirubin levels about every 3 months is advisable during treatment with carbamazepine.

DISULFIRAM

Kristensen (1981) has reported 11 cases of suspected disulfiram hepatotoxicity. In 5 of these cases, the hepatotoxicity recurred on rechallenge. Most cases occur within 2 months of beginning treatment, and women are more often affected (Bass & Ockner, 1990). The liver changes are reversible if the drug is promptly discontinued.

NALTREXONE

Naltrexone is an opioid antagonist that is used orally primarily in the treatment of opiate addition. When used in therapeutic doses (50 mg/day), this drug appears to be safe; however, in large doses naltrexone has the potential to be hepatotoxic (Mitchell, Knopman, Levin, & Morley, 1985). Elevations in serum transaminases have been observed in up to 20% of patients treated with naltrexone in doses between 200–300 mg/day.

BENZODIAZEPINES

Benzodiazepines are relatively free of hepatotoxic potential. However, a few reports exist of cholestasis associated with chlordiazepoxide, diazepam, and flurazepam (Fang, Ginsberg, & Dobbins, 1978; Zimmerman, 1978).

VALPROIC ACID

Valproic acid is being increasingly used as an alternative in the treatment of bipolar disorders. Treatment with valproid acid is frequently associated with minor elevations of transaminases (ALT, AST). These appear to be dose-related. Elevations in serum bilirubin and alteration in other liver function tests may occasionally occur and should raise suspicion of serious hepatotoxicity (Willmore, Wilder, Bruni, & Villarreal, 1978). Fatal hepatic failure has been described with use of valproic acid. The incidence is highest during the first 6 months of treatment; children under the age of 2 years and those with hepatic disease are at increased risk. Laboratory tests may not always be abnormal. When hepatic dysfunction is suspected, the drug should be immediately discontinued. Screening for liver function before and periodically after beginning valproic acid treatment is important in prevention of this complication.

REFERENCES

Bass NM, Ockner RK, 1990: Drug induced liver disease. In: *Hepatology,* edited by D Zakin and T Boyer, Philadelphia, PA: W. B. Saunders.

Deanstag JL, Wands JR, Isselbacher KJ, 1991: Acute hepatitis. In: *Harrison's principles of internal medicine,* edited by JD Wilson, Braunwald E, Isselbacher KJ, Petersdorf RG, Martin JB, Fauci AS, and Root RK. New York: McGraw-Hill.

Dossing M, Andreasen B, 1982: Drug-induced liver disease in Denmark. An analysis of 572 cases of hepatotoxicity reported to The Danish Board of Adverse Reactions to Drugs. *Scandinavian Journal of Gastroenterology, 17,* 205–211.

Ebert MH, Shader RI, 1970: Hepatic effects. In: *Psychotropic drug side effects,* edited by RI Shader and A Dimascio. Baltimore: Williams and Wilkins.

Fang MH, Ginsberg AL, Dobbins WO III, 1978: Cholestatic jaundice associated with flurazepan hydrochloride. *Annals of Internal Medicine, 89,* 363–364.

Ishak KG, Irey NS, 1972: Hepatic injury associated with the phenothiazines. Clinicopathologic and follow-up study of 36 patients. *Archives of Pathology, 93,* 283–304.

Jones JK, 1981: Suspected drug-induced hepatic reactions reported to the FDA's adverse reactions system: An overview. *Seminars on Liver Disease, 1,* 157.

Kristensen M, 1981: Toxic hepatitis induced by disulfiram in alcoholics. *Acta Medica Scandinavia, 209,* 335–336.

Levy M, Goodman MW, Van Dyne BJ, Summer HW, 1981: Granulomatous hepatitis secondary to carbamazepine. *Annals of Internal Medicine, 95,* 64;ne65.

Medical Economics Company, 1989: *Physician's desk reference,* 43rd edition. Oradell NJ: Author.

Mitchell J, Knopman D, Levin AS, Morley JE, 1985: *Gastroenterology, 88,* 1646.

Sellers EM, Bendayan R, 1987: Pharmacokinetics of psychotropic drugs in selected patient populations. In: *Psychopharmacology, the third generation of progress,* edited by HY Meltzer. New York: Raven Press.

Sheehan DV, Claycomb JB, Kauretas N, 1980–1981: Monoamine oxidase inhibitors: Prescription and patient management. *International Journal of Psychiatry in Medicine, 10,* 99–212.

Sherlock S, 1972: Progress report. Hepatic reactions to drugs. *Gut, 20,* 634–648.

Willmore LJ, Wilder BJ, Bruni J, Villarreal HJ, 1978: Effect of valproic acid on hepatic function. *Neurology, 28,* 961–964.

Zimmerman HJ, 1978: *Hepatotoxicity.* New York: Appleton-Century-Crofts.

23

Adverse Cardiovascular Effects

Matcheri S. Keshavan

Psychotropic drugs, notably tricyclic antidepressants (TCAs), have been reported to be responsible for a number of adverse cardiovascular effects. These adverse reactions may occasionally be fatal (Risch, Groom, & Janowsky, 1981). This chapter will review the literature on three areas of concern: postural hypotension caused by a variety of psychotropic drugs, hypertensive reactions mainly noticed in relation to monoamine oxidase inhibitor (MAOI) treatment, and the risk of disturbances of cardiac function caused by psychotropic drugs.

POSTURAL HYPOTENSION

Postural hypotension is defined as a drop in systolic blood pressure of over 20 mm Hg or an increase in pulse rate of over 20 beats per minute. Among the antipsychotic drugs, postural hypotension is most common with aliphatic or piperidine phenothiazines. Preexisting cardiovascular disease, use of large doses, and parenteral administration are predisposing factors. Postural hypotension may manifest as dizziness or lightheadedness and could lead to sudden fainting and falls, often leading to fractures and lacerations. Up to 40% of patients on phenothiazines have this problem (Jefferson, 1974).

About 20% of patients receiving therapeutic doses of imipramine develop postural hypotension. The problem is more frequent with imipramine and amitriptyline, and less common with secondary amine TCAs such as nortriptyline (Roose et al., 1981). Depressed patients are more likely to have this side effect. The use of TCAs has been associated with an increased risk of fractures in the elderly (Ray, Griffin, Schaffner, Baugh, & Melton, 1987) and with precipitation of myocardial infarction and cerebrovascular accidents (Muller, Goodman, & Bellek, 1961). Postural hypotension is also common with MAOIs, although the incidence is variable. This is particularly common when MAOIs are combined with antihypertensives, meperidine, or inhalation anesthetics. The second generation antidepressants such as bupropion and fluoxetine may be less prone to cause postural hypotension.

Pathophysiology

Postural hypotension has been thought to be caused by blockade of alpha adrenergic receptors, which results in increased venous pooling by inhibiting the normal reflex vasoconstriction that occurs on standing. With MAOIs, postural hypotension is thought to be caused by gradual displacement of noradrenaline by indirectly acting amines or "false" neurotransmitters such as octopamine.

Prevention

It is helpful to check postural changes in blood pressure (recumbent and standing) before beginning antidepressants; there is evidence that pretreatment postural hypotension predicts drug-induced postural hypotension (Glassman, Roose, Giardina, & Bigger, 1987). Wherever possible, use drugs that are less prone to cause postural changes, such as nortriptyline or desipramine. A careful history to identify possible predisposing factors such as low salt diet, hypothyroidism, cardiac disease, or concurrent antihypertensive drug use will also help avoid drug-induced hypotension.

Management

Management of postural hypotension has been well reviewed recently by Pollock and Rosenbaum (1987). An important first step in the treatment of postural hypotension is patient education (i.e., informing the patient about the side effect and the need to get up slowly from a recumbent to a seated position). Starting the medication with small doses and increasing slowly will help the patient to cope better with any postural effects. In the elderly, the use of divided doses during the day will help reduce the risk of falls and fractures. The use of elastic stockings can help prevent pooling of blood in the extremities. If the systolic blood pressure falls below 90 mm Hg, it is important to withhold or reduce the dose of the medication. In the event of profound hypotension, one may place the patient in the shock Trendelenberg position (i.e., legs elevated). The use of a footboard or other form of exercise to strengthen calf muscles may also help prevent pooling of blood in the extremities. For older patients who are nutritionally depleted, attention to diet and blood protein concentrations (albumin) is also important.

Although these nonpharmacological measures may temporarily benefit the symptoms of postural hypotension, they may often be insufficient and justify the need for pharmacological approaches. Fludrocortisone has been used as an effective drug in the treatment of antidepressant-induced hypotension. Used orally in doses of .1 to .4 mg per day, this drug benefits many cases of postural hypotension. However, this drug may cause sodium and fluid retention and thus increase the risk of edema, hypertension, and hypokalemia. Additionally, its long-term use is associated with pigmentation changes in the skin and osteoporosis. Salt tables (600–1800 mg b.i.d.) can also be used to treat postural hypotension (Munjack, 1984). However, this should be avoided in patients with impaired cardiovascular or renal functioning, since it may worsen edema and hypertension.

DRUG-INDUCED HYPERTENSION

The simultaneous ingestion of MAOIs and substances containing certain sympathomimetic amines has been known to result in potentially serious hypertensive crises. Commonly referred to as "the cheese reaction," this complication can be caused by concomitant ingestion of certain foods and drugs (Table 1).

Table 1 Foods, beverages, and drugs causing hypertensive reactions with MAOIs

Foods

Cheese[a] with high tyramine content, such as boursalt, blue cheese, cheddar, stilton, mozzarella, romano, and parmesan
Aged meats: chicken liver, fermented sausages (bologna, pepperoni, salami); meat extracts ("Marmite" or "Bovril," etc.)
Fish: pickled herring, dried salted fish
Vegetables: canned or overripe figs, stewed whole bananas[b] or banana peels, avocado, fava, broadbeans, plums, raisins, spinach, tomatoes
Other: yeast products, sour cream, licorice, soy sauce

Beverages[c]

Beer
Wines: chianti, sherry, Italian red wine, Riesling, Sauterne, champagne

Drugs

Sympathomimetic agents such as amphetamine and its congeners, procaine preprations, epinephrine, dopamine, methyldopa, ephedrine, psudoephedrine, phenylephrine, methylphenidate, heterocylic antidepressants, other MAOIs, levodopa, metaraminol, mephenteramine, buspirone, chlorphenitramine
Meperidine and congeners
Additives such as cyclamates and monosodium glutamate

[a]Nonmature cheeses such as cottage cheese, farmer's cheese, and cream cheese are safe.
[b]Banana pulp is allowed.
[c]Clear alcohol such as vodka and white wine are relatively safe.

Pathophysiology

Inhibition of the monoamine oxidase results in accumulation of tyramine, which then circulates peripherally and is taken up by adrenergic nerve terminals. In these terminals, MAOIs have already caused an increased presynaptic concentration of neurotransmitters. Tyramine displaces this norepinephrine causing a excessive pressor response.

Clinical Features

Symptoms begin usually within several hours after ingestion of a contraindicated drug or food substance. The symptoms include headaches, nausea, vomiting, stiff neck, rapid heartbeat, fever, sweating, elevated blood pressure, photophobia, and dilated pupils. The headache is often described by the patient as "the worst headache I have ever experienced." Other symptoms include retrosternal chest pain, breathlessness, and flushing. This complication may occasionally be fatal.

Management

The first step in the management of MAOI-induced hypertensive reaction is to discontinue the MAOI. The other major therapeutic goal is to reduce the hypertension. The traditional treatment of choice has been phentolamine, an alpha adrenergic blocker, used in doses of 2–5 mg IV. The limitations of this treatment include side effects such as angina, nausea, vomiting, diarrhea, and confusion. Chlorpromazine in doses of 100-mg has also been recommended orally in emergency settings. Some advocate that patients on MAOI treatment carry 100 mg tablets of chlorpromazine with them at all times and to take this drug in the event of a severe headache. Since blood pressure could drop precipitously and other side effects such as sedation could ensue, this should be avoided if possible.

MAOI-induced hypertensive crises can also be effectively treated by newer drug treatments used in the treatment of hypertension. Potentially useful treatments include diazoxide 100–150 mg IV given Q 5 to 15 minutes; sodium nitroprusside 200 μg per minute IV given up to 3 mg per kilogram body weight; and nifedipine 10 to 20 mg p.o.

Prevention

MAOI treatment should be avoided in debilitated patients and those with a history of hypertension, cardiovascular disease, or cerebrovascular disease. MAOIs may be of benefit to older patients but should be used with extra caution particularly focused on concerns about postural hypotension and drug-associated hypertensive reactions. Hypertensive reactions are more common with tranylcypromine than with other MAOIs. In patients prone to the reaction, it is helpful to switch to an MAOI less likely to cause the adverse reaction. Patients being started on MAOI should be placed on low tyramine diets for at least 24 hours before initiating therapy and must avoid any over-the-counter cold medications including indirect-acting sympathomimetic drugs such as ephedrine, phenylephrine, or asthma preparations containing epinephrine. When switching from one MAOI to another, at least a 10-day washout period should be observed to minimize the potential risk of hypertensive crises. The same principle would apply to treatment with a TCA. An even longer period of washout is necessary when switching to MAOIs from antidepressants with prolonged halflife such as fluoxetine.

DISTURBANCES IN CARDIAC FUNCTION

Conduction Disturbances

Conduction defects represent the most common adverse cardiac effects caused by psychotropic drugs. Among the antipsychotics, low-potency drugs such as chlorpromazine and thioridazine have significant effects on cardiac conduction. The TCAs, notably tertiary amines such as imipramine and amitriptyline, are associated with the most pronounced conduction effects that can occur at therapeutic plasma concentrations; these are followed by secondary amine TCAs such as nortriptyline and desipramine. MAOIs do not significantly affect conduction. Amoxapine, alprazolam, mianserin, maprotiline, and trazodone appear to be less prone to cause conduction defects at therapeutic doses. Similarly, fluoxetine and bupropion have been considered to be devoid of significant adverse cardiac side effects at therapeutic doses (Halper & Mann, 1988).

Using his bundle electrocardiography (ECG), attempts have been made to isolate the components of AV conduction and evaluate them separately. The atrioventricular nodal conduction is unaffected by TCAs whereas the H-V (intraventricular) conduction is prolonged (see Glassman et al., 1987, for a review). In vitro studies of cultured cardiac cells suggest that TCAs mainly affect the inward sodium current, which mediates the depolarization of the cardiac action potential. This results in prolongation of PR, QRS, and QT intervals.

Electrocardiographic changes with TCAs include increased PR, QRS, or QT interval; depressed or flattened ST segment; T wave changes; and appearance of U waves—changes that resemble the effects produced by quinidine and procainamide. For these reasons, TCAs have been classified as type Ia (quinidine like) antiarrhythmic agents (Giardina et al., 1979; Stoudemire & Atkinson, 1988).

In otherwise healthy subjects, these conduction changes may be benign and do not need to cause concern in therapeutic doses. However, some patients with preexisting cardiac conduction disease may develop further atrioventricular block when treated with tricyclics.

Psychotropic drug effects on cardiac conduction and repolarization have been implicated as a possible cause for some cases of sudden death noticed in patients receiving antipsychotic drugs. Thioridazine has been blamed the most, since this calcium-channel blocking drug often causes ECG changes, notably T wave abnormalities. However, the causal relationship between antipsychotics and the rare occurrence of sudden death in psychiatric patients is not established (Levinson & Simpson, 1987).

Lithium rarely causes significant cardiac effects in therapeutic doses. The most notable effect is suppression of automaticity, especially of the sinus node. ECG changes are common, and include inversion of T waves, appearances of U waves, and QT prolongation; bundle branch block and complete heart block may occur rarely (Crowley & Colodner, 1983).

Cardiac Rhythm

Although it is clear that TCAs are actually potent antiarrhythmic agents similar to those of type I antiarrhythmics such as quinidine, large doses of TCAs can produce ventricular irritability and potential arrthymias (Giardina et al., 1983). Furthermore, in patients with already compromised cardiac function, TCAs may cause premature ventricular contractions or supraventricular or ventricular tachycardias or both. In particular, patients with congenital long QT syndrome and those with Wolff-Parkinson-White (WPW) syndrome (characterized by short PR intervals) are at risk for ventricular arrhythmias included by TCAs.

Torsade de pointes, also known as polymorphic ventricular tachycardia, is a malignant form of ventricular tachycardia that frequently results in ventricular fibrillation. TCAs and phenothiazines are among the common causes of this syndrome.

Cardiac Rate

TCAs and low-potency antipsychotic agents often cause a slight increase in heart rate of about 8–10 beats per minute, but this is rarely of any clinical significance. Preexisting cardiovascular disease, older age, and rapid increase in dose are associated with more frequent occurrence of this side effect. Tertiary amine antidepressants (e.g., imipramine) are more likely to cause tachycardia than secondary amine tricyclics (e.g., nortriptyline and desipramine). Usually, tolerance develops after a few weeks of treatment. The tachycardia probably results from the anticholinergic effects of medications. However, such tachycardia is undesirable in patients with ischemic heart disease because this increases the cardiac oxygen need. Fluoxetine causes a small and clinically insignificant reduction in heart rate.

Ventricular Function

Controlled studies directly assessing ventricular function using radionuclide scans, cardiac catheterization, and Swan-Ganz readings in patients on TCAs have revealed no evidence of impairment. Cardiac function appears to be preserved while taking TCAs, even in patients with congestive heart failure (Glassman et al., 1983).

Prevention and Management

A detailed medical history and physical examination before beginning psychotropic medication will help screen patients potentially at risk for cardiac complications. A routine ECG may not be indicated in all young healthy subjects, but should be carried out in the elderly, those with significant cardiovascular disease, and wherever large doses are used. A careful review of systems is very important before starting antidepressant treatment. Patients should also be educated about the possible side effects. Patients with a prolonged QT interval before treatment with a tricyclic antidepressant are at a higher risk of ventricular tachycardia, and these drugs may cause a further prolongation of the QT interval. Patients with preexisting conduction disease may often develop heart block when treated with tricyclic antidepressants. Isolated first degree A-V block or hemiblock appear to pose less risk than bundle branch block and bifascicular block (Dietsch & Fine, 1990). For this reason, caution should be exercised in using these medications in such patients. The decision to use a heterocyclic antidepressant in such patients should be made in consultation with a cardiologist, and treatment should be closely monitored, preferably in an inpatient setting. Trazodone and fluoxetine may be safer alternatives. Use of relatively small doses and gradual titration with ECG monitoring are important. In patients at higher risk, a detailed cardiac workup including 24-hour holter monitoring, echocardiography, ventriculography, and exercise ventriculography may be required. Monitoring plasma levels of the antidepressant is also quite helpful. In patients whose total TCA level exceeds 500 ng/ml, the dose should be lowered; patients with unusually high blood levels (i.e., 300–500 ng/ml) should be monitored with frequent ECGs (i.e., every 2 days).

If significant cardiac complications have already occurred, the offending medication should be discontinued and alternative, less cardiotoxic medications and/or electroconvulsive therapy should be considered. Concurrent administration of drugs that affect the cardiovascular system, such as anticholinergic agents, should be avoided when posisble. Low-potency antipsychotics and TCAs can have additive adverse effects on cardiac function and should be avoided if possible. If the patient has taken an overdose, immediate hospitalization and continuous monitoring are necessary. Management of TCA overdose is discussed further in Chapter 3.

If patients who already have a second or third degree conduction disturbance have to be treated with a TCA, a permanent pacemaker insertion should be considered before beginning treatment. In such patients, type I antiarrhythmics such as procainamide and disopyramide should be avoided. Appropriate agents useful in the treatment of TCA-induced arrhythmias include lidocaine and phenytoin. Acid imbalance, which may predispose to ventricular irritability, can be corrected by sodium bicarbonate administered intravenously. When severe arrhythmias persist, cardioversion and cardiac pacing may be required.

REFERENCES

Crowley IS, Colodner RM, 1983: The effects of psychotropic drugs on the heart. In: *Clinical essays on the heart,* edited by JW Hurst. New York: McGraw-Hill.

Dietsch JJ, Fine M, 1990: The effect of nortriptyline in elderly patients with cardiac conduction disease. *Journal of Clinical Psychiatry, 51,* 67–67.

Giardina EGV, Bigger JT, Glassman AH, Perel JM, Kantor SJ, 1979: The electrocardiographic and antiarrhymthmic effects of imipramine hydrochloride at therapeutic plasma concentrations. *Circulation, 60,* 1045–1052.

Giardina EGV, Bigger JT, Glassman AH, Perel JM, Saroff AL, Roose SP, Siris SC, Davis JC, 1983: Effects of desmethylimipramine and imipramine on left ventricular function and the ECG: A randomized crossover design. *International Journal of Cardiology, 2,* 375–385.

Glassman AH, Jounson LL, Giardina ECV, Walsh BT, Roose SP, Cooper TB, Bigger JT, 1983: The use of imipramine in depressed patients with congestive heart failure. *Journal of the American Medical Association, 250,* 1997–2001.

Glassman AH, Roose SP, Giardina EV, Bigger JT, 1987: Cardiovascular effects of tricyclic antidepressants. In: *Psychopharmacology, the third generation of progress,* edited by HY Meltzer. New York: Raven Press.

Halper JP, Mann JJ, 1988: Cardiovascular effects of antidepressant medications. *British Journal of Psychiatry, 153*(Suppl 3), 87–98.

Jefferson J, 1974: Hypotension from drugs. *Diseases of the Nervous System, 35,* 66–71.

Levinson DF, Simpson GM, 1987: Serious nonextrapyramidal adverse effects of antipsychotics: Sudden death, agranulocytos, and hepatotoxicity. In: *Psychopharmacology, the third generation of progress,* edited by HY Meltzer. New York: Raven Press.

Muller OF, Goodman N, Bellek S, 1961: The hypotensive effect of imipramine hydrochloride in patients with cardiovascular disease. *Clinical Pharmacology and Therapeutics, 2,* 300–307.

Munjack D, 1984: The treatment of phenelzine induced hypotension with salt tablets: Case report. *Journal of Clinical Psychiatry, 45,* 89–90.

Pollock MH, Rosenbaum JF, 1987: Management of antidepressant induced side effects: A practical guide for the clinician. *Journal of Clinical Psychiatry, 48,* 3–8.

Risch SC, Groom GP, Janowsky DS, 1981: Interfaces of psychopharmacology and cardiology. *Journal of Clinical Psychiatry, 42,* 23–34.

Ray WA, Griffin MR, Schaffner W, Baugh DK, Melton LJ, 1987: Psychotropic drug use and the risk of hip fracture. *New England Journal of Medicine, 316,* 363–369.

Roose SP, Glassman AH, Siris S, Walsh GT, Bruno RL, Wright LB, 1981: Comparison of imipramine and nortriptyline induced orthostatic hypotension: A meaningful difference. *Journal of Clinical Psychopharmacology, 1,* 316–319.

Stoudemire A, Atkinson P, 1988: Use of cyclic antidepressants in patients with cardiac conduction disturbances. *General Hospital Psychiatry, 10,* 389–397.

24

Sexual Dysfunction

Brian K. Toone

Drug treatment may produce unwanted alterations in sexual desire (libido), activity, or performance. Psychotropic drugs (i.e., drugs that are prescribed primarily for their beneficial psychological effects) act principally through the central nervous system (CNS), but also affect the peripheral nervous system (PNS). Effects on either system may powerfully influence sexual function. This chapter will attempt to review and, where possible, explain these side effects in terms of the neuropharmacological actions of the causative drugs. One unique type of sexual dysfunction, priapism, is discussed in more detail in Chapter 25. Drugs, other than alcohol, that are abused for their psychotropic effects, will also be discussed.

It will be apparent that most published work, whether animal, experimental, or clinical, is concerned only with males. It cannot be assumed that observation limited to males applies equally, or even at all, to females.

PHYSIOLOGY OF SEXUAL FUNCTION

Our understanding of the structure and function of the sexual end organs and the neurological and vascular elements that subserve them has increased considerably in recent years. A brief account is essential to any understanding of neuropharmacological actions.

Peripheral Pathways

In humans, sympathetic preganglionic fibers arise in the intermediolateral grey matter of the spinal cord (11th thoracic to second lumbar) and descend via the paravertebral chain ganglia or the prevertebral chain and hypogastric nerves. The fibers then join with parasympathetic presynaptic elements emanating from the second, third, and fourth sacral spinal cord segments (the nervi erigentes) to form the pelvic nerves, which then expand to constitute the pelvic plexus. Some preganglionic fibers make synaptic contact with ganglion cells in the pre- and paravertebral chains; others reach the pelvic plexus before doing so.

The pelvic plexus thus serves as a relay and integration center within which sympathetic and parasympathetic preganglionic neurones make synaptic contact with postganglionic neurones, which then form the cavernous nerve and directly supply the penis. There are also important somatic pathways. The penile skin, prepuce, and glans, which form the afferent limb of the sacral erectile, reflex. Severance of these fibers results in reflex but not psychogenic erectile failure.

Central Mechanisms

The supraspinal pathways have been studied in animal experimental models using lesioning and stimulation techniques, and in humans more inferentially through observations of the consequences of surgery. The preeminence of the medial preoptic-anterior hypothalamic area in the control of sexual activity, penile erection, and ejaculation seems well established. Efferent pathways from the medial preoptic area descend in the medial forebrain bundle through the brainstem, pons, and medulla to occupy an anterolateral position in the spinal cord. Branches project to make contact with autonomic nuclei in the brainstem and lumbosacral centers. Efferent fibers conveying sexual sensation (e.g., orgasmic experience) pass upward in the same tracts and can eventually be traced to the caudal thalamic intralaminar nuclei. Less is known of neurotransmitter/modulator mechanisms, but a peptidergic pathway utilizing oxytocin descends from the supraventricular nucleus through the medial forebrain bundle.

Other higher centers—the medial frontal limbic cortex, anterior thalamus, mamillary bodies, and hippocampus—may also be relevant, but their exact contribution is still uncertain. The amygdaloid complex and adjacent pyriform cortex may have an inhibitory function.

Adequate levels of sex hormone are essential for normal sexual activity, although the significance of variations in levels within the normal range remains uncertain. Sex hormone receptors, situated directly on neuronal membranes and able thereby to modulate neurotransmitter function and synaptic transmission, are widely distributed throughout the nervous system in those areas that subserve sexual behavior.

Central Neurotransmission

Monoamines have received much attention. Again, knowledge is largely derived from animal experimental work and may not necessarily have the same implications for human behavior. The serotonergic pathways would appear to be generally inhibitory, although seminal emission may be enhanced. Clonidine, an alpha-2 adrenergic receptor (i.e., an autoreceptor) agonist, inhibits erections and copulatory activity, whereas yohimbine, an alpha-2 antagonist, increases sexual behavior. These findings suggest that the noradrenergic system may also be inhibitory. Dopamine precursors and other dopamine receptor agonists facilitate male copulatory behavior.

In animal research, opiate and gamma-aminobutyric acid (GABA)-receptor stimulation may produce erection and ejaculation, and antagonists the converse. Oxytocin injected into the hippocampus or paraventricular nucleus causes penile erection. These findings are broadly consistent with the effects of opiate addiction in humans.

Peripheral Neurotransmission

In humans, stimulation of the parasympathetic pathways (bilateral stimulation of the second and third sacral spinal roots) elicits maximum penile erection. Acetylcholine is the transmitter in the ganglia on the sacral parasympathetic pathways to the penis, and there is ample evidence of postganglionic cholinergic fibers and terminal vesicles lying in close proximity to penile blood vessels and corporeal trabecular smooth muscles. However, the mechanisms underlying vasodilatation and, in particular, the transmitters that mediate that response have yet to be clearly established. Pharmacological research, particularly an observed inconsistent response to atropine, suggests that cholinergic pathways may be of secondary importance or may only act in conjunction with a cotransmitter. The neuropeptide vasoactive intestinal polypeptide (VIP) is the leading candidate for this role as it is found in cholinergic ganglia. VIP-immunoreactive nerve fibers are present in the human penis within the smooth muscle of the corpus cavernosus and the penile arteries, and VIP-immunoreactive vesicles are colocalized with cholinergic vesicles. VIP acts directly on smooth muscle causing relaxation or acts synergistically with acetylcholine as in other neuroeffector systems.

The role of the sympathetic pathways is even more complex. Stimulation of sympathetic pathways in the lumbar sympathetic chain, hypogastric, or pudendal nerves produces detumescence, but erection in response to psychic stimulation may persist after surgical interruption of the sacral parasympathetic pathways to the penis, only to be abolished by removal of the lumbar sympathetic or inferior mesenteric ganglia. In the first condition, reflex erection in response to penile manipulation does not occur. Therefore, although reflex erection is dependent on the integrity of the sacral parasympathetic pathways, psychogenic erection is mediated by higher lumbar sympathetic routes.

The role of noradrenergic mechanisms in maintaining penile smooth muscle tone would seem firmly established. Noradrenergic receptors, beta and particularly alpha, are densely distributed in relation to smooth muscle structures. Alpha receptor stimulation, which induces and maintains smooth muscle contraction, can be activated by electrical stimulation and by exogenous drugs and is probably of greater importance physiologically. Postsynaptic alpha-1 and alpha-2 receptors may both be relevant, but presynaptic alpha-2 receptors may also contribute by inhibiting cholinergic and peptidergic pathways. Peptidergic mechanisms may be more directly involved as there is some evidence that neuropeptide Y can act as a cotransmitter with noradrenaline in the enervation of penile structures.

The Vascular Mechanisms Underlying Erection

Penile erection commences when the arterial inflow of blood to the corpora cavernosa exceeds the venous outflow. At full erection the intracorporeal pressure may be greater than the systolic blood pressure, and blood flow through the structures virtually ceases. The contents of the corpora cavernosa are encased within the tunica albuginea, a tough but elastic collagen fibrous sheath, and comprise most essentially a system of sinusoidal spaces fed by the cavernosine arterioles and drained by venules that run between the sinusoidal walls and the tunica albuginea. In the placid state, smooth muscle tonic contraction ensures that the arterioles are vasoconstricted and sinusoidal spaces shrunken. With relaxation, the sinusoids expand, blood is drawn in through the dilating arteriolar system, and the venules are compressed against the relatively noncompliant tunica.

Emission and Ejaculation

The deposition into the posterior urethra of the secretions of the seminal vesicles and prostate gland, accompanied by sperm from the vas deferens, constitutes emission. This is under alpha adrenergic control. For anterograde ejaculation to take place, first the bladder neck must close (to prevent retrograde ejaculation into the bladder), then the external urethral sphincter muscle must relax, and the bulbourethral muscles contract—propelling the semen out of the urethra. The former is also under alpha adrenergic control; the latter is under somatic control, receiving enervation from a branch of the pudendal nerve. Orgasm is essentially a subjective culminating experience accompanying, or occasionally even in the absence of, ejaculation. Its determinants are probably of central origin.

The earlier description of peripheral mechanisms subserving sexual arousal is based principally on observations of the human male. There have been fewer studies of females, but it seems likely that the essential pattern of enervation and neurotransmission will be the same.

THE ACTION OF PSYCHOTROPIC DRUGS

Sexual side effects of psychotropic drugs are reviewed here according to patterns of neurotransmission. Many drugs act on more than one system. In this instance, categorization will be according to the neurotransmitter action deemed responsible for the unwanted effect.

Drugs That Act on the Dopamine System

Animal experimental studies suggest that central dopaminergic activity has a facilitatory effect on sexual behavior. In humans, clinical observations attest to the effect of dopamine agonists on the sexual activity of parkinsonian patients. Although much of this literature is anecdotal, it is also remarkably consistent. The response is unlikely to be solely a result of the mobilizing effect of antiparkinsonian agents. The decline in libido associated with prolactinomas is probably a result of the high levels of circulating prolactin (PRL). The restoration of sexual function with bromocriptine is unlikely to be completely accounted for by the consequent fall in PRL but may reflect bromocriptine's central dopamine agonism. This observation is in keeping with the drug's ability to improve sexual function in uraemic patients.

Dopamine agonists are rarely used in psychiatric practice. For obvious reasons, in management of the psychotic patient, anticholinergic agents are preferred to dopamine agonist therapy in the treatment of drug-induced parkinsonism. Apomorphine has been used in the treatment of alcoholism, and it was the incidental observation that penile erection occurred following sublingual administration (Schlatter & Lal, 1972) that led to a series of studies by Lal and associates that clearly demonstrated that this effect could only be explained by central dopamine agonism. Lal et al. (1987) also reported that a subgroup of impotent patients may be responsive to bromocriptine treatment. Dopamine reuptake inhibitors such as amphetamine and cocaine are widely used as drugs of addiction. There is some limited evidence that in the short term these drugs may enhance penile erectile capacity but that chronic usage may lead to diminution.

Antipsychotic drugs exert their action through postsynaptic dopamine (predominantly DA2) receptor antagonism. A low level of sexual interest and awareness has often been noted in patients treated with these drugs, but interpretation of this observation is rendered more difficult by the extreme and changing mental state of the patients at the time that such drugs are introduced and by the complex action that drugs belonging to this category have on neurotransmitter systems (most exhibit alpha adrenergic, cholinergic, and histaminic antagonism). Any apparent change in sexual interest or activity may also be attributable to the rise in PRL concentrations that invariably follows the introduction of antipsychotic agents.

As well as loss of libido, erectile dysfunction may also occur. This has been attributed to the antialpha, adrenergic activity of antipsychotic drugs. This explanation may not be complete, since it has also been observed to occur with sulpiride and with pimozide, two antipsychotics with relatively specific DA2 receptor antagonism. One double-blind study with chlorpromazine and haloperidol failed to demonstrate any impairment of erectile function, but doses employed were lower than are commonly used in clinical practice (Tennet, Bancroft, & Cass, 1974).

Drugs That Act on the Adrenergic System

The effect on sexual function of central adrenergic neurotransmission remains unclear. The role of alpha adrenergic activity in the control of penile erection, emission, and ejaculation is better understood (see previous discussion). Drugs that oppose alpha adrenergic action may increase penile erectile capacity, and it is this that forms the basis for the highly effective treatment of erectile impotence with intracavernosal papaverine. However, other drugs that contain within their profile antiadrenergic activity may inadvertently induce priapism. These include a number of antipsychotic drugs (e.g., chlorpromazine, thioridazine, fluphenazine, and the atypical antidepressants trazodone and prazosin). Anticholinergic drugs such as benztropine may reverse this effect. Many antidepressants including most of the commonly prescribed tricyclic antidepressants, monoamine oxidase inhibitors (MAOIs), phenelzine, tranylcypromine, and the atypical antidepressant maprotiline may cause erectile impotence. Symptoms appear early in treatment and may be abolished by reduction in dosage. The evidence is based for the most part on case history studies, and one placebo-controlled study of phenelzine and imipramine was unable to confirm earlier reports (Harrison et al., 1985). An early effect (within 2 weeks) of both amitriptyline and mianserin on nocturnal penile tumescence has been demonstrated (Kowalski, Stanley, Dennerstein, Burrows, & Maguire, 1985). Beta-blocking agents that cross the blood-brain barrier such as propranolol may also cause erectile impotence presumably because of a central action.

Alpha adrenergic antagonists predictably impair emission, ejaculation, and the experience of orgasm. A number of psychotropic agents including chlorpromazine, thioridazine, trifluoperazine, phenelzine, amitriptyline and clomipramine have been reported as causing impaired ejaculation. It cannot be assumed that this is exclusively or even predominantly a result of an alpha adrenergic action. Many of these drugs also have an anticholinergic or antidopamine action. Some (e.g., clomipramine) are potent 5-HT reuptake inhibitors, and it is suggested (see next discussion) that these actions may also impair ejaculation. Phenoxybenzamine, an alpha antagonist that was administered by intracavernosal injection to treat erectile impotence but has now been superseded by papaverine, may also delay ejaculation. Of the commonly prescribed antipsychotics, thioridazine is the drug most frequently implicated in ejaculatory difficulties, and these may occur in up to 20% of treated subjects. In low doses it may retard ejaculation; in higher doses orgasm occurs in the absence of ejaculation. The mechanisms that underlie this are unclear but probably involve a failure of emission rather than retrograde ejaculation into the bladder, as was once thought. It may also cause anorgasmia, particularly in women. Beta blockers do not appear to have any adverse effects on emission or ejaculation.

Drugs That Act on the Serotonergic System

A number of commonly prescribed antidepressants including imipramine, amitriptyline, and isocarboxazid may be associated with ejaculatory impairment or failure. By reuptake blockade or MAO inhibition, each of these agents increases levels of 5-HT or noradrenaline. There is reason to believe that the effect on 5-HT is more relevant. The greatest risk is attached to clomipramine, a 5-HT reuptake blocker. In one double-blind study (Monteiro, Noshirvani, Marks, & Lelliott, 1987), 22 of 24 patients treated for 2 weeks became anorgasmic. Males and females were equally affected. Cyproheptadine hydrochloride, a drug with antiserotonergic properties, has been used successfully to reverse anorgasmia induced by imipramine, nortriptyline, and MAOIs. A central action is presumed, since serotonergic mechanisms do not appear to be implicated in the peripheral control of emission and ejaculation. The distribution of serotonergic axons on the medial forebrain bundle enhances ejaculatory activity in experimental animals, but no consistent pattern has emerged from pharmacological studies, perhaps reflecting the complexities of 5-HT receptor subtyping. There is little evidence to suggest that serotonergic agonists or antagonists significantly influence erectile function.

Recently, fluoxetine, a serotonin reuptake inhibitor, has been reported to cause sexual dysfunction (anorgasmia and/or delayed orgasm) in patients treated with this drug (Herman et al., 1990). Fenfluramine, a centrally acting anorectic, releases 5-HT and is reported to decrease libido in a substantial proportion of women treated for obesity.

Drugs That Act on the Cholinergic System

The significance of cholinergic innervation in the control of sexual function remains debatable. The importance of the cholinergic parasympathetic fibers in the nervi erigentes may have been overemphasized. Among those drugs that are associated with erectile and ejaculatory impotence, many (e.g., the tricyclic antidepressants, most antipsychotic drugs to a varying degree) possess an anticholinergic effect along with other neurotransmission actions. The cholinergic drug bethanechol has been successfully used on different occasions to reverse erectile impotence resulting from MAOIs (tranylcypromine, isocarboxazid) (Gross, 1982) and tricyclic antidepressants (protriptyline) (Yager, 1986). Bethanechol may act by opposing the anticholinergic action of tricyclic antidepressants, but MAOIs possess little muscarinic action. Muscarinic receptors have been identified on adrenergic nerve terminals in the penis, and it may be that through "cross-talk" mechanisms of this type the cholinergic system exercises a modulatory role in adrenergic transmission.

Drugs That Act on the Opiate System

Heroin and methadone each may reduce sexual interest, cause erectile difficulties, and delay ejaculation—methadone to a lesser extent than heroin. Drug withdrawal may lead temporarily to increased ejaculatory activity and to premature ejaculation. The administration of the opiate antagonist naloxone in conjunction with yohimbine, an adrenergic alpha-2 antagonist, has been shown to result in full erections in normal volunteers. These findings suggest that in humans the opiate system impairs sexual awareness and responsiveness. The mechanisms by which it does so are unclear. Endocrinological abnormalities, in particular lower plasma luteinizing hormone (LH) and testosterone levels, have been reported by some authorities but not replicated by others.

Other Psychotropic Drugs

Benzodiazepines, although widely prescribed, rarely give rise to sexual difficulties. There is one case report of ejaculatory failure occurring in the course of treatment with chlordiazepoxide and remitting on its withdrawal. More recently, single dose diazepam has been shown to delay female orgasm.

Carbamazepine, an anticonvulsant that has also been shown to have an antidepressant and mood-stabilizing effect may, in common with other commonly prescribed anticonvulsants, lower plasma free testosterone, leading to a compensatory rise in LH (Toone, Wheeler, & Fenwick, 1980). The fall in testosterone is most probably a result of the direct action of the anticonvulsant on the testes. Libido is diminished, sexual activity reduced, and erectile impotence frequently described. Two reports, one a double-blind study, refer to the effect of lithium carbonate on erectile function. The reasons for this are unknown. Marijuana may enhance the subjective experience of sexual activity, but there is little to suggest a pharmacological role.

REFERENCES

Gross MD, 1982: Reversal by bethanechol of sexual dysfunction caused by anticholinergic antidepressants. *American Journal of Psychiatry, 139,* 1193–1194.

Harrison WM, Stewart J, Ehrhardt AA, Rabkin J, McGrath P, Liebowitz M, Quitkin FM, 1985: A controlled study of the effects of antidepressants on sexual function. *Psychopharmacology Bulletin, 21,* 85–88.

Herman JB, Brotman AW, Pollock MH, Falk WE, Biederman J, Rosenbaum JF, 1990: Fluoxetine induced sexual dysfunction. *Journal of Clinical Psychiatry, 51,* 25–27.

Kowalski A, Stanley RO, Dennerstein L, Burrows G, Maguire KP, 1985: The sexual side effects of antidepressant medication: Double blind comparison of two antidepressants in a nonpsychiatric population. *British Journal of Psychiatry, 147,* 13–418.

Lal S, Laryea E, Thavundayil JX, Nir NP, Negrete J, Ackman D, Blundell P, Gardiner RJ, 1987: Apomorphine-induced penile tumescence in impotent patients—preliminary findings. *Progress in Neuropsychopharmacology and Biological Psychiatry, 11,* 235–242.

Monteiro WO, Noshirvani HF, Marks IM, Lelliott PT, 1987: Anorgasmia from clomipramine in obsessive compulsive disorder: A controlled trial. *British Journal of Psychiatry, 151,* 107–112.

Schlatter EKE, Lal S, 1972: Treatment of alcoholism with Dent's oral apomorphine method. *Quarterly Journal of Studies on Alcohol, 33,* 430–436.

Tennet G, Bancroft J, Cass J, 1974: The control of deviant sexual behavior by drugs: A double blind controlled study of benperidol, chlorpromazine, and placebo. *Archives of Sexual Behavior, 3,* 261–271.

Toone BK, Wheeler M, Fenwick PBC, 1980: Sex hormone changes in male epileptics. *Clinical Endocrinology, 12,* 391–395.

Yager J, 1986: Bethanechol chloride can reverse erectile and ejaculatory dysfunction induced by tricyclic antidepressants and mazindol: Case report. *Journal of Clinical Psychiatry, 47,* 210–211.

25

Priapism

Vikram K. Yeragani

Priapism is a painful and prolonged erection unrelated to sexual activity. The word "priapism" comes from Priapus, a mythical Greek god of fertility. Priapism differs from natural erection in that only the corpora cavernosa are involved, and the corpus spongiosum remains flaccid (Sagalowsky, 1982). It is a rare but serious condition that may need surgical intervention and may sometimes lead to erectile impotence. Priapism is known to occur with several psychotropic agents, mainly the antipsychotic group of drugs. Recently, there have been several reports on the association of priapism with the antidepressant trazodone, and this has kindled a renewed interest in iatrogenic priapism.

Priapism has been classified as type I and type II based on the findings of cavernography and arteriography (Bruhlman, Pouliadis, Hauri, & Zollikofer, 1982; Hauri, Spycher, & Bruhlmann, 1983). Type I is caused by the obstruction of the venous outflow from corpus cavernosum associated with painful erection; if not treated early, this may result in fibrosis. In type II, the obstruction of venous outflow is not remarkable, and priapism is caused by an abnormal increase of arterial blood inflow; usually there is no pain and the penis is relatively elastic. Priapism may occur in the proximal corpora cavernosa, and the distal corpora can be flaccid; this condition has been described as partial priapism (Johnson & Corriere, 1980). Technically, priapism also can occur in the female—clitoral priapism has been described (Lozano & Castaneda, 1981).

ETIOLOGY

Of the reported cases of priapism, about 50% have been classified as idiopathic (Darrish, Atassi, & Clark, 1974; Nelson & Winter, 1987). Etiological factors include a direct obstructive effect as produced by local pelvic pathology, blood dyscrasias such as sickle cell disease (which facilitate thrombosis), trauma, neurological lesions, and several pharmacological agents. Priapism has also been described in association with renal dialysis (Singhal, Lynn, & Scharschmidt, 1986) and total parenteral nutrition (Ekstrom & Olsson, 1987). The pharmacological agents known to be associated with priapism include antihypertensive drugs such as prazosin (Bhalla, Hoffbrand, & Phatak, 1979) and labetalol (Abramowicz, 1987); vasodilators such as hydralazine (Abramowicz, 1987), phenoxybenzamine (Funderburk, Philippart, Dale, Cederbaum, & Vyden, 1974), and papaverine (Nellans, Ellis, & Kramer-Levien, 1987); anticoagulants such as heparin (Burke, Smith, Scott, & Wakerly, 1983); and psychotropic agents such as phenothiazines (Kogeorgos & Alwis, 1986), butyrophenones (Morera, Estrada & Velanciano, 1988), and antidepressants such as trazodone (Warner, Peabody, Whitefore, &

Hollister, 1987). The potential for this side effect is estimated to be greater for trazodone than for other drugs for which priapism reports have been submitted to the Food and Drug Administration (Mead-Johnson Pharmaceutical Division, 1985).

PATHOPHYSIOLOGY

A detailed discussion of the physiology of erection appears in Chapter 25. It appears that there is a balance between the adrenergic, serotonergic, cholinergic, and peptidergic mechanisms for the states of flaccidity and erection of the penis. When there is a persistent disruption of this balance—especially due to pharmacological agents—this may result in prolonged erection. However, the final mechanism of priapism may be the obstruction of venous drainage, leading to stagnation of blood, decreased oxygen content, rising viscosity, and sludging, which further impair drainage. Persistence of this condition often leads to fibrosis of the corpora and impotence (Hinman, 1960). Venous stasis and increased viscosity appear to prolong the erection, and factors such as platelet aggregation may also play some role in this regard (Burke et al.; 1983).

PSYCHOTROPICS AND PRIAPISM

Antipsychotic Drugs

Mitchell and Popkin (1982) reviewed the literature on male sexual dysfunction associated with antipsychotic drug treatment and found that these agents are associated with both erectile impotence and priapism. They found 19 cases of priapism in which an antipsychotic drug may have been responsible. Six patients were receiving thioridazine (minimum dose of 100 mg), six were taking chlorpromazine (minimum dose of 100 mg), one received mesoridazine at a dose of 400 mg per day, and one was treated with a single intramuscular injection of 25 mg of chlorpromazine. There have also been reports of an association of priapism with molindone, perphenazine (Mitchell & Popkin, 1982), haloperidol (Morera et al., 1988), triflupromazine, and chlorprothixene (Mitchell & Popkin, 1982; Pryor, 1982).

Priapism during antipsychotic treatment may result from the alpha-adrenergic effects of these drugs. Almost all antipsychotics also possess anticholinergic activity, and this may be one of the reasons why priapism is not a common side effect. As suggested by Lawrence, Stewart, & Frankel (1984), priapism may occur in those patients who are specially sensitive to the alpha-adrenergic blocking effects of these drugs.

Antidepressants

Since the introduction of trazodone in 1982, there have been several reports linking it to priapism (Gershon, Yeragani, & Aleem, 1986; Warner et al., 1987). Warner et al. (1987) report that, as of April 1986, there had been at least 57 cases of priapism in patients whose only medication was trazodone. Their ages ranged from 14–64 years. The dosage of trazodone associated with priapism ranged from

50–400 mg per day, and the treatment duration ranged from 1 day to 18 months. Based on the reports received by the pharmaceutical company, the incidence of priapism while receiving trazodone is between 1 in 1,000 and 1 in 10,000. Approximately one half of the trazodone-related cases resolved spontaneously, one third resolved with surgery, and approximately one eighth of the cases resolved with nonsurgical medical intervention. In the portion of cases that needed surgical intervention, permanent impairment of erectile function or impotence resulted (Mead-Johnson Pharmaceutical Division, 1985).

Several mechanisms have been suggested regarding trazodone-induced priapism. Trazodone has alpha-1 blocking activity, which has been implicated in prazosin and phenothiazine-induced priapism. Trazodone has very little direct anticholinergic activity. There is evidence of cholinergic factors in the pathophysiology of priapism. Bethanechol, a cholinergic agent, is useful in treating erectile impotence secondary to antidepressant treatment (Gross, 1982), and benztropine, an anticholinergic agent, has been found useful in the treatment of priapism secondary to thioridazine (Greenberg & Lee, 1987). In monkeys, m-chlorophenyl piperazine, a serotonin receptor agonist and a metabolite of trazodone, has been found to induce penile erection that was blocked by metergoline, a serotonin antagonist (Aloi, Insel, Mueller, & Murphy, 1984).

Yeragani and Gershon (1987) have reported a patient who developed priapism while taking 30 mg per day of the monoamine oxidase inhibitor, phenelzine. This effect was attributed to the sympatholytic activity of the drug as the patient also developed a hypotensive effect from phenelzine. Yeragani, Aleem, Pohl, & Gershon (1987) have hypothesized that alpha-1 blocking, serotonin, and cholinergic mechanisms may be linked to the pathophysiology of priapism by different psychotropic drugs.

Other Psychotropic Agents

Pryor (1982) has mentioned the possible association of diazepam with priapism. In addition to the drug effects, other factors such as alcohol and cannabis abuse may also play a role in the development of priapism (Winter, 1981).

MANAGEMENT

In cases where priapism is secondary to another disease, treatment should be focused at the primary disease process. Techniques that have been tried with some success are epidural anesthesia (Wasmer, Carrion, Mekras, & Politano, 1981), inhalation of amyl nitrate (Parrillo & Manfrey, 1983), ketamine and physostigmine (Ravindran, Dryden, & Somerville, 1982), benztropine (Greenberg & Lee, 1987), and different surgical techniques such as drainage of corpora cavernosa and cavernous spongiosum shunts.

Brindley (1984) has found that 0.4 mg of metaraminol, an alpha adrenoceptor agonist, caused conspicuous shrinkage of the penis. He has reported a definite improvement of iatrogenic priapism caused by phenoxybenzamine and papaverine in 4 impotent patients treated with metaraminol. Stanners and Colin-Jones (1984) also reported on the effectiveness of metaraminol in treating priapism. They used 1 mg of metaraminol intracavernously followed by another 1 mg 1 hour later.

Other pharmacologic agents such as norepinephrine, phenylephrine, and epinephrine also cause smooth muscle contraction by acting on postjunctional alpha receptors (Padma-Nathan, Goldstein, & Krane, 1986).

Padma-Nathan et al. (1986) have reported in detail the procedure of intracavernosal adrenergic irrigation. After a clinical evaluation, penile doppler pulsations are recorded to make sure that nonischemic priapism exists. The patient is hooked on to a continuous electrocardiographic monitor, and a 19-gauge sterile butterfly needle is inserted laterally into each corpus cavernosum at mid-shaft. Arterial blood gases are performed on the first sample of corporal blood. For corporal aspiration, 1 ml of epinephrine is added to 1 L of normal saline. About 20–30 ml of blood is aspirated and an equal volume of the epinephrine solution is used for irrigation. This cycle is continued only a few times after the onset of corporal drainage. If systemic adrenergic symptoms develop, the aspiration/irrigation procedure should be terminated.

This procedure was very effective in 9 patients with priapism secondary to phentolamine and/or papaverine. There were also no significant complications reported. Padma-Nathan et al. (1986) suggest that if the duration of priapism exceeds 6–8 hours, more conventional shunting techniques should be used. The long duration results from the possible development of corporal ischemia, smooth muscle necrosis, and acidosis. These authors also mention that this technique may be effectively used in idiopathic priapism or priapism secondary to sickle cell anemia within 24–48 hours after the development of the condition.

Lue, Hellstrom, McAnninch, & Tanagho (1986) stress the need for intracorporal blood gas and pressure monitoring to differentiate ischemic (low-flow) from nonischemic (high-flow) priapism. They have described the use of norepinephrine in doses of less than 15 mg at intervals of more than 5 minutes. They recommend a shunt procedure in late and severely ischemic cases. They also suggest larger shunts if the intracorporal pressure remains greater than 50 mm Hg. Kits are now available for the outpatient treatment of priapism (Canton Medical Incorporation, Massachusetts).

Priapism, although a rare side effect of psychotropic medication, should be promptly diagnosed and treated. Early diagnosis and pharmacological treatment appear to prevent the serious sequelae of priapism such as erectile impotence.

REFERENCES

Abramowicz M, 1987: Drugs that cause sexual dysfunction. *Medical Letters, 29,* 65–68.

Aloi JA, Insel TR, Mueller EA, Murphy DL, 1984: Neuroendocrine and behavioral effects of m-chlorophenyl-piperazine administration in rhesus monkeys. *Life Sciences, 34,* 1325–1331.

Bhalla AK, Hoffbrand BI, Phatak PS, 1979: Prazosin and priapism. *British Medical Journal, 2,* 1039.

Brindley G, 1984: New treatment for priapism. *Lancet, i,* 220–221.

Bruhlmann W, Pouliadis G, Hauri D, Zollikofer CH, 1982: A new concept of priapism based on the results of angiography and cavernosography. *Urologic Radiology, 5,* 31–36.

Burke BJ, Smith PJB, Scott GL, Wakerly GR, 1983: Heparin-associated priapism. *Postgraduate Medical Journal, 59,* 332–333.

Darrish ME, Atassi B, Clark SS, 1974: Priapism: Evaluation of treatment regimens. *Journal of Urology, 112,* 92–94.

Ekstrom B, Olsson AM, 1987: Priapism in patients treated with total parenteral nutrition. *British Journal of Urology, 59,* 170–171.

Funderburk SJ, Philippart M, Dale C, Cederbaum SD, Vyden JK, 1974: Priapism after phenoxybenzamine in a patient with Fabry's disease. *New England Journal of Medicine, 190,* 630–631.

Gershon S, Yeragani VK, Aleem A, 1986: Tolerance et pharmacovigilance de la trazodone. *L'Encephale, 12,* 249–257.

Greenberg WM, Lee KK, 1987: Priapism treated with benztropine. *American Journal of Psychiatry, 144,* 384–385.

Gross MD, 1982: Reversal by bethanechol of sexual dysfunction caused by anticholinergic antidepressants. *American Journal of Psychiatry, 139,* 1193–1194.

Hauri D, Spycher M, Bruhlmann W, 1983: Erection and priapism: A new physiopathological concept. *Urologia Internationalis, 38,* 138–145.

Hinman F Jr, 1960: Priapism: Reasons for failure of therapy. *Journal of Urology, 83,* 420–423.

Johnson GR, Corriere JN, 1980: Partial priapism. *Journal of Urology, 124,* 147–148.

Kogerorgos J, de Alwis C, 1986: Priapism and psychotropic medication. *British Journal of Psychiatry, 149,* 241–243.

Lawrence J, Stewart T, Frankel F, 1984: Alpha blockade and priapism. *American Journal of Psychiatry, 141,* 6.

Lozano GBL, Castaneda PF, 1981: Priapism of the clitoris. *British Journal of Urology, 53,* 390.

Lue TF, Hellstrom WJG, McAninch JW, Tanagho EA, 1986: Priapism: A refined approach to diagnosis and treatment. *Journal of Urology, 136,* 104–108.

Mead-Johnson Pharmaceutical Division Newsletter. Evansville, Indiana. October, 1985.

Mitchell JE, Popkin MK, 1982: Antipsychotic drug therapy and sexual dysfunction in men. *American Journal of Psychiatry, 139,* 633–637.

Morera A, Estrada AG, Velanciano R, 1988: Priapism and neuroleptics: A case report. *Acta Psychiatrica Scandinavica, 77,* 111–112.

Nellans RE, Ellis LR, Kramer-Levien D, 1987: Pharmacological erection: Diagnosis and treatment applications in 69 patients. *Journal of Urology, 138,* 52–54.

Nelson JH III, Winter CC, 1987: Priapism: Evolution of management in 48 patients in a 22 year series. *Journal of Urology, 117,* 455–458.

Padma-Nathan H, Goldstein I, Krane RJ, 1986: Treatment of prolonged or priapistic erections following intracavernosal papaverine therapy. *Seminars in Urology, 4,* 236–238.

Parrillo SJ, Manfrey S, 1983: Idiopathic priapism treated with inhalation of amyl nitrate. *Annals of Emergency Medicine, 12,* 226–227.

Pryor JP, 1982: Priapism. *Practitioner, 226,* 1873–1879.

Ravindran RS, Dryden GE, Somerville GM, 1982: Treatment of priapism with ketamine and physostigmine. *Anesthesia and Analgesia, 61,* 705–707.

Sagalowsky AI, 1982: Priapism. *Urologic Clinics of North America, 9,* 255–257.

Singhal PC, Lynn RI, Scharschmidt LA, 1986: Priapism and dialysis. *American Journal of Nephrology, 6,* 358–361.

Stanners A, Colin-Jones D, 1984: Metaraminol for priapism. *Lancet, i,* 978.

Warner MD, Peabody CA, Whitefore HA, Hollister LE, 1987: Trazodone and priapism. *Journal of Clinical Psychiatry, 48,* 244–245.

Wasmer JM, Carrion HM, Mekras G, Politano VA, 1981: Evaluation and treatment of priapism. *Journal of Urology, 125,* 204–207.

Winter C, 1981: Priapism. *Journal of Urology, 125,* 212.

Yeragani VK, Gershon S, 1987: Priapism related to phenelzine therapy. *New England Journal of Medicine, 317,* 117–118.

Yeragani VK, Aleem A, Pohl R, Gershon S, 1987: Neuropharmacological basis of priapism. *Clinical Neuropharmacology, 10,* 93–95.

26

Adverse Hematological Effects

Rudra Prakash

Numerous hematological disturbances, mostly rare and clinically inconsequential, have been reported during various psychopharmacotherapies (Balon & Berchou, 1986). However, the latter may occasionally be complicated by serious and even fatal hematological changes. Therefore, recognition of the psychotropic drug as an etiological factor is imperative. The existing body of knowledge is largely based on various anecdotal reports. Polypharmacy, rare occurrence, and lack of rechallenge data preclude an unconditional acceptance of the findings. Leukocytic changes are the most widely reported hematological side effects of psychopharmacotherapy. Leukocytosis induced by lithium makes it unique among psychotropic drugs insofar as this hematological disturbance has been exploited to therapeutic advantage. Pervasive hematological changes in bone marrow and thrombocytopenia are two other frequent hematological complications of the treatment with psychotropic drugs. Tables 1–6 summarize information as classified according to drugs and hematological disturbances.

ETIOLOGY AND PATHOGENESIS

Although various hematological changes have been observed during psychopharmacotherapy, the etiological mechanisms are little known. The most common and clinically significant blood dyscrasia is agranulocytosis. In vitro studies have led to identification of three basic etiological mechanisms—immune complex, hapten, and autoimmune. The subject has been reviewed by Class (1989). According to the immune complex theory, the drug molecule is too small to be immunogenic on its own. Together with noncellular soluble plasma macromolecules, the drug molecule forms a complex that in turn induces antibodies and binds the drug. The newly formed drug-antibody complex is absorbed by the granulocytes and leads to granulocytopenia. Occasionally the drug-induced antibodies may destroy the hematopoietic precursor cells, resulting in bone marrow suppression. Peripheral and bone marrow destruction are likely caused by the same mechanisms. Another type of neutropenia may be related to the dose of drug. It is caused by interference with protein synthesis or cell replication. The effect is often nonselective and can involve pluripotential stem cells or other cells. Phenothiazines may cause this type of neutropenia. There is some evidence to suggest that a variable degree of cross-tolerance to other drugs within the same family may develop. However, occasionally immunogenic reaction can be evoked by a metabolite and no cross reactivity with the parent compound may exist. For instance, Salama and Mueller-Eckhardt (1986) observed metabolite-specific antibodies in immune hemolytic anemia related to nomifensine.

Table 1 Anemia

Type	Drugs of treatment
Anemia	Clonazepam, fluoxetine, haloperidol, thioridazine, trifluoperazine
Hemolytic anemia	Chlorpromazine, chlorprothixene, perphenazine, prochlorperazine
Megaloblastic anemia	Lithium

Phenothiazines, especially chlorpromazine, have been implicated in hemolytic anemia. Immune complex mechanisms may destroy erythrocytes leading to intravascular hemolysis and renal failure resulting from hemoglobinuria. A rising incidence of immune hemolytic anemia with increasing use of nomifensine led to its withdrawal from the market. The immune complex mechanism was also hypothesized in a case of hemolytic anemia and thrombocytopenia during doxepin therapy. A similar mechanism has been considered in thrombocytopenic processes. Additionally, impairment of platelet-aggregating property has been observed.

The precise mechanism of the granulopoietic effect of lithium is unknown. In vitro studies indicate that lithium promotes granulopoiesis by boosting colony-stimulating activity. Other putative mechanisms include increase in the absolute number of committed granulocyte precursors, direct effect on pluripotential stem cell, and production of colony-stimulating factor. That such granulopoietic effect of lithium may go unarrested to a leukemogenic effect is theoretically plausible but remains unsubstantiated. There are only a few anecdotal reports of leukemia in which lithium has been implicated and the causal relationship is far from established. Mechanisms for the thrombocytopenic effect of lithium are poorly understood. A negative balance for vitamin B12 and folate as a cause of megaloblastic anemia may be related to entrapment of these vitamins by binding proteins, which are released by granulocytes in the presence of lithium. Only one case of megaloblastic anemia related to lithium therapy has been reported (Prakash, 1985).

Barbiturates are notorious for precipitating porphyria. Virtually all antiseizure medications with the exception of bromides have some potential for precipitating an acute attack of porphyria. Generally, these drugs induce aminolevulinic acid synthetase and heme synthesis.

CLINICAL FEATURES AND DIAGNOSIS

Three clinically significant hematological disturbances associated with psychopharmacotherapy are: agranulocytosis, bone marrow suppression, and thrombocytopenia (Tables 1–6).

Table 2 Pervasive disturbances

Type	Drugs of treatment
Aplastic anemia	Chlorpromazine, diphenhydramine, glutethimide, lithium, meprobamate, methyprylon, prochlorperazine, thioridazine
Bone marrow depression	Amitriptyline, desipramine, imipramine, maprotiline, nortriptyline, protriptyline, trimipramine
Pancytopenia	Bupropion, chlorpromazine, chlorprothixene, fluphenazine, perphenazine, prochlorperazine, thioridazine, trifluoperazine

Table 3 Platelets

Type	Drugs of treatment
Thrombocytopenia	Amitriptyline, buspirone, carbamazepine, clonazepam, desipramine, diphenhydramine, ethchlorvynol, imipramine, loxapine, meprobamate, nortriptyline, protriptyline, tranylcypromine, trifluoperazine, trimipramine
Thrombocytosis	Haloperidol, fluoxetine
Thrombocytopenic purpura	Chlorpromazine, chlorprothixene, fluphenazine, glutethimide, meprobamate, methyprylon, perphenazine, propranolol

Agranulocytosis

The incidence of agranulocytosis related to antipsychotic drugs ranges from 0.1 to 1.0 per 1,000. A review of 46 cases revealed that the complication did not appear until 10 or more days after commencement of phenothiazine treatment; in most cases, agranulocytosis developed after at least 20 days of treatment; if it did not develop within the initial 90 days of treatment, agranulocytosis was not likely to develop later (Pisciotta, 1969). Granulocytopenia usually presents clinically with signs of infection such as fever, sore throat, and myalgia. Stomatitis, lymphadenopathy, fatigue, malaise, and pharyngitis may also accompany granulocytopenia. Examination of peripheral blood film will show few or absent neutrophils. Granulocytopenia and agranulocytosis with phenothiazines and the newly introduced antipsychotic, clozapine, are discussed in further detail in Chapter 28.

Bone Marrow Suppression

Clinically, psychotropic drug-induced anemia may present with fatigue, pallor, lassitude, palpitation, breathlessness, bleeding tendency, and signs of infection or jaundice in case of hemolysis. Pancytopenia or aplastic anemia is the main hemato-

Table 4 White blood cells

Condition	Drugs of treatment
Agranulocytosis	Amitriptyline, amoxapine, bupropion, chlorpromazine, chlorprothixene, clozapine, desipramine, diphenhydramine, fluphenazine, glutethimide, imipramine, loxapine, meprobamate, mesoridazine, methyprylon, perphenazine, prochlorperazine, protriptyline, thioridazine, trifluoperazine
Eosinophilia	Amitriptyline, buspirone, chlorpromazine, chlorprothixine, clonazepam, fluphenazine, imipramine, maprotiline, nortriptyline, perphenazine, prochlorperazine, protriptyline, tryptophan
Leukemia (?)	Lithium
Leukocytosis	Haloperidol, lithium
Leukopenia	Amantadine, amitriptyline, amoxapine, buspirone, chlorpromazine, chlorprothixine, clonazepam, fluphenazine, fluoxetine, flurazepam, glutethimide, haloperidol, loxapine, mesoridazine, oxazepam, perphenazine, prochlorperazine, promethazine, protriptyline, thioridazine, thiothixene, tranylcypromine
Neutropenia	Amantadine, diazepam, methylprylon, trazodone
Lymphocytosis	Fluoxetine

Table 5 Miscellaneous disturbances

Type	Drugs of treatment
Decreased hematocrit	Alprazolam, chlorazepate
Decreased hemoglobin	Alprazolam
Decreased red cell count	Haloperidol
Decreased bleeding time	Valproic acid
Increased bleeding time	Fluoxetine
Petechiae	Fluoxetine, valproic acid
Increased sedimentation rate	Fluoxetine
Purpura	Amitriptyline, desipramine, fluoxetine, imipramine, maprotiline, nortriptyline protriptyline, trimipramine

Table 6 Class of psychotropic drugs and hematological changes

Class	Change
Antipsychotic	
Aliphatic	Agranulocytosis, eosinophilia, aplastic, anemia, pancytopenia, hemolytic anemia, T purpura
Piperazine	Agranulocytosis, aplastic anemia, pancytopenia, anemia, T purpura
Piperidine	Agranulocytosis, leukopenia, pancytopenia, anemia
Thioxanthenes	Eosinophilia, leukopenia, T purpura
Indoles	
Butyrophenones	Leukocytosis, leukopenia, thrombocytosis
Clozapine	Agranulocytosis
Lithium	Leukocytosis, leukemia, aplastic anemia, megaloblastic anemia
Antidepressant	
Tricyclics	Bone marrow depression
Monoamine oxidase inhibitors	Leukopenia, anemia
Tetracyclics	Eosinophilia
Fluoxetine	Thrombocytosis
Bupropion	Anemia, pancytopenia
Anxiolytic	
Benzodiazepines	Aplastic anemia, anemia, T purpura
Anticonvulsant	
Carbamazepine	Agranulocytosis, aplastic anemia, bone marrow depression, eosinophilia, leukocytosis, leukopenia, pancytopenia, thrombocytopenia
Valproic acid	Anemia, bone marrow suppression, eosinophilia, hypofibrinogenemia, leukopenia, lymphocytosis, thrombocytopenia
Miscellaneous	
Tryptophan	Eosinophilia

T purpura = thrombocytopenic purpura.

logical finding. As a result, low red cell count, hematocrit, hemoglobin, and fatty bone marrow are commonly observed.

Thrombocytopenia

When symptomatic, thrombocytopenia presents within one or another form of bleeding; epistaxis, ecchymoses, petechial hemorrhage, and easy bruising are some of the common symptoms. Internal bleeding may be seen in severe cases. Reduced platelet count, prolonged bleeding time, and impaired clot retraction are the cardinal laboratory findings.

Eosinophilia

A transient eosinophilia occurs with tricyclic antidepressant treatment during the first few weeks of therapy; this is of little clinical significance. As a psychotropic agent, L-tryptophan, a serotonin precursor, has been used in a variety of clinical situations. A flurry of cases have recently linked tryptophan to a potentially life-threatening blood dyscrasia characterized by severe eosinophilia, myalgia, swelling of extremities, skin rash, and fever. This topic is discussed in further detail in this book.

Porphyria

The most common symptom of acute porphyric episode is acute abdominal pain. Other gastrointestinal symptoms (nausea, vomiting), tachycardia, hypertension, mental symptoms, and pain may also be seen. A significantly high level of urinary porphobilinogen (PBG) is usually diagnostic in porphyria. Watson-Schwartz test is frequently used. Some of the psychotropic drugs that precipitate porphyria (acute intermittent, hereditary coproporphyria, and variegata porphyria) include: barbiturates, carbamazepine, ethchlorvynol, glutethimide, meprobamate, phenytonin, and valproic acid. After a positive qualitative test, a quantitative test should be done that would generally show the PBG level in the range of 50–200 mg/day.

TREATMENT AND PREVENTION

The value of early detection and immediate discontinuation of the offending agent cannot be overemphasized. Fever, sore throat, rash, and signs of bleeding or infection in the absence of an apparent cause must alert the physician to the possibility of iatrogenesis. Risk of infection is directly proportional to duration and severity of neutropenia. A close watch for these heralding signs must be kept, particularly during the first 3 months of psychotropic treatment. Beyond 3 months of therapy, periodic monitoring of blood cellular elements may not be a cost-effective exercise—except in case of clozapine where a periodic monitoring of blood is required.

Because a hematological disturbance may be a potentially fatal complication, a thorough and immediate medical evaluation, preferably in an inpatient setting and in consultation with a hematologist, is strongly warranted. Examination of blood and bone marrow films, microbial cultures, restoration of electrolyte balance and nutrition, as well as antibiotic therapy and other supportive measures are some of the essential elements of therapeutic plan. Granulocyte transfusion may be desirable but generally is not necessary. There are conflicting reports on the therapeutic role of lithium in neutropenic states caused by nonpsychotropic drugs; its therapeutic potential resulting from granulopoietic side effect has not been properly assessed in neutropenia related to psychotropic drugs. A few anecdotal reports have, however, claimed an antileukopenic effect of lithium in leukopenia induced by antipsychotics and carbamazepine.

Transfusion of packed red cells may be indicated in aplastic anemia. In thrombocytopenia, glucocorticoids have a debatable specific therapeutic role. Generally, platelet transfusions are ineffective because of rapid destruction. However, in life-threatening situations, platelet transfusion is indicated. If recovery occurs, it usually does so within the first 2 weeks of initiating treatment. If the bone marrow shows normal appearing promyelocytes and myelocytes, neutrophils will reappear within 4–7 days after stopping the offending agent. There is also some evidence to suggest that thrombocytosis may herald recovery from drug-induced agranulocytosis.

In general, hematological disturbances may be prevented from becoming severe by early detection. Fortunately, these disturbances are rare, reversible, and usually not life threatening, if diagnosed early. One should be cognizant of potentially hematotoxic effects of a psychotropic drug that is being prescribed. Reexposure to the same drug or a drug of the same family should be avoided. Prolonged periodic white blood cell count is of questionable clinical yield except in the case of clozapine, a special high-risk clinical situation. If a history of porphyria is known, certain psychotropic drugs, as described here, should be avoided. Leukocytosis is a common and benign side effect of lithium therapy with some therapeutic potential in select leukopenic states.

REFERENCES

Balon R, Berchou R, 1986: Hematologic side effects of psychotropic drugs. *Psychosomatics, 27,* 119–127.

Class FHJ, 1989: Drug-induced agranulocytosis: Review of possible mechanisms, and prospects for clozapine studies. *Psychopharmacology, 99,* S113–S117.

Prakash R, 1985: A review of hematological side effects of lithium. *Hospital and Community Psychiatry, 356,* 127–128.

Salama A, Mueller-Eckhardt C, 1986: Rh blood group-specific antibodies in immune hemolytic anemia induced by nomifensine. *Blood, 68,* 1285–1288.

27

Adverse Endocrine Effects

Viktoria R. Erhardt and Morris B. Goldman

Endocrine disorders are caused by many commonly prescribed psychotropic drugs. The physician must be particularly alert for their occurrence, since the disorders can undermine patient progress, erode compliance, and be mistaken for an exacerbation of the psychiatric illness. Problems can be minimized by routine laboratory testing and by remaining alert to signs and symptoms of the disorders. Even if symptoms occur, the disorder can often be treated without stopping the psychotropic medication.

This chapter focuses on clearly established and clinically significant drug-induced disorders. Some drug-induced alterations are omitted. Rare reports (less than 1%) of possible endocrine-mediated dysfunction (e.g., galactorrhea and gynecomastia with verapamil or valproic acid; menstrual irregularities with alprazolam, buspirone, chlordiazepoxide, valproic acid, or verapamil) are not included since their relationship to the psychotropic medication is unclear. Similarly, minimal endocrine changes that are well established but of no apparent clinical consequence (e.g., tricyclic antidepressant-induced increases in growth hormone, prolactin, and cortisol levels; lithium-induced increases in cortisol levels) are not addressed (Meltzer, 1980; Meltzer, Gudelsky, & Koenig, 1987).

PROLACTIN

Dopamine, the putative prolactin release inhibiting factor (PRIF), is secreted from tuberoinfundibular dopamine neurons (TIDA) at the median eminence and transported by the portal venous system to the anterior pituitary. Prolactin secretion and release from pituitary lactotroph cells is inhibited by tonic dopamine suppression, except during lactation. Although the most dramatic physiological function of prolactin is to stimulate lactation, it likely has other physiological actions that we do not as yet understand.

Classic antipsychotics elevate prolactin by antagonizing the effect of dopamine on pituitary lactotroph cells and also probably in the hypothalamus. Methylphenidate and dextroamphetamine diminish prolactin secretion by augmenting dopaminergic activity (Greenhill et al., 1984; Shaywitz et al., 1982). The latter effects have been postulated to account for the diminished growth rate in children treated with psychostimulants. This, however, seems unlikely since prolactin's minimal growth-inducing effects are apparent only when growth hormone production is diminished.

ELEVATED PROLACTIN LEVELS

Etiology and Pathophysiology

Prolactin levels rise within hours after antipsychotics are first given and reach a peak within several days (Meltzer et al., 1987). In single dose trials, maximal increases are obtained with subtherapeutic doses (Gruen et al., 1978); with sustained treatment, levels continue to rise as dose increases. Tolerance appears to develop in some patients during the first several weeks of treatment, and many patients on long-term antipsychotic drug therapy have normal prolactin levels.

Excess prolactin stimulates breast tissue leading to breast tenderness, gynecomastia, and galactorrhea. Hyperprolactinemia causes mammary tumors in laboratory animals, although there appears to be no increased risk to patients on antipsychotic drugs (Overall, 1978). Long-term carcinogenic effects have not, however, been thoroughly assessed.

Prolactin also inhibits gonadotropin releasing hormone (GnRH) release, thereby decreasing luteinizing hormone (LH) and follicle stimulating hormone (FSH) secretion. LH and FSH are the major gonadotropins involved in regulating ovarian and testicular function. In women, even mild hyperprolactinemia may cause irregular menses, whereas higher levels generally cause amenorrhea. In men, hyperprolactinemia lowers testosterone levels, leading to infertility and sexual dysfunction. Other factors likely play a role.

Decreased bone density has been found in women with hyperprolactinemia caused by CNS disease (Klibanski, Neer, & Beitans, 1981; Koppelmann et al., 1984). Two small studies found no correlation between hyperprolactinemia and bone density in women taking antipsychotics (Ataya, Mercado, Kartaginer, Abbasi, & Maghissi, 1988; Rogers & Burke, 1987). Further studies are needed in the psychiatric population.

Clinical Picture

Breast Tenderness, Gynecomastia, and Galactorrhea

These are common. The incidence of galactorrhea ranging from a few drops on expression to spontaneous soaking of clothes, varies from 10–57% (Plante & Roy, 1967; Robinson, 1957). Since prolactin levels were not determined in these studies, the association with hyperprolactinemia was only inferred. Men develop gynecomastia and breast tenderness much less frequently.

Menstrual Changes

Oligomenorrhea, irregular menses, and amenorrhea have been reported to occur in over 50% of subjects studied (Ghadirian, Chouinard, & Annabel, 1982; Sandison, Whitelaw, & Currie, 1960). In one study, higher prolactin levels were clearly correlated with menstrual irregularities.

Sexual Symptoms

A wide range of sexual dysfunction has been reported, but rarely systematically studied. Eight percent of male patients on antipsychotics report diminished libido and quality of orgasm (Haider, 1966; Witton, 1962). Serum prolactin levels were slightly but significantly correlated with complaints of sexual dysfunction (i.e., erectile dysfunction, changes in ejaculation, ability to achieve orgasm, and quality of orgasm) in male, but not female, outpatients (Ghadirian, et al., 1982). Women do not appear to be as likely as men to complain of sexual dysfunction.

Pretreatment Evaluation and Diagnosis

Since many patients are hesitant to discuss disturbances in sexual and reproductive function, or are ignorant of the possible relationship to drug treatment, the clinician must directly inquire. The incidence of complaints in reported studies seems much higher than expected, and suggests that many patients fail to spontaneously report problems. A baseline history will help evaluate the significance of later complaints.

Normal prolactin levels vary between laboratories, but in general are 0 to 20 ng/ml for women and 0 to 15 ng/ml for men. Levels are higher during the night, may rise during the midmenstrual cycle, and are sensitive to stress. Thus levels should be drawn at least 2 hours after awakening, at times other than midcycle, and borderline high values should be repeated to exclude stress effects. Basal prolactin levels may help the clinician interpret subsequent values.

Prolactin elevations secondary to antipsychotics are rarely above 100 ng/ml, and thus a higher level suggests other sources. Other causes such as pregnancy, hypothyroidism, hypothalamic disease, prolactinoma, and medications including oral contraceptives, cimetidine, methyldopa, metoclopramide, and methadone should be considered.

Prevention and Treatment

Dose Reduction

The correlation between clinical potency and ability to stimulate prolactin secretion has been shown to be highly significant for most drugs (Meltzer et al., 1987). Two exceptions are clozapine, which causes less stimulation, and thioridazine, which appears to cause more. Theoretically, dose reduction should be effective in at least some patients, although no published studies were found.

Amantadine

This is a dopamine agonist that reverses antipsychotic-induced hyperprolactinemia (Siever, 1981). Amantadine treatment (200–300 mg daily) significantly affected six target areas: elevated prolactin levels, breast tenderness, gynecomastia, galactorrhea, decreased libido, amenorrhea, and weight gain (Correa, Opler, Kay, & Birmaher, 1987).

Bromocriptine

This dopamine agonist has also been successful in doses of 2.5 mg b.i.d. in treating antipsychotic-induced galactorrhea and amenorrhea. Complete resolution of symptoms may not occur for 12 weeks (Gioia & Asnis, 1988).

Both bromocriptine and amantadine can exacerbate psychosis during concurrent antipsychotic treatment (Frye, Pariser, & Kim, 1982; Hauser, 1980). Even though no studies have compared the efficacy of bromocriptine and amantidine, the side effects (depression, nausea, hypotension) and cost of bromocriptine may make amantadine the treatment of choice.

THYROID HORMONE

Thyroid hormone regulates growth and maturation by modulating oxidative phosphorylation, genomic expression, and transmembrane transport of ions and substrates. Thyroid hormone is required for the development of the nervous system, and furthermore, thyroid dysfunction in the adult routinely induces psychiatric symptoms, particularly depression. The mechanism of neuropsychiatric symptom induction is unknown, but may be related to thyroid hormone's modulation of CNS β-adrenergic receptors or selective processing and binding to both nuclear and synaptosomal receptors (Dratman & Crutchfield, 1989).

Lithium and carbamazepine lower thyroid hormone levels, whereas in hyperthyroid patients, haloperidol and perphenazine induce a state resembling thyroid storm and neuroleptic malignant syndrome. Minor tranquilizers and antipsychotics may alter total hormone levels, but free hormone, and hence thyroid function, is not affected (Jefferson & Marshal, 1981).

DIMINISHED THYROID HORMONE

Etiology and Pathophysiology

Lithium's net effect is to decrease release of thyroid hormone (Salata & Klein, 1987). Numerous steps in thyroid hormone synthesis are inhibited including iodine uptake, iodination of tyrosine, thyroid hormone release, and response to thyroid-stimulating hormone (TSH). The resulting decrease in serum levels of thyroxine (T4) and triiodothyronine (T3) leads to a physiological compensatory rise in TSH levels that may be insufficient to reestablish a euthyroid state.

In addition, thyroid antibodies are present in increased titer in some patients with affective disorders before lithium treatment (Lazarus, et al., 1986) and may further increase as a result of lithium treatment (Crowe, Lloyd, Bloch, & Rosser, 1973). These patients with limited thyroid reserve may be particularly prone to develop hypothyroidism.

Carbamazepine routinely decreases levels of T4, T3, and free thyroxine index (FTI) (Strandjord, Aanderud, Myking, & Johannesen, 1981). Peripheral catabolism and clearance are increased in a manner analogous to the effects of phenytoin on thyroid hormone (Bentsen & Graml, 1983; Yeo et al., 1983). Carbamazepine may also inhibit the thyrotropin (TSH) response to thyroid-releasing hormone (TRH) (Joffe, Gold, Uhde, & Post, 1984).

Clinical Picture

Common signs and symptoms of hypothyroidism include decreased energy, depression, poor appetite, weight gain, intellectual and psychomotor slowing, cold intolerance, constipation, menorrhagia, and dry skin. Lithium-treated patients present with various forms of thyroid dysfunction including clinical hypothyroidism, elevated TSH with normal free thyroxine, goiter (with or without hypothyroidism), and rarely, hyperthyroidism. The sum of the incidence of clinical and asymptomatic hypothyroidism and goiter is about 9% (Wolff, 1979). The incidence of hypothyroidism is similar in the first and second years of therapy (Myers et al., 1985), with a mean incidence occurring at 3.4 years in patients followed for 10 years (Yassa, Saunders, Nastase, & Camille, 1988a).

Women and patients with limited thyroid reserve are significantly more at risk to develop thyroid dysfunction (Maarbjerg, Vestergaard, & Schou, 1987). Another important risk factor is rapid-cycling illness, which has a higher incidence of both basal and lithium-induced hypothyroidism. The incidence in rapid cycling patients on lithium is between 30 and 50% (Cho, Bone, Dunner, Colt, & Fieve, 1979). Increased age may also be a risk factor (Transbol, Christiansen, & Baastrup, 1978).

In contrast to lithium, carbamazepine-induced decreases in T3, T4, and FTI occur early on and do not appear to progress. Frank hypothyroidism is rarely seen (Aanderud & Strandjord, 1980), whereas the incidence of more subtle clinical changes has not been carefully assessed. Investigators have avoided treating patients with low thyroid hormone levels because TSH has remained normal (Strandjord et al., 1981); however, as noted previously, carbamazepine may also inhibit the compensatory TSH increase.

Pretreatment Evaluation and Diagnosis

To optimize diagnosis and treatment of lithium-induced hypothyroidism, an endocrine history and laboratory evaluation should be obtained before beginning treatment. The pretreatment assessment includes T4, FTI, TSH, and where there is heightened concern, antithyroid antibodies. During lithium treatment, symptom monitoring and a periodic physical exam should be performed. TSH is a readily available and relatively sensitive test for primary hypothyroidism and should be checked every 6 to 12 months, but more often in rapid cyclers and those with elevated antibody levels. Frequent assessment in rapid cyclers is particularly important (Bauer & Whybrow, 1990).

Patients receiving carbamazepine should probably have T4 and T3 levels checked before starting treatment and 1 month later. Patients should be carefully observed for subtle signs of hypothyroidism.

Prevention and Treatment

If clinical hypothyroidism develops, thyroxine or triiodothyronine therapy is efficacious and allows continued treatment with lithium. Treatment should be initiated slowly, particularly in the elderly, to avoid a rapid change in metabolic rate. Both T3 and TSH levels (the latter alone is adequate if the high sensitivity assay is available) should be monitored to assure appropriate dosing.

In many cases transient increases in TSH may adequately compensate for the antithyroid effects of lithium, following which T3 returns to normal. If the TSH remains elevated in the absence of clinical symptoms, treatment should probably be initiated. Cooper, Rachelle, Wood, Levin, & Ridgway (1984) found in medical patients that very mild symptoms of hypothyroidism with normal T4 but elevated TSH improve with thyroxine therapy.

ELEVATED THYROID HORMONE

Etiology and Pathophysiology

The addition of the butyrophenone, haloperidol, or the phenothiazine perphenazine to patients with hyperthyroidism can induce a neurotoxic state (Jefferson & Marshall, 1981; Weiner, 1979). The mechanism is unknown but may be related to the finding that laboratory animals given low-dose thyroxine and haloperidol often die, whereas controls receiving just haloperidol do not (Selye & Szabo, 1971).

Clinical Picture

Patients present within days after beginning treatment with fever, rigidity, and tremor. Dyspnea and difficulty swallowing are common, as are diarrhea and diaphoresis. Elevated white blood count has been described, but other laboratory values (i.e., elevated creatinine phosphokinase levels) that might suggest a concurrent or alternative diagnosis of neuroleptic malignant syndrome have not been reported.

Pretreatment Evaluation and Diagnosis

This syndrome is not widely known and may easily be missed. Before starting treatment with high-potency antipsychotics, the physician should examine and inquire about signs and symptoms of hyperthyroidism. Although the disorder is rare, if symptoms of hyperthyroidism are apparent, baseline thyroid hormone measurements should be considered before initiating drugs. If neurotoxic symptoms occur, thyroid hormone levels should be obtained along with other laboratory tests.

Prevention and Treatment

Haloperidol, perphenazine, and probably other high-potency antipsychotics should not be prescribed to hyperthyroid patients. If the syndrome is identified, it will usually respond within 48 hours to stopping the antipsychotic and treating the hyperthyroidism (e.g., propranolol, propylthiouriacil, iodine, glucocorticoids, supportive measures). However, one fatality occurred even when appropriate treatment measures appeared to be instituted (Weiner, 1979).

VASOPRESSIN (ANTIDIURETIC HORMONE)

Vasopressin is released from the posterior pituitary into the bloodstream. It acts on receptors in the distal tubule and collecting duct of the kidney to stimulate reabsorption of water, thereby concentrating the urine. The main physiological stimulant for vasopressin is an elevated concentration of plasma osmolality or sodium. If vasopressin does not produce sufficient water reabsorption, then thirst is perceived.

Besides elevated plasma sodium and osmolality, the other physiological stimulants for vasopressin (and thirst) are hypovolemia, hypotension, nausea, and hypoglycemia.

Clinical problems can occur when vasopressin's actions are either augmented or blocked. The syndrome of inappropriate antidiuresis (SIAD) is present when the patient has dilute plasma (i.e., hyponatremia) and relatively concentrated urine (in the absence of physiological stimulants). If the hyponatremia is sufficiently severe, or occurs sufficiently rapidly, the patient will become water intoxicated. In contrast, drugs or disorders that block vasopressin action produce excessively dilute urine, and a secondary thirst (i.e., nephrogenic diabetes insipidus).

Carbamazepine, several classes of antidepressants, and rarely antipsychotics cause SIAD. Lithium is the most common cause of nephrogenic diabetes insipidus.

AUGMENTED VASOPRESSIN ACTIVITY

Etiology and Pathophysiology

Controversy exists whether the mechanism of carbamazepine-induced SIAD is the result of increased levels (Kimura, Matsui, & Sato, 1974), or enhanced action of vasopressin on renal receptors (Gold et al., 1983b). In unselected manic depressive patients carbamazepine appears to have no effect on basal vasopressin levels, and if anything, diminishes vasopressin secretion following osmotic stimulation (Gold et al., 1983b). On the other hand, carbamazepine commonly diminishes water excretion, indicating that some aspect of antidiuretic function is impaired (Yassa, Iskandar, Nastase, & Camille, 1988b). Studies directly examining carbamazepine's effects on water excretory capacity are needed to resolve this question.

The mechanism of antidepressant-induced SIAD is unknown, and the role of altered vasopressin secretion has not been clarified. Likewise, the two cases of SIAD clearly related to antipsychotic treatment (with haloperidol and thiothixene) (Aljouni, Kern, Tures, Theil, & Hagan, 1974; Peck & Shenkman, 1979) did not provide vasopressin levels. Investigations suggest that antipsychotics do not cause SIAD either in normals or psychiatric patients (in the absence of drug-induced hypotension) (Kendler, Weitzman, & Rubin, 1978; Raskind, Courtney, & Mursburg, 1987; Sarai & Matsunaga, 1989) and do not account for the increased incidence of enhanced vasopressin secretion in schizophrenic patients (Emsley, Potgieter, Taljaard, Joubert, & Gledhill, 1989; Goldman, Luchins, & Robertson, 1988).

Clinical Picture

Patients with drug-induced hyponatremia may be asymptomatic and exhibit subtle cognitive changes, deteriorated behavior, or frank water intoxication (lethargy, confusion, irritability, tremulousness, seizures, nausea, ataxia, coma, and death) (Yassa et al., 1988b).

A low plasma sodium was reported in 25% of a small sample of patients within 3 months of beginning carbamazepine (Yassa et al., 1988b). Risk factors include elevated carbamazepine levels (>6 $\mu g/ml$), age above 30 years, primary polydipsia, and basal hyponatremia (Lahr, 1985; Uhde & Post, 1983; Yassa et al., 1988b). Antidepressant-induced hyponatremia has been reported with several structural classes, including tricyclics, MAO inhibitors, serotonin reuptake inhibitors such as fluoxetine, and atypical agents like bupropion. The elderly seem to be particularly at risk (Abbot 1983; Cohen, Mahelsky, & Adler, 1990). Although most structural classes of antipsychotics have been reported to cause hyponatremia, the actual role of the drugs, as noted previously, is unclear. Only the dibenzoxapines (loxapine, clozapine) and the indole derivative molindone (Raskind et al., 1987; Sandifer, 1983) have not been associated with hyponatremia, but this may simply be because these drugs are prescribed less often.

Diagnosis and Pretreatment Evaluation

A basal sodium level and urine specific gravity should be obtained in all patients receiving carbamazepine. Plasma sodium should be obtained monthly for 3 months in all polydipsic or hyponatremic patients. Patients and families should also be taught to identify prodromal signs of water intoxication. Patients with persistent hyponatremia should be carefully tested for subtle cognitive impairments, and switched if possible, to other agents.

No special measures are required for patients receiving antidepressants, but the physician should remain alert, particularly in the elderly, for symptoms of hyponatremia. Sodium levels should be obtained when there are any changes in cognition or alertness.

Prevention and Treatment

Carbamazepine-induced SIAD may resolve spontaneously. If the patient develops symptomatic hyponatremia, and it is not advisable to stop the drug, addition of lithium or demeclocycline may normalize the sodium level (Ringel & Brick, 1986). Patients given demeclocycline (600 mg b.i.d.) must be periodically evaluated for both renal and hepatic toxicity. Alternatively, if the patient is cooperative, he or she can adjust fluid intake to maintain a constant body weight known to be associated with normal sodium levels (Goldman & Luchins, 1987). Patients who become hyponatremic on antidepressants or antipsychotics can often tolerate agents from other structural classes (Abbot, 1983).

DIMINISHED VASOPRESSIN ACTIVITY

Etiology and Pathophysiology

Lithium causes acute nephrogenic diabetes insipidus by interfering with the generation of the second messenger, cyclic adenosine monophosphate (cAMP), in renal tubular cells. In addition, long-term lithium treatment causes a further decline in concentrating ability. This second defect may be related to structural deformities in the renal cortex, in particular tubular dilatation and microcysts (Bendz, 1983). Although vasopressin's actions on the kidney are inhibited by lithium, its release from the hypothalamus is actually augmented (Gold et al., 1983a), but this is inadequate to overcome the renal defect.

Lithium also causes minor changes in glomerular filtration rate that have been of great concern to clinicians. The impairment appears to be reversible (Bendz,

1985) and unrelated to the length of treatment on lithium (Boton, Gaviria, & Batlle, 1987). The mechanism is unknown, but may be at least partly the result of diminished delivery of filtrate from mild volume contraction. In any event, the changes are rarely of clinical concern. Although there have been reports of chronic marked impairments in patients on lithium, the significance of lithium therapy (in the absence of lithium intoxication) is unknown (Boton, Gaviria, & Batlle, 1987). Other changes in renal function, including acidification defects and mild protein loss, do not appear to be of clinical concern.

Clinical Picture

Up to 40% of patients on lithium complain of polyuria, excessive thirst, and polydipsia (Lee, Jampol, & Brown, 1971). The most disturbing complaint to the patient is usually nocturia, which occurs in about 30% of patients. Water deprivation tests show that concentration impairments exist in over 50% of patients, although frank polyuria (>3 L/day) occurs in only 20% (Boton et al., 1987). Urine volumes of up to 8 L have been associated with lithium-induced nephrogenic diabetes insipidus; higher values suggest some component of primary (psychogenic) polydipsia. Hypernatremia and its associated neurological symptoms are very rare as long as the thirst mechanism is intact. It is unclear if antipsychotics aggravate the polyuria (Bendz, 1983; Bucht, Wahlin, Wentzel, & Winblad, 1980; Vestergaard & Amdisen, 1981). Patients with lithium-induced polyuria appear to be particularly prone to obesity, presumably because of increased intake of high-calorie liquids (Vendsborg, Bech, & Rafaelsen, 1976).

Pretreatment Evaluation and Diagnosis

Blood urea nitrogen (BUN), creatinine, sodium, and a urinalysis should be obtained before initiating lithium and annually thereafter. Complaints of polyuria or nocturia are not necessarily reliable indicators of urine volume (Baylis & Heath, 1978), and thus objective measures should be obtained. Although 24-hour urine collections are preferred, single-urine samples that demonstrate low specific gravity (<1.005), low urine osmolality (>250 mOsm/kg), or low urine creatinine concentration (<50 mg/dl) (Goldman, unpublished data; Viewig, Godlesky, & Hundley, 1988) are easily obtained and useful for diagnosis. The latter is more precise since creatinine excretion is more constant than the others.

A renal concentrating defect can be confirmed by the patient's inability to concentrate urine above 500 mOsm/kg during a 16-hour fluid deprivation. This procedure should be performed in the hospital, and body weight followed closely, to prevent excess water loss. Many patients have primary (psychogenic) polydipsia, and as a consequence also fail to concentrate urine normally (presumably because of "medullary washout"). Thus it is helpful to have basal indexes of urine volume to help distinguish these two conditions. This is particularly important since thiazides reverse lithium-induced polyuria, but may induce fatal water intoxication if the patient has a primary polydipsia (Beresford, 1970).

Lithium should be given cautiously to patients with renal disease, since it may aggravate the condition. In patients with normal kidneys, it is important to monitor serum creatinine not because lithium is likely to significantly alter glomerular filtration, but as a routine screen for renal impairment of any etiology. Some have suggested serum B2-microglobulin be obtained, since it is more sensitive to changes in glomerular function than serum creatinine (Samiy & Rosnick, 1987).

Prevention and Treatment

Intervention should be considered for those with symptomatic polyuria or nocturia and for the polyuric patient who becomes obese on lithium. If lithium treatment is stopped, the concentrating defect will improve rapidly over the first 8 weeks, although some defect is still seen in 50% of polydipsic patients after one year (Bendz, 1985; Bucht & Wahlin, 1980). Lowering the lithium dose (Conte, Vazzola, & Sacchetti, 1988) or changing to a once-daily regimen may reduce urine volume (Plenge et al., 1982).

Alternatively the defect can be "bypassed" by prescribing thiazide diuretics (Crawford, Kennedy, & Hill, 1960). By enhancing the proximal reabsorption of water, thiazides diminish maximal urine flow rates. Thiazides, however, can produce hypokalemia, lithium toxicity, and water intoxication. Lithium toxicity can be prevented by reducing the lithium dose by one third before starting the thiazide. Hypokalemia can be prevented by providing potassium supplements or adding a potassium sparing diuretic like amiloride. Water intoxication can be prevented by excluding those patients who had significant polydipsia before lithium treatment.

Amiloride alone is frequently effective, reducing urine volume by about one third (Batlle et al., 1985) and carries a lower risk of lithium toxicity, hypokalemia, and water intoxication. Furthermore, since amiloride works, at least in part, by directly inhibiting uptake of lithium into renal tubular cells, it may help prevent long-term impairment (Boton et al., 1987). With either agent, BUN, lithium, and other electrolyte levels should be monitored closely during the first few weeks. Patients should also be reminded about maintaining a constant salt intake and avoiding dehydration.

PARATHYROID HORMONE

Parathyroid hormone (PTH) increases serum calcium by increasing calcium release from bone and absorption from the gut and kidney, and increasing phosphate excretion. PTH release is regulated by serum calcium, and to a lesser extent, serum magnesium. Lithium commonly elevates serum calcium levels but symptoms rarely occur.

ELEVATED PARATHYROID HORMONE

Etiology and Pathophysiology

Lithium appears to raise PTH and serum calcium levels by directly lowering the set point for PTH release (Brown, 1981), and perhaps through an indirect effect on bone and kidney (Mallette & Eichhorn, 1986). Lithium also appears to enhance the growth of parathyroid adenomas (Mallette & Eichhorn, 1986). The elevations in serum calcium occur in two phases—acutely over several weeks and subsequently over months to years.

Osteopenia has been linked to lithium-induced hypercalcemia (Christiansen, Bastrup, & Transbol, 1975), a result not only of elevated PTH, but perhaps also direct inhibition of osteoid synthesis (Mallette & Eichhorn, 1986) and washout of calcium from lithium-induced polyuria (Delva, Crammer, & Jarzylos, 1989).

Clinical Picture

Patients are usually asymptomatic with mild elevations, but higher levels cause fatigue, weakness, anorexia, nausea, vomiting, thirst, and headache. Neuropsychiatic symptoms are common (depression, anxiety, psychosis) and may be indistinguishable from an exacerbation of the underlying illness (Cervi-Skinner, 1977; Gammon & Docherty, 1980; Mallette & Eichhorn, 1986).

Serum calcium and PTH increase in approximately 80% of patients after one month on lithium, but usually remain within the normal range (Christiansen, Bastrup, & Transbol, 1980). Hypercalcemia occurs in 10%. In a smaller subset this progresses and usually correlates with both length of treatment and total cumulative lithium dose (Christiansen et al., 1975).

Pretreatment Evaluation and Diagnosis

Calcium levels should be obtained before starting lithium treatment to rule out a preexisting problem—one month after starting treatment and annually thereafter. Calcium and thyroid hormone levels should be obtained during exacerbations of the psychiatric illness.

Prevention and Treatment

If hypercalcemia is detected, it is important to rule out lithium toxicity, since the two ions are handled similarly by the kidney. Also other drugs (e.g., thiazide diuretics) raise calcium levels. If the level is mildly elevated (<11.0 mg/dl) and the patient is stable, the serum calcium can simply be monitored. Otherwise, the patient should be switched to another medication (e.g., carbamazepine), and the calcium level followed for several weeks. Even if the calcium level returns to normal after discontinuation of lithium, it may rise again, indicating the presence of a parathyroid adenoma. Once the adenoma is removed, the patient can take lithium again (Mallette & Eichhorn, 1986).

GROWTH HORMONE/SOMATOMEDINS

Growth hormone is necessary for normal linear growth. Its growth-stimulating effects appear to be modulated by the somatomedins. Methylphenidate, pemoline, and dextroamphetamine affect growth hormone secretion and somatomedin activity.

ELEVATED GROWTH HORMONE

Etiology and Pathophysiology

Methylphenidate and dextroamphetamine increase growth hormone levels, both acutely (Aarskog, Fevang, Klove, Stoa, & Thorsen, 1977; Brown, 1977) and chronically (Aarskog et al., 1977; Greenhill et al., 1984). In particular, the magnitude of the nocturnal growth hormone release, which appears closely related to growth velocity, is increased with methylphenidate (but not dextroamphetamine) (Greenhill et al., 1984). Although these changes might be expected to increase, not decrease, growth velocity, the latter appears to be the more common effect. In addition, both drugs inhibit the action of somatomedin on cartilage (Van Wyk et al., 1974).

Clinical Picture

Reduced growth velocity and diminished weight gain are frequently reported. The reduction in height is generally small (i.e., 0.8 cm/year) but continues throughout treatment in the absence of drug holidays. The diminished weight velocity is more marked (0.5 kg/yr), but appears to disappear over 2 years of treatment (Mattes & Gittleman, 1983). Diminished growth velocity appears to be dose related (Mattes & Gittleman, 1983) and less marked with methylphenidate than dextroamphetamine (Greenhill et al., 1984). It is unclear, however, if comparisons were made between equivalent doses. Also, the difference between agents has been attributed to methylphenidate's shorter half-life, and methylphenidate is now often used in a slow release form (Greenhill et al., 1984).

Two studies with methylphenidate suggest that ultimate adult height is not diminished despite a lower growth velocity (Hechtman, Weiss, & Perlman, 1984; Klein & Mannuzza, 1988). However, these patients were treated for variable periods of time with the short-acting methylphenidate, had drug holidays, and were withdrawn from treatment before epiphyseal closure (thus allowing for "rebound" growth). Although preliminary data suggest treatment in adolescents has less marked effects on growth than treatment started in childhood (Vincent, Varley, & Legar, 1990), many clinical issues remain unresolved.

Pretreatment Evaluation and Diagnosis

Height and weight should be monitored before and at 6-month intervals during therapy. Although individual growth velocities vary greatly over time, making it difficult to identify drug effects, any sustained decrease of 10 percentile points or greater suggests a significant drop.

Prevention and Treatment

Drug holidays restore height velocity (Klein & Mannuza, 1988), presumably by allowing for a rebound period. One would anticipate that lower doses or changing from dextroamphetamine to methylphenidate might help. Psychostimulant treatment should be stopped before epiphyseal closure, if possible, if diminished growth velocity is a concern.

BODY WEIGHT REGULATION

The regulation of food intake is poorly understood, but the endocrine system likely plays a major role. Cholecystokinin (CCK), insulin, glucagon, thyrotropin-releasing hormone (TRH), and oxytocin have all been shown to influence satiety (Steffens, Scheurink, Luiten, & Bohus, 1988). Metabolic factors controlling energy consumption are clearly under endocrine control and are likely to account for part of the drug-induced weight gain.

Many of the tricyclic, heterocyclic, and monoamine oxidase inhibitor antidepressants and antipsychotics, as well as lithium, induce weight gain. There is considerable variability between the weight-inducing properties within each type of psychotropic, enabling the physician, in most instances, to choose an agent with minimal effects.

WEIGHT GAIN

Lithium has insulin-like effects (Clausen, 1968), increases appetite, diminishes thyroid hormone activity, and increases fluid retention and intake. The significance of each these factors has not been determined, although one study suggests that increased thirst is more important than increased appetite (Vendsborg, Bech, & Rafaelsen, 1976). Antipsychotics produce marked increases in appetite (Robinson, McHugh, & Folstein, 1975) and diminish activity (Gordon & Groth, 1964). Antidepressants increase carbohydrate craving in a dose-related fashion (Bernstein, 1988; Paykel, Mueller, & De La Vergne, 1973). Carbohydrate metabolism is only subtly affected.

Clinical Picture

Lithium

Weight gains of up to 10 kg in 60% of patients treated with lithium for over 5 years have been reported (Vendsborg et al., 1976). Average weight gain is about 4 kg and tends to stabilize after 2 years. Patients with prior obesity and polydipsia are most at risk (Vendsborg et al., 1976).

Antipsychotic

Weight gain averages 15 kg in patients on chlorpromazine. High-potency antipsychotics are less likely to produce weight increases (Klett & Caffey, 1960), whereas depot and oral forms appear equivalent (Korsgaard & Skausig, 1979). Molidone is the one antipsychotic that does not cause significant weight gain. Weight gain appears to parallel clinical response with antipsychotics but not antidepressants (Bernstein, 1988).

Antidepressants

Weight gain with antidepressants averages about 2 kg/year (Paykel et al., 1973), at least some of which compensates for weight lost from depression. Weight increases of nearly 10 kg are seen with amitriptyline (Paykel et al., 1973); maprotiline and phenelzine appear to induce intermediate increases; and nortryptiline, amoxapine, and desipramine induce little. Bupropion, zimelidine, fluoxetine, and tranylcypromine induce no consistent weight gain and may cause weight loss (Bernstein, 1988; Fernstrom & Kupfer, 1988).

Pretreatment Evaluation and Diagnosis

Lithium should be prescribed cautiously to patients with a history of obesity, although there appears to be no increased risk of diabetes mellitus (Vestergaard & Schou, 1987). Concerns about weight gain are serious, because of both implications for general health and drug compliance. Weight gain in several studies was the most common reason given for stopping medication.

Treatment

Patients who gain large amounts of weight on lithium should be assessed for hypothyroidism, polydipsia, and peripheral edema. In the absence of these reversible factors, dose reduction or carbamazepine should be considered. Carbamazepine has been reported to induce less appetite stimulation and weight gain than lithium (Bernstein, 1988).

Similarly, dose reduction of antipsychotics and antidepressants can induce weight loss (Bernstein, 1988; Klett & Caffey, 1960), as can switching to an agent like molindone (Gardos & Cole, 1977) or fluoxetine (Asberg, Erikson, & Martensson, 1986).

REFERENCES

Aanderud S, Strandjord RE, 1980: Hypothyroidism induced by anti-epileptic therapy. *Acta Neurologica Scandinavica, 61,* 330–332.

Aarskog D, Fevang FO, Klove H, Stoa KF, Thorsen T, 1977: The effect of the stimulant drugs, dextroamphetamine and methylphenidate, on secretion of growth hormone in hyperactive children. *Journal of Pediatrics, 90,* 136–139.

Abbot R, 1983: Hyponatremia due to antidepressant medication. *Annals of Emergency Medicine, 12,* 708–710.

Aljouni K, Kern MW, Tures JF, Theil GB, Hagan TC, 1974: Thiothixene induced hyponatremia. *Archives of Internal Medicine, 134,* 1103–1105.

Ataya K, Mercado A, Kartaginer J, Abbasi A, Moghissi KS, 1988: Bone density and reproductive hormones in patients with neuroleptic-induced hyperprolactinemia. *Fertility and Sterility, 50,* 876–881.

Asberg M, Eriksson B, Martensson B, 1986: Therapeutic effects of serotonin uptake inhibitors in depression. *Journal of Clinical Psychiatry, 47,* 23–35.

Batlle DC, von Riotie AB, Gaviria M, Grupp M, 1985: Amelioration of polyuria by amiloride in patients receiving long term lithium treatment. *New England Journal of Medicine, 312,* 408–414.

Bauer MS, Whybrow PC, 1990: Rapid cycling bipolar affective disorder. *Archives of General Psychiatry, 47,* 435–440.

Baylis PH, Heath DA, 1978: Water disturbances in patients treated with oral lithium carbonate. *Annals of Internal Medicine, 88,* 607–609.

Bendz H, 1983: Kidney function in lithium treated patients. *Acta Psychiatrica Scandinavica, 68,* 303–324.

Bendz H, 1985: Kidney function in a selected lithium population. *Acta Psychiatrica Scandinavica, 72,* 451–463.

Bentsen KD, Graml VA, 1983: Serum thyroid hormones and blood folic acid during monotherapy with carbamazepine or valproate. *Acta Neurologica Scandinavica, 67,* 235–241.

Beresford HR, 1970: Polydipsia, hydrochlorothiazide, and water intoxication. *Journal of the American Medical Association, 214,* 879–883.

Bernstein JG, 1988: Psychotropic drug induced weight gain: Mechanisms and management. *Clinical Neuropharmacology, 11*, S195–S206.

Boton R, Gaviria M, Batlle D, 1987: Prevalence, pathogenesis, and treatment of renal dysfunction associated with chronic lithium therapy. *American Journal of Kidney Disease, VX*, 3329–345.

Brown WA, 1977: Psychologic and neuroendocrine response to methylphenidate. *Archives of General Psychiatry, 34*, 1103–1108.

Brown EM, 1981: Lithium induced abnormal calcium-regulated PTH release in dispersed bovine parathyroid cells. *Journal of Clinical Endocrinology and Metabolism, 52*, 1046–1048.

Bucht G, Wahlin A, 1980: Renal concentrating capacity in long term lithium treatment and after withdrawal of lithium. *Acta Medica Scandinavica, 207*, 309–314.

Bucht G, Wahlin A, Wentzelt T, Winblad B, 1980: Renal function and morphology in long-term lithium and combined lithium neuroleptic treatment. *Acta Medica Scandinavica, 208*, 381–385.

Cervi-Skinner SJ, 1977: Lithium carbonate induced hypercalcemia. *Western Journal of Medicine, 127*, 527–528.

Cho JT, Bone S, Dunner DL, Colt E, Fieve RR, 1979: The effect of lithium treatment on thyroid function in patients with primary affective disorder. *American Journal of Psychiatry, 136*, 115–116.

Christiansen C, Baastrop PC, Transbol I, 1975: Osteopenia and dysregulation of divalent cations in lithium treated patients. *Neuropsychobiology, 1*, 344–354.

Christiansen C, Baastrop PC, Transbol I, 1980: Development of primary hyperparathyroidism during lithium therapy: Longitudinal study. *Neuropsychobiology, 6*, 280–283.

Clausen T, 1968: The relationship between the transport of glucose and cations across cell membranes in isolated tissues. IV. The insulin-like effect of lithium. *Biochimica et Biophysica Acta, 150*, 66–72.

Cohen BJ, Mahelsky M, Adler L, 1990: More cases of SIADH with fluoxetine (letter). *American Journal of Psychiatry, 147*, 948–949.

Conte G, Vazzola A, Sacchetti E, 1988: Renal function in chronic lithium-treated patients. *Acta Psychiatrica Scandinavica, 79*, 503–504.

Cooper DS, Rachelle H, Wood LC, Levin AA, Ridgway EC, 1984: L-thyroxine therapy in sub-clinical hypothyroidism. *Annals of Internal Medicine, 101*, 18–24.

Correa N, Opler LA, Kay SR, Birmaher B, 1987: Amantadine in the treatment of neuroendocrine side effects of neuroleptics. *Journal of Clinical Psychopharmacology, 7*, 91–95.

Crawford JD, Kennedy JC, Hill LE, 1960: Clinical results of treatment of diabetes insipidus with drugs of the chlorothiazide series. *New England Journal of Medicine, 262*, 737–743.

Crowe MJ, Lloyd GG, Bloch S, Rosser RM, 1973: Hypothyroidism in patients treated with lithium: A review and 2 case reports. *Psychological Medicine, 3*, 337–342.

Delva NJ, Crammer JL, Jarzylos V, 1989: Osteopenia, pathological fractures and increased urinary calcium excretion in schizophrenic patients with polydipsia. *Biological Psychiatry, 26*, 781–793.

Dratman MB, 1978: The mechanism of thyroxine action. In: *Hormonal proteins and peptides*, volume 6. New York: Academic Press.

Dratman MB, Crutchfield FL, 1989: Thyroxine, tri-iodothyronine, and reverse triiodothyronine processing in the cerebellum: Autoradiographic studies in adult rats. *Endocrinology, 125*, 1723–1733.

Emsley R, Potgieter A, Taljaard F, Joubert G, Gledhill R, 1989: Water excretion and plasma vasopressin in psychotic disorders. *American Journal of Psychiatry, 146*, 250–253.

Fernstrom MH, Kupfer DJ, 1988: Antidepressant-induced weight gain: A comparison study of four medications. *Psychiatry Research, 26*, 265–271.

Frye P, Pariser SF, Kim MH, 1982: Bromocriptine associated with symptom exacerbation during neuroleptic treatment of schizoaffective schizophrenia. *Journal of Clinical Psychiatry, 43*, 252–253.

Gammon GD, Docherty JP, 1980: Thiazide induced hypercalcemia in a manic depressive patient. *American Journal of Psychiatry, 137*, 1453–1454.

Gardos G, Cole JO, 1977: Weight reduction in schizophrenics by molindone. *American Journal of Psychiatry, 134*, 302–304.

Ghadirian A, Chouinard G, Annabel L, 1982: Sexual dysfunction and plasma prolactin levels in neuroleptic treated schizophrenic outpatients. *Journal of Nervous and Mental Disease, 170*, 463–467.

Gioia D, Asnis G, 1988: Serial plasma prolactin levels in neuroleptic induced galactorrhea: A case report. *Journal of Clinical Psychiatry, 49*, 29–31.

Gold P, Robertson GL, Ballenger JC, Kaye W, Chen J, Rubinow DR, Goodwin FK, Post RM, 1983b:

Carbamazepine diminishes the sensitivity of the plasma arginine vasopressin response to osmotic stimulation. *Journal of Clinical Endocrinology and Metabolism, 57,* 592–597.

Gold PW, Robertson GL, Post RM, Kaye W, Ballenger J, Rubinow D, Goodwin FK, 1983a: The effect of lithium on the osmoregulation of arginine vasopressin secretion. *Journal of Clinical Endocrinology and Metabolism, 56,* 295–299.

Goldman MB, Dratman MB, Crutchfield FL, Jennings AS, Maruniak JA, Gibbons R, 1985: Intrathecal triiodothyronine administration causes greater heart rate stimulation in hypothyroid rats than intravenously delivered hormone. *Journal of Clinical Investigation, 76,* 1622–1625.

Goldman MB, Luchins DJ, 1987: Prevention of episodic water intoxication with target weight procedure. *American Journal of Psychiatry, 144,* 365–366.

Goldman MB, Luchins DJ, Robertson GL, 1988: Mechanism of abnormal water metabolism in psychotic patients with polydipsia and hyponatremia. *New England Journal of Medicine, 318,* 397–403.

Gordon HL, Groth C, 1964: Weight change during and after hospital treatment. *Archives of General Psychiatry, 10,* 187–191.

Greenhill LL, Puig-Antich J, Novacenko H, Solomon M, Anghern C, Florea J, Goetz R, Fiscina B, Sachar EJ, 1984: Prolactin, growth hormone and growth response in boys with attention deficit disorder and hyperactivity treated with methylphenidate. *Journal of the American Academy of Child Psychiatry, 23,* 58–67.

Gruen PH, Sachar EJ, Altman N, Langer G, Tabrizi MA, Halpern FS, 1978: Relation of plasma prolactin to clinical response in schizophrenic patients. *Archives of General Psychiatry, 35,* 1222–1227.

Haider I, 1966: Thioridazine and sexual dysfunction. *International Journal of Neuropsychiatry, 5,* 255–257.

Hauser R, 1980: Amantadine associated recurrence of psychosis. *American Journal of Psychiatry, 137,* 240–242.

Hechtman L, Weiss G, Perlman T, 1984: Young adult outcome of hyperactive children who received long-term stimulant treatment. *Journal of the American Academy of Child and Adolescent Psychiatry, 23,* 261–269.

Jefferson JJ, Marshal JR, 1981: *Neuropsychiatric features of medical disorders.* New York: Plenum.

Joffe RT, Gold PW, Uhde TW, Post RM, 1984: The effects of carbamazepine on the thryotropin response to thyrotropin releasing hormone. *Psychiatry Research, 12,* 161–166.

Kendler KS, Weitzman RE, Rubin RT, 1978: Lack of arginine vasopressin response to central dopamine blockade in normal adults. *Journal of Clinical Endocrinology and Metabolism, 47,* 204–207.

Kimura T, Matsui K, Sato Y, 1974: Mechanism of carbamazepine induced antidiuresis: Evidence for release of antidiuretic hormone and impaired excretion of a water load. *Journal of Clinical Endocrinology and Metabolism, 38,* 356–362.

Klett CJ, Caffey EM, 1960: Weight changes during treatment with phenothiazine derivatives. *Journal of Neuropsychiatry, 2,* 102–108.

Klein RG, Mannuzza S, 1988: Hyperactive boys almost grown up, III: Methylphenidate effects on ultimate height. *Archives of General Psychiatry, 45,* 1131–1134.

Klibanski A, Neer R, Beitins I, 1981: Decreased bone density in hyperprolactinemic women. *New England Journal of Medicine, 303,* 1511–1514.

Koppelmann MC, Kurtz DW, Morrish KA, Bou E, Susser J, Shapiro J, Loriaux D, 1984: Vertebral body bone mineral content in hyperprolactinemic women. *Journal of Clinical Endocrinology and Metabolism, 59,* 1050–1055.

Korsgaard S, Skausig S, 1979: Increase in weight after treatment with depot neuroleptics. *Acta Psychiatrica Scandinavica, 59,* 139–144.

Lahr MB, 1985: Hyponatremia during carbamazepine therapy. *Clinical Pharmacology and Therapeutics, 37,* 693–696.

Lazarus J, McGregor AM, Ludgate M, Darke C, Creagh FM, Kingswood CJ, 1986: Effect of lithium carbonate therapy on thyroid immune status in manic depressive patients: A prospective study. *Journal of Affective Disorders, 11,* 155–160.

Lee RV, Jampol LM, Brown VW, 1971: Nephrogenic DI and lithium intoxication—complications of lithium carbonate therapy. *New England Journal of Medicine, 284,* 93–94.

Maarbjerg K, Vestergaard P, Schou M, 1987: Changes in serum thyroxine (T4) and serum thyroid stimulating hormone (TSH) during prolonged lithium therapy. *Acta Psychiatrica Scandinavica, 75,* 217–221.

Mallette LE, Eichhorn E, 1986: Effects of lithium carbonate on human calcium metabolism. *Archives of Internal Medicine, 146,* 770–776.

Mattes JA, Gittelman R, 1983: Growth of hyperactive children on maintenance regimen of methylphenidate. *Archives of General Psychiatry, 40,* 317–321.

Meltzer H, 1980: Effect of psychotropic drugs on neuroendocrine function. *Advances in Psychoneuroendocrinology, 3,* 277–297.

Meltzer H, Gudelsky GA, Koenig J, 1987: Antipsychotics, tricyclic antidepressants, and lithium. In: *Handbook of clinical psychoneuroendocrinology,* edited by CB Nemeroff and PT Loosen. New York: Guilford.

Myers DH, Carter RA, Burns BH, Armond A, Hussain SB, Chengapa VK, 1985: A prospective study of the effects of lithium on thyroid function and on the prevalence of antithyroid antibodies. *Psychological Medicine, 15,* 55–61.

Overall J, 1978: Prior psychiatric treatment and the development of breast cancer. *Archives of General Psychiatry, 35,* 898–899.

Paykel ES, Mueller PS, De La Vergne PM, 1973: Amitriptyline, weight gain and carbohydrate craving: A side effect. *British Journal of Psychiatry, 123,* 501–507.

Peck P, Shenkman L, 1979: Haloperidol induced syndrome of inappropriate secretion of antidiuretic hormone. *Clinical Pharmacology and Therapeutics, 26,* 442–444.

Plante N, Roy P, 1967: Galactorrhoea and neuroleptics. *Laval Medical, 38,* 103–107.

Plenge P, Mellerup ET, Bolwig TG, Brun C, Hetmar O, Ladefoged J, Larsen S, Rafelsen OJ, 1982: Lithium treatment: Does the kidney prefer one daily dose instead of two? *Acta Psychiatrica Scandinavica, 66,* 121–128.

Raskind MA, Courtney N, Mursburg MM, 1987: Antipsychotic drugs and plasma vasopressin in normals and acute schizophrenic patients. *Biological Psychiatry, 22,* 453–462.

Raskind MA, Weizman RE, Orientstein H, 1978: Is antidiuretic hormone elevated in psychosis: A pilot study. *Biological Psychiatry, 13,* 385–390.

Ringel RA, Brick JF, 1986: Perspective on carbamazepine induced water intoxication: Reversal by demeclocycline. *Neurology, 36,* 1505–1507.

Robinson B, 1957: Breast changes in the male and female with chlorpromazine or reserpine therapy. *Medical Journal of Australia, 44,* 239–241.

Robinson RG, McHugh PR, Folstein MF, 1975: Measurement of appetite disturbance in psychiatric disorders. *Journal of Psychiatric Research, 12,* 59–68.

Rogers GA, Burke G, 1987: Neuroleptics, prolactin and osteoporosis. *American Journal of Psychiatry, 144,* 388–389.

Salata R, Klein I, 1987: Effects of lithium on the endocrine system: A review. *Journal of Laboratory Clinical Medicine, 110,* 130–136.

Samiy AH, Rosnick PB, 1987: Early identification of renal problems in patients receiving chronic lithium treatment. *American Journal of Psychiatry, 144,* 670–672.

Sandifer MG, 1983: Hyponatremia due to psychotropic drugs. *Journal of Clinical Psychiatry, 44,* 301–303.

Sandison RA, Whitelaw E, Currie JD, 1960: Clinical trials with Mellaril in the treatment of schizophrenia. *Journal of Mental Science, 106,* 732–741.

Sarai M, Matsunaga H, 1989: ADH secretion in schizophrenic patients on antipsychotic drugs. *Biological Psychiatry, 26,* 576–580.

Selye H, Szabo S, 1972: Protection against haloperidol by catatoxic steroids. *Psychopharmacologica, 24,* 430–434.

Shaywitz SE, Hunt RD, Jatlow P, Cohen DJ, Young JG, Pierce RN, Anderson GM, Shaywitz BA, 1982: Psychopharmacology of attention deficit disorder: Pharmacokinetic, neuroendocrine, and behavioral measures following acute and chronic treatment with methylphenidate. *Pediatrics, 69,* 688–694.

Siever LJ, 1981: Effects of amantadine on prolactin levels and galactorrhea on neuroleptic treated patients. *Journal of Clinical Psychopharmacology, 1,* 2–7.

Steffens AB, Scheurink AJ, Luiten PG, Bohus B, 1988: Hypothalamic food intake regulating areas are involved in the homeostasis of blood glucose and plasma FFA level. *Physiological Behavior, 44,* 581–589.

Strandjord S, Aanderud S, Myking OL, Johannessen SI, 1981: Influence of carbamazepine on serum thyroxine and triidothyronine in patients with epilepsy. *Acta Neurologica Scandinavica, 63,* 111–121.

Transbol I, Christiansen C, Baastrup PC, 1978: Endocrine effects of lithium I: Hypothyroidism, its prevalence in long term treated patients. *Acta Endocrinologica, 87,* 759–767.

Uhde TW, Post RM, 1983: Effects of carbamazepine on serum electrolytes: Clinical and theoretical implications. *Journal of Clinical Psychopharmacology, 3,* 103–106.

Van Wyk JJ, Underwood LI, Hintz RL, Clendons DR, Voina SJ, Weaver RP, 1974: The somatomedins: A family of insulin-like hormones under growth hormone control. *Recent Progress on Hormonal Research, 30,* 259–318.

Vendsborg P, Bech P, Rafaelsen OJ, 1976: Lithium treatment and weight gain. *Acta Psychiatrica Scandinavica, 53,* 139–147.

Vestergaard P, Amdisen A, 1982: Lithium treatment and kidney function: A follow-up study of 237 patients in long term treatment. *Acta Psychiatrica Scandinavica, 63,* 333–345.

Vestergaard P, Schou M, 1987: Does long-term lithium treatment induce diabetes mellitus? *Neuropsychobiology, 17,* 130–132.

Viewig WVR, Godleski LS, Hundley PL, 1988: Diurnal weight gain as an index of polyuria and hyponatremia among chronically psychotic patients. *Psychiatric Medicine, 6,* 13–28.

Vincent J, Varley CK, Leger P, 1990: Effects of methylphenidate on early adolescent growth. *American Journal of Psychiatry, 147,* 501–502.

Weiner M, 1979: Haloperidol, hyperthyroidism, and sudden death. *American Journal of Psychiatry, 16,* 717–718.

Witton K, 1962: Sexual dysfunction secondary to Mellaril. *Disorder of the Nervous System, 23,* 175.

Wolff J, 1979: Lithium's interactions with the thyroid gland. In: *Lithium controversies and unresolved issues,* edited by TB Cooper and S Gershon. Princeton: Excerpta Medica.

Yassa R, Iskandar H, Nastase C, Camille Y, 1988b: Carbamazepine and hyponatremia in patients with affective disorder. *American Journal of Psychiatry, 145,* 339–342.

Yassa R, Saunders A, Nastase C, Camille Y, 1988a: Lithium induced thyroid disorders: A prevalence study. *Journal of Clinical Psychiatry, 49,* 14–16.

Yeo PPB, Bates D, Howe JG, Ratcliffe WA, Schardt CW, Heath A, Evered DC, 1978: Anticonvulsants and thyroid function. *British Medical Journal, 1,* 1581–1583.

28

Immunological Alterations

K. N. Roy Chengappa, Vishwajit L. Nimgaonkar,
and Rohan Ganguli

The function of the immune system is to protect the organism from both external and internal pathogens. The immune system learns what is "self" in early development, and this prevents the organism from mounting an immune response against its own organ systems. The immune system is organized into stationary organs (thymus, lymph nodes, tonsils, appendix, Peyer's patches, the lymphatic vessels) and circulating components, phagocytes and lymphocytes. These cells arise from precursors in the bone marrow.

There are three main types of lymphocytes: T cells, B cells, and natural killer (NK) cells. Phagocytes that process the pathogen and present it on their surface are called antigen-presenting cells (macrophages and dendritic cells). Killer T cells have receptors that recognize the foreign antigen and multiply to kill the antigen-presenting cells. Subsets of T cells (helpers or suppressors) help modify this response. This is termed "cell-mediated immunity." In contrast, in humoral immunity, B cells are stimulated when antigens bind to specific receptors and no antigen-presenting cell is required. Stimulated B cells, in the presence of factors derived from T cells and phagocytes, multiply and release antibodies to the various body fluids or at tissue sites. Antibodies bind antigens, and these complexes are cleared by phagocytes. The presence of intact skin and mucosa, as well as the production of antibodies at mucosal sites, provides protection against pathogens. This is called "local immunity."

There is increasing evidence that brain, behavior, and immune function are interrelated (Ader, 1981). There are several neuropsychiatric diseases where the immunological functions go awry. Studies have found that immune parameters are disturbed in stress, as well as in subsets of depressed and schizophrenic patients. Psychotropic drugs also have significant immunological effects.

The effects of psychotropic drugs on the individual components of the immune system have not been investigated thoroughly. Indeed, it is not known if these drugs consistently alter the primary function of the immune system (i.e., defense against internal and external pathogens). On the other hand, psychotropic drugs, like most others, can cause serious and even fatal idiosyncratic reactions (e.g., agranulocytosis), some of which are presumably immune-mediated. A wide range of purported immune effects on different organs have been described.

ANTIPSYCHOTIC AGENTS

Antibody-Mediated Immune Changes

Chlorpromazine is known to induce antibodies to various nuclear proteins (antinuclear and antihistone antibodies), cardiolipin (anticardiolipin antibodies, ACA), and lupus anticoagulant (Canoso, de Oliveria, & Nixon, 1990). Only a small fraction of patients with antibodies will go on to develop the associated clinical syndrome (e.g., drug-induced lupus or thrombosis). Although the frequency of thrombosis in patients with systemic lupus erythematosus (SLE) increases from 15% to 50% when lupus anticoagulant is present, chlorpromazine-induced lupus anticoagulant and IgM-ACA are not associated with an increased risk of thrombosis (Canoso & de Oliveira, 1988). In SLE, the disease activity and ACA of the IgG class (as opposed to IgM-ACA raised by antipsychotics) may be responsible for the thrombotic episodes. It has been suggested that phenothiazines stabilize membranes and thus exert a protective effect against thrombosis at the endothelial cell level. The clinical significance of elevated levels of serum IgM remains unclear (Zarrabi et al., 1979).

Cell-Mediated Immune Changes

The following cellular immune changes are induced by chlorpromazine: decreased percentage of T lymphocytes (Zarrabi et al., 1979), production of atypical lymphocytes (Hirata-Hibi & Fessel, 1964; Fieve, Blumenthal, & Little, 1966); inhibition of phytohemagglutination-induced leucocyte cell proliferation (Sakalis, Curry, Mould, & Lader, 1972), and hypersensitivity reactions. Hypersensitivity reactions include maculopapular and photosensitive skin rashes, exfoliative dermatitis and the Stevens-Johnson syndrome, contact dermatitis in people handling chlorpromazine (an occupational hazard), agranulocytosis, and hepatitis. In this chapter, we provide details of a serious complication, agranulocytosis. Details of other adverse reactions are discussed in Chapters 20, 22, and 26.

Clozapine-Induced Agranulocytosis and Neutropenia

Epidemiology

U.S. data suggest that the annual rate of clozapine-induced agranulocytosis is around 2% (Lieberman, 1987, cited in Lieberman et al., 1988). Lower rates have been reported in Europe (Grohmann, Schmidt, Spieb-Kiefer, & Ruther, 1989). A cluster of 16 cases with 8 fatalities occurred in Finland in 1975 (Amsler, Teerenhovi, Barth, Harjula, & Vuopio, 1977). Clozapine induces neutropenia probably at a higher rate than agranulocytosis. The peak period of risk for agranulocytosis seems to be between 3 to 18 weeks, although it can occur both earlier and later. Reviewing the 185 cases of clozapine-associated granulocytopenia reported to Sandoz Ltd., Krupp and Barnes (1989) suggest that 77% of all cases and 85% of all fatalities occurred in the first 18 weeks of treatment. Nearly twice as many women as men were affected, with the mean age for both sexes being in the 40s. Nearly 75% of patients were receiving concomitant medication. Recently, Lieberman et al. (1990) reported a strong association of HLA-B38, DR4, DWQ 3, and clozapine-induced agranulocytosis in Jewish patients with schizophrenia.

Pathogenesis

In addition to a possible direct toxic effect of the drug or its metabolite on the bone marrow, immunologic mechanisms have been strongly suspected (Claas, 1989). Clozapine is a small molecule and may not be immunogenic by itself. However, as a hapten it may form a complex with a protein on the granulocyte or a precursor cell, and this may become immunogenic, leading to the formation of antibodies that then destroy the granulocyte or the precursor cell in the marrow. In another immune model, the drug may induce an autoimmune response by the anomalous triggering of a lymphocyte, and the resultant antibodies may destroy granulocytes or their stem cells by no longer recognizing these as "self." It is also possible that a metabolite of clozapine but not clozapine itself is immunogenic. Finally, clozapine may trigger the production of cytotoxic lymphocytes that destroy granulocytes and their precursors. In all these conditions, clozapine acts as a trigger or stimulus and hence has to be discontinued immediately for recovery to occur. Lieberman et al. (1988) have identified an antibody in the IgM fraction from the sera of patients who developed agranulocytosis on clozapine; they (Lieberman et al., 1990) postulate that gene products contained in the haplotype of Jewish patients with schizophrenia may be involved in mediating clozapine-induced agranulocytosis.

Clinical Features, Course, and Outcome

Although the clinical course varies, in most patients, previously normal peripheral white blood cell (WBC) counts fall acutely to less than 2,000/mm^3 in a few days. There is a near total absence of polymorphonuclear leucocytes, relative lymphopenia with normal erythrocyte, and platelet values (Lieberman et al., 1988). Many of the patients have a sore throat, fever, and weakness at the onset of agranulocytosis. The bone marrow reveals a selective loss of granulocyte precursors with preservation of other cells. Discontinuation of clozapine, institution of supportive care, and antibiotics resulted in recovery of all five patients with clinical and hematological improvement seen in 14 to 21 days (Lieberman et al., 1988). The outcome is favorable when the diagnosis of granulocytopenia is made early and secondary infections have not yet occurred (Farina, Krupp, & Tobler, 1978, cited by Krupp & Barnes, 1989). Age and sex, daily or cumulative dose of clozapine, duration of treatment, and concomitant use of other drugs do not appear to predict outcome.

Phenothiazine-Induced Agranulocytosis

Epidemiology

Phenothiazine-induced agranulocytosis usually appears between 10 and 90 days after initiating the offending drug, although later onset cases have been seen (Pisciotta, 1969). Older females and whites may be more vulnerable (Mandel & Gross, 1968). Doses of the drugs used have been variable. Two studies done when high doses of low-potency phenothiazines were the mainstay of antipsychotic therapy found rates of 1:1,240 and 1:2,000 for phenothiazine-induced agranulocytosis, although a higher number of patients had phenothiazine-induced leukopenia (Litvak & Kaelbling, 1971; Pisciotta, 1969). Since these studies, reports of antipsychotic-related agranulocytosis (except clozapine) have become less frequent, presumably because the high-potency and nonphenothiazine antipsychotic drugs have become the main mode of drug treatment for the psychoses (Levinson & Simpson, 1987). Levinson and Simpson (1987) point out that many of the early cases occurred in large institutions with heterogenous patients who had serious concurrent medical illnesses. Hence, some cases of agranulocytosis that have been attributed to phenothiazines may have to be reconsidered.

Pathogenesis

Pisciotta (1973) has suggested that a toxic mechanism may be involved in chlorpromazine-induced agranulocytosis rather than an immunogenic one. Bone marrow cells from patients who had recovered from chlorpromazine-induced agranulocytosis were found to have a defect in the final stage of DNA synthesis; patients sensitive to other drugs lacked this defect (Pisciotta, 1971). Pisciotta (1971) hypothesizes that phenothiazine-sensitive patients may have a defect in DNA synthesis that is usually quiescent, but in the presence of phenothiazines for sufficient periods of time, they may be predisposed to cessation of granulocyte production.

Clinical Features and Outcome

Leukopenia or agranulocytosis may be clinically silent, and when they come to attention, signs of infection may often be present. Complete blood counts should be done immediately and the drug discontinued pending confirmation of the results and determination of the causes of the infection. Recovery generally occurs in 1 to 3 weeks; death occurs in a minority of cases.

LITHIUM

Changes in Humoral Immunity

Lithium can induce antinuclear antibodies (ANA, anti-DNA) and has been implicated in drug-induced lupus (Presley, Kahn, & Williamson, 1976; Shukla & Borrison, 1982; Whalley et al., 1981). Test of thyroid function and titers of thyroid antibodies were measured in 133 patients before they received lithium treatment. Of the 12 patients who subsequently became hypothyroid, 9 had thyroid autoantibodies and an exaggerated thyroid-stimulating hormone (TSH) response to thyrotropin-releasing hormone (TRH) before the commencement of lithium (Myers et al., 1985). This study also found that lithium administration was accompanied by a rise in thyroid antibody titers in 20 patients and a fall in 5 patients.

Autoimmune Disorders

Although uncommon, the induction or exacerbation of autoimmune disorders has been reported as a side effect of lithium therapy: hypothyroidism and hyperthyroidism (Crowe, Lloyd, Bloch, & Rosser, 1973; Pohl, Berchou, & Gupta, 1979), diabetes mellitus (Craig, Abu-Saleh, & Smith, 1977; Johnston, 1977), myasthenia gravis (Neil, Himmelhoch, & Licta, 1976), psoriasis (Carter, 1972; Evans & Martin, 1979), and alopecia and arthritis (Black & Waziri, 1984). This provides indirect evidence for the immunomodulating role of lithium.

Immunopotentiating Role

On a more positive note, lithium's immunopotentiating and antiviral properties are reported to cause remission of recurrent herpes virus infection, allergic rhinitis, purpura, poison ivy dermatitis, and recurrent upper respiratory infections (Gilis, 1983; Leib, 1979).

Cellular Immunity

Lithium has numerous effects on hematopoietic cells: proliferation of lymphocytes in response to mitogens, enhanced phagocytosis by macrophages and rosette formation by T cells, peripheral leucocytosis, increased number of granulocytic colonies in the bone marrow, decreased suppressor T cell activity, and enhanced helper T cells activity (Shenkman, Borkowsky, & Holtzman, 1978; *Biomedicine,* 1978; *Lancet,* 1980; Dosch, Matheson, & Schuurman, 1980; Pisciotta, Westring, & DePray, 1967). Although some reports suggest that lithium may induce or ameliorate leukemia (Orr & McKernan, 1979; Paladine, Price, & Williams, 1981; Visca et al., 1979), other investigators have not found any association between lithium therapy and leukemia (Lyskowski & Nasrallah, 1981; Resek & Olivieri, 1983). The ability of lithium to cause neutrophil leucocytosis and increase bone marrow granulocyte colony-stimulating activity has been exploited as a supplement to chemotherapy for acute leukemia, hairy cell leukemia, and small cell carcinoma of the lung. Lithium is also used in patients who fail to respond to traditional therapy in aplastic anemia, cyclic neutropenia, neutropenic children, Felty's syndrome, recurrent staphylococcal skin infections, recurrent fever, and neutropenia (Blum, 1979, 1980; Chan, Freedman, & Saunders, 1981; Charron, Barret, & Faille, 1977; Gerner, Wolff, & Fauci, 1981; Gupta, Robinson, & Smith, 1975; Lyman, Williams, & Preston, 1980; Scanni, Tomirotti, & Berrar, 1980; Shenkman, Borkowsky, & Shopsin, 1980; Steinherz, Rosen, & Ghavini, 1980). Kontozoglou and Mambo (1983) have presented histopathological evidence of lithium-induced, cellular-immune mediated thyroiditis in a case report.

ANTIDEPRESSANTS

There are probably more studies of immune function in depression than in any other psychiatric disorder. Although the results of all these studies are far from unanimous, the following changes (as compared to controls) have been reported consistently: lowered proliferative response to mitogens (Kronfol, Silva, & Greden, 1983; Schleifer, Keller, Myerson, & Stein, 1984) and lowered in-vitro NK cell activity. Not surprisingly, these immune parameters have also been studied in relation to antidepressant drug actions.

A lowering of the proliferative response to mitogens is generally reported (Audus & Gordon, 1982; Baker et al., 1977). However, the effects were invariably observed in dose ranges well above those that are therapeutically relevant.

Albrecht et al. (1985) found that the mean mitogen response for a group of 22 depressed patients was lower following treatment compared with their baseline. However, this study is difficult to interpret as patients received a variety of treatments including tricyclics, lithium, and electroconvulsive therapy. The value of mitogen stimulation tests has also been questioned as this in-vitro technique may not have physiological relevance.

NK cell activity does appear to be inhibited in the physiological dose range at least by desmethylimipramine (Miller, Anis, & Van Praag, 1986). Amitryptiline and imipramine were also reported to have similar effects. Some inhibition of mitogen stimulation was also observed by these investigators.

The aforementioned data suggest that tricyclics do have measurable effects on in-vitro tests. However, little can be inferred about the clinical significance of these changes. Studies need to be done employing better immunological measures as well as examining actual clinical outcomes such as infection in patients on antidepressants. The interactions with physiological alterations such as lymphocyte subsensitivity to corticosteroids (Lowy, Reder, Antel, & Meltzer, 1984) should also be included in the designs of such studies.

Heterocyclic antidepressants may occasionally produce maculopapular rashes or a photosensitivity reaction, which may be an allergic response. Less than 1% of patients on heterocyclics develop liver toxicity, which seems to be a hypersensitivity reaction (Schoonover, 1987). Most often, there is evidence of abnormal liver function tests without overt jaundice. In a few patients, fever, anorexia and eosinophilia may accompany mild and transient jaundice, usually during the first 2 months of treatment.

Agranulocytosis seems to an allergic reaction, usually appearing within 40 to 70 days after initiating treatment, and patients with advancing age and concomitant physical illnesses seem to be at greater risk (Schoonover, 1987). The onset is sudden, accompanied by fatigue, malaise, normal red cell count, low white cell count with reduced granulocyte numbers, and infections of the oropharnyx.

Immune alterations (Table 1) with the monoamine oxidase inhibitor (MAOI) antidepressants are less well known. The occasional occurrence of liver damage may result from a direct toxic effect or a hypersensitivity reaction.

Nomifensine and Autoimmune Hemolytic Anemia

Nomifensine, a nontricyclic antidepressant, was withdrawn by the manufacturer in the United States after reports in the United Kingdom and other European countries linked it to fatal hypersensitivity associated hemolytic anemia (*FDA Drug Bulletin,* 1986; Morton, Yu, Waldek, Holmes, & Mundy, 1986; Ross, 1985). Earlier reports had linked it to autoimmune hemolytic anemia and other hypersensitivity reactions, hyperpyrexia, liver injury, and eosinophilia. Two different immune mechanisms have been implicated in nomifensine-induced hemolysis: (1) an "innocent bystander" mechanism, in which the drug and antibody combine and then bind to the red cells, which in turn activate complement and cause acute, often fatal intravascular hemolysis and hemoglobulinuria; and (2) similar to the mechanism with methyldopa, the antibody is directed against a red cell antigen and not the drug. In this case there is no intravascular hemolysis; the Coombs's test may remain positive for months and the patient may have mild

Table 1 Psychotropic drug-induced immune alterations

Organ system	Effects	Drugs often implicated
Hematological (see details in Chapter 26)	Leukopenia	Chlorpromazine, clozapine, fluphenzaine, heterocyclic and MAOI antidepressants
	Agranulocytosis	Clozapine, chlorpromazine, other neuroleptics, heterocyclic antidepressants
	Eosinophilia	Clozapine, chlorpromazine, heterocyclic antidepressants
	Basophilia	Clozapine
	Autoimmune hemolytic anemia	Nomifensine
	Thrombocytopenic purpura	Chlorpromazine, fluphenazine
	Lymphocytosis	Fluoxetine
	Leucocytosis	Lithium
Cutaneous	Itching, erythema, urticaria, photosensitivity, maculopapular rash, Stevens-Johnson syndrome, exfoliative dermatisis, angioneurotic edema	Chlorpromazine, carbamazepine, benzodiazepines
	Worsening of psoriasis, vitiligo	Lithium
Thyroid	Autoimmune thyroiditis	Lithium
Neurological	Guillain-Barre syndrome	Zimelidine
Hepatic	Cholestatic jaundice	Chlorpromazine, thioridazine, haloperidol, thiothixene, loxapine, molindone
Multisystem	Drug induced lupus	Chlorpromazine, lithium
	? Exacerbation/induction of leukemia	Lithium
	Eosinophilia-myalgia syndrome	Altered manufacturing process of L-tryptophan

chronic hemolysis leading to anemia (Ross, 1985). Interstitial pneumonitis presumably mediated by immune measures has also been reported in a patient on nomifensine (Patel & Keshavan, 1987).

Zimelidine and Guillain-Barre Syndrome

Zimelidine, a selective serotonin reuptake blocker, was also withdrawn by the manufacturer after it was shown that the risk of developing Guillain-Barre syndrome was increased 25-fold among patients receiving zimelidine (Fagius, Osterman, Siden, & Wiholm, 1985). Eighteen months after its introduction, the Swedish Adverse Drug Reactions Advisory Committee received 13 reports of cases of Guillain-Barre syndrome, occurring within 6 to 17 days after starting zimelidine. The initial influenza-like symptoms—fever, myalgia, sore throat—gave way to widespread symmetrical dysfunction of peripheral nerves in an additional 1 to 20 days. This was seen clinically as limb weakness, paresthesia, cranial nerve palsies, areflexia in the arms and legs, ataxia, and sometimes sensory loss. Bladder paresis and respiratory paralysis rarely were noted. Cerebrospinal fluid findings were consistent with the diagnosis, and nerve conduction studies showed reduced velocity. The cumulative doses used at the start of the symptoms were 900 to 3400 mg, and at the beginning of the neurological signs and symptoms they were 1200 to 4400 mg of zimelidine. Five of the 13 cases recovered in 5 to 8 weeks, whereas others showed moderate to marked improvement over a longer period (up to 31 weeks). Given the temporal sequence of events and clinical features that could not be attributed to other viral illnesses, it was thought that zimelidine was the causative agent, and that the syndrome was mediated by an immune mechanism. It was believed that a neurotoxic mechanism was less likely, since many patients had used much larger doses of the drug for longer periods without developing any symptoms.

BENZODIAZEPINES

Benzodiazepines are alleged to cause "depression of humoral and cellular immune response" (Descotes, Tedone, & Evreux, 1982). As with the literature on tricyclics, this assertion is based mainly on animal studies that employed high doses of medication. A more recent study (Zavala & Lenfant, 1987) reported that benzodiazepines enhanced the humoral response to sheep red blood cells (SRBC) in mice. The latter may be a more physiologically relevant measure than the more commonly used mitogen response tests. Since stress reduces the SRBC response, the observed effect with benzodiazepine may be the result of "stress reduction."

At this point, little can be said about the clinical significance of the effects of benzodiazepines on the immune system. Allergic skin rashes, hepatic injury, and agranulocytosis have been rarely reported with this group of drugs. Since stress (and, by implication, anxiety) has measurable immunologic effects, further studies are undoubtedly needed.

MISCELLANEOUS DRUGS

L-tryptophan

The use of L-tryptophan has been associated with the increased occurrence of the eosinophilia-myalgia syndrome (EMS) with some fatalities. This resulted in the drug being taken off the market in the United States (Eidson, Philen, Sewell, Voorhees, & Kilbourne, 1990).

Using a case-control design, surveillance (health practitioners and media announcements) and a telephone survey of households, Belongia et al. (1990) estimated that the attack rate increased from 54 in 1988, to 268 per 100,000 female tryptophan users in 1989 and from 0 in 1988 to 144 per 100,000 male tryptophan users in 1989. Most cases have been reported in non-Hispanic whites with the median age being 45 years (range 4 to 77 years), and most affected patients are women. Most of the subjects were taking the drug for insomnia, and a smaller number for premenstrual syndrome, depression or anxiety, headache, behavior disorder, and so forth. Although most had been taking the drug when the syndrome occurred, it has also occurred 3 weeks to 4 months after stopping the drug. Although the majority of cases occur a few months after starting the drug, a small number of cases do occur during the first month of treatment.

Pathogenesis

Among the subjects for whom the source of tryptophan was known, the majority had used a product produced by one company (Showa Denko K.K., Tokyo, Japan). Belongia et al. (1990) suggested that altered manufacturing conditions (using a new strain of *Bacillus amyloliquefaciens* and using reduced amounts of powdered carbon) led to the formation of a trace chemical constituent that may contribute to the pathogenesis of this syndrome. The exact mechanisms by which this constituent contributes to the inflammatory changes is not known. Muscle biopsies have revealed evidence of perimyositis, perivasculitis, or fasciitis. Despite some clinical similarities between the toxic oil syndrome and the EMS, the serum IgE levels were normal in EMS (unlike toxic oil syndrome, where it was elevated in almost 50% of the patients). The clinical syndrome, eosinophilia, and the temporal sequence of events suggest an allergic-type immune pathogenesis.

Clinical Features

Eosinophilia (more than 1,000/μL), disabling myalgia which often prevents the patient from being able to work, muscle weakness requiring assistance to walk, muscle cramps, muscle tenderness, edema, paraesthesia, rash, arthralgia, pruritis, fever, dyspnea, tight and shiny hard skin, dry mouth, cough and an abnormal chest x ray have all been reported (Belongia et al., 1990; Eidson et al., 1990). A third of the patients studied by Belongia et al. (1990) were hospitalized.

Carbamazepine

It is unclear whether agranulocytosis, thrombocytopenia, aplastic anemia, and leukopenia—which occur with the use of carbamazepine—result from a direct toxic effect on the bone-marrow precursor cells or if an immune mechanism is involved. Skin rashes and other cutaneous conditions (Stevens-Johnson syndrome, lupus-like reactions, exfoliative dermatitis, photosensitivity) have been reported in about 3% of patients (Weilburg, 1987). Post (1990) described rashes to be one of the most common side effects (12%) in his patients on carbamazepine. He stated that it often occurs in the first 3 weeks of treatment and often required that the drug be discontinued. Serious blood dyscrasias (agranulocytosis and aplastic anemia) occur at the rate of 1 per 125,000 individuals receiving the drug (Pellock, 1987).

MANAGEMENT OF DRUG-INDUCED REACTIONS

A high index of suspicion is required because it is in the first few weeks of treatment with psychotropic drugs that many of the serious and even fatal reactions occur. General management consists of discontinuing the offending drug, instituting supportive measures, and consulting the appropriate medical specialist for continued management, especially if the situation demands transfer of care to the other specialist.

Clozapine

Because of the risk of agranulocytosis, the availability of clozapine in the United States is contingent on patient and physician participation in a monitoring system called the Clozaril Patient Management System (CPMS). This "bundling" of a drug with a mandatory monitoring system is unique in the history of therapeutics. CPMS consists of a case administrator who organizes blood draws and drug delivery. Patients must first be enrolled in the system by their doctors who mail in enrollment forms. Patients receive weekly whole blood counts (WBC) and are given a 1-week supply of clozapine. All subsequent supply of the drug is contingent on the patient having blood drawn. The system is expensive ($25 per day). Recently, the manufacturer has revised the labeling of clozapine to allow other "systems" for patient treatment in a more traditional manner. CPMS is no longer the mechanism of clozapine availability.

In response to the changes in the WBC count of patients on clozapine, the following clinical guidelines are recommended:

1. If the WBC count falls to between 3,500 and 3,000/mm^3 or the granulocyte count falls to between 1,500 and 1,000/mm^3, then WBC monitoring is stepped up to twice a week.

2. If the WBC count falls to between 3,000 and 2,000/mm^3 or the granulocyte count falls to between 1,000 and 500/mm^3, then clozapine should be stopped and biweekly WBC monitoring should be continued. If the count goes above 3,500/mm^3 and the granulocytes above 1,500/mm^3, clozapine may be reinstituted with biweekly monitoring.

3. If the WBC count falls below 2,000/mm^5 or the granulocyte count below 500/mm^3, clozapine should be stopped. The patient should not be rechallenged with clozapine as the onset of agranulocytosis could be very rapid. It is advisable to consult a hematologist and if signs of infection (e.g., fever and sore throat) are present, the patient should be transferred to a medical service.

4. If the drug is discontinued (for whatever reason), weekly WBC and granulocyte counts should be performed for an additional 4 weeks.

Since CPMS monitoring system was instituted, 55 cases of agranulocytosis have been detected in the United States (as of February, 1991). One fatality has recently occurred, but this patient was also receiving carbamazepine, a drug known to cause blood dyscrasias (Sandoz Ltd., personal communication).

Chlorpromazine

In the rare case of chlorpromazine-induced SLE, the drug should be discontinued; if symptoms persist, consultation with a specialist will help decide further clinical management. Treatment of psychotic symptoms will require another antipsychotic from a different chemical class of drugs.

Lithium

Lithium may need to be discontinued if it exacerbates other autoimmune disorders. However, in consultation with experts in their respective specialities, it may be possible to continue lithium while the patient receives therapy for the other autoimmune disorder. The management of thyroid disease during lithium treatment is discussed further in Chapter 27.

L-Tryptophan

Centers for Disease Control guidelines (Kilbournet, Swygert, & Philen, 1990) recommend that L-tryptophan be discontinued when eosinophilia-myalgia syndrome is suspected or diagnosed and glucocorticoids be used to reduce eosinophilia counts. In addition, a nonsteroidal antiinflammatory agent or narcotic analgesic may be used to relieve severe muscle pain. However, many patients continue to be symptomatic despite medical treatment.

Carbamazepine

It has been suggested that patients who must take carbamazepine despite skin rashes can be retried under the cover of prednisone. However, Post (1990) points out that this may work as long as there is no evidence of systemic allergy. He suggested that an absolute neutrophil count of 1,500 be used as a cutoff to discontinue carbamazepine. It is important to monitor the patient to make sure this is a "benign" process rather than a serious one before deciding to either discontinue the drug or add lithium with a view to augment neutrophil production. One clue might be that in the absence of infection, if the absolute neutrophil count levels off above 1,500 and the red cells and platelets are unaffected, then the addition of lithium may augment the neutrophil production.

REFERENCES

Ader R, 1981: *Psychoneuroimmunology.* Orlando: Academic Press.

Albrecht J, Helderman JH, Schlesser MA, Rush AJ, 1985: A controlled study of cellular immune function in affective disorders before and during somatic therapy. *Psychiatry Research, 15,* 185–193.

Amsler HA, Teerenhovi L, Barth E, Harjula K, Vuopio P, 1977: Agranulocytosis in patients treated with clozapine. A study of the Finnish epidemic. *Acta Psychiatrica Scandinavica, 56,* 241–248.

Audus KL, Gordon MA, 1982: Tricyclic antidepressant effects on the immune system lymphocyte response. *Journal of Immunopharmacology, 4,* 13–27.

Baker GA, Santalo R, Blumenstein J, 1977: Effect of psychotropic agents upon the blastogenic response to human t-lymphocytes. *Biological Psychiatry, 12,* 159–169.

Belongia EA, Hedberg CW, Gleich GJ, White KE, Mayeno AN, Loefering DA, Dunnette SA, Pirie PL, MacDonald KL, Osterholm MT, 1990: An investigation of the cause of the Eeosinophilia-Myalgia syndrome associated with tryptophan use. *New England Journal of Medicine, 323,* 357–365.

Biomedicine, 1978: Immunologic function in man receiving lithium carbonate *(editorial). Biomedicine, 29,* 223–225.

Black DW, Waziri R, 1984: Arthritis associated with lithium toxicity: Case report. *Journal of Clinical Psychiatry, 45,* 135–136.

Blum SF, 1979: Lithium therapy of aplastic anemia. *New England Journal of Medicine, 300,* 677.

Blum SF, 1980: Lithium in hairy-cell leukemia. *New England Journal of Medicine, 303,* 464–465.

Canoso RT, de Oliveira RM, 1988: Chlorpromazine-induced anticardiolipin antibodies and lupus anticoagulant. Absence of thrombosis. *American Journal of Hematology, 2,* 272–275.

Canoso RT, de Oliveira RM, Nixon RA, 1990: Neuroleptic-associated autoantibodies. A prevalence study. *Biological Psychiatry, 27,* 863–870.

Carter TN, 1972: The relationship of lithium carbonate to psoriasis. *Psychosomatics, 13,* 325–327.

Chan HSL, Freeeman MH, Saunders EF, 1981: Lithium therapy of children with chronic neutropenia. *American Journal of Medicine, 70,* 1073–1077.

Charron D, Barrett AJ, Faille A, 1977: Lithium in acute myeloid leukaemia. *Lancet, i,* 1307.

Claas FHJ, 1989: Drug-induced agranulocytosis: Review of possible mechanisms, and prospects for clozapine studies. *Psychopharmacology, 99*(suppl), 113–117.

Craig J, Abu-Saleh M, Smith B, 1977: Diabetes mellitus in patients on lithium. *Lancet, ii,* 1028.

Crowe MJ, Lloyd GG, Bloch S, Rosser RM, 1973: Hypothyroidism in patients treated with lithium: A review and two case reports. *Psychological Medicine, 3,* 337–342.

Descotes JR, Tedone R, Evreux JC, 1982: Suppression of humoral and cellular immunity in normal mice by diazepam. *Immunology Letters, 5,* 41–43.

Dosch HM, Matheson D, Schuurman RKB, 1980: Anti-suppressor cell effects of lithium in vitro and invivo. In: *Lithium effects on granulopoiesis and immune function,* edited by AH Rossof and WA Robinson. New York: Plenum Press.

Eidson M, Philen RM, Sewell CM, Voorhees R, Kilbourne EM, 1990: L-tryptophan and eosinophilia-myalgia syndrome in New Mexico. *Lancet, 335,* 645–648.

Evans DL, Martin W, 1979: Lithium carbonate and psoriasis. *American Journal of Psychiatry, 136,* 1326–1327.

Fagius J, Osterman PO, Siden A, Wiholm BE, 1985: Guillain-Barre syndrome following zimelidine treatment. *Journal of Neurology, Neurosurgery and Psychiatry, 48,* 65–69.

Farina JC, Krupp P, Tobler HJ, 1978: Computer tools in spontaneous reporting of adverse drug reactions: A multinational company approach. In: *Conference on computer aid to drug therapy and to drug monitoring,* edited by H Ducrot, M Goldberg, R Hoigne, and P Middleton. Amsterdam: North-Holland Publishing.

FDA Drug Bulletin, 1986: Nomifensine withdrawn by manufacturer. *FDA Drug Bulletin, 16,* 7–8.

Fieve RR, Blumenthal B, Little B, 1966: The relationship of atypical lymphocytes, phenothiazines and schizophrenia. *Archives of General Psychiatry, 15,* 529–534.

Gerner RH, Wolff SM, Fauci AS, 1981: Lithium carbonate for recurrent fever and neutropenia. *Journal of the American Medical Association, 246,* 1584–1586.

Gilis A, 1983: Lithium in herpes simplex. *Lancet, ii,* 516.

Grohmann R, Schmidt LG, Spieb-Kiefer C, Ruther E, 1989: Agranulocytosis and significant leucopenia with neuroleptic drugs: Results from the AMUP program. *Psychopharmacology, 99*(suppl), 109–112.

Gupta RC, Robinson WA, Smyth CJ, 1975: Efficacy of lithium in rheumatoid arthritis with granulocytopenia (Felty's syndrome). *Arthritis and Rheumatism, 18,* 179.

Hirata-Hibi M, Fessel WJ, 1964: The bone marrow in schizophrenia. *Archives of General Psychiatry, 10,* 414–419.

Johnston BB, 1977: Diabetes mellitus in patients on lithium. *Lancet, ii,* 935–936.

Kilbourne EM, Swygert LA, Philen RM, 1990: Interim guidance on the eosinophilia-myalgia syndrome. *Annals of Internal Medicine, 112,* 85–88.

Kontozoglou T, Mambo N, 1983: The histopathologic features of lithium-associated thyroiditis. *Human Pathology, 14,* 737–739.

Kronfol Z, Silva J, Greden J, 1983: Impaired lymphocyte function in depressive illness. *Life Sciences, 33,* 241–247.

Krupp P, Barnes P, 1989: Leponex-associated granulocytopenia: A review of the situation. *Psychopharmacology, 99*(suppl), 118–121.

Lancet, 1980: Lithium in hematology *(editorial). Lancet, ii,* 626–627.

Levinson DF, Simpson GM, 1987: Serious non-extrapyramidal adverse effects of neuroleptics—sudden death, agranulocytosis and hepatotoxicity. In: *Psychopharmacology: The third generation of progress,* edited by HY Meltzer. New York: Raven Press.

Lieb J, 1979: Remission of recurrent herpes infection during therapy with lithium. *New England Journal of Medicine, 301,* 942.

Lieberman JA, 1987: *Neuropharmacologic and immunologic effects of clozapine in chronic schizophrenia.* Presented at the American College of Neuropsychopharmacology Meeting, San Juan, Puerto Rico.

Lieberman JA, Johns CA, Kane JM, Kanti R, Pisciotta AV, Saltz BL, Howard A, 1988: Clozapine-induced agranulocytosis: Non-cross-reactivity with other psychotropic drugs. *Journal of Clinical Psychiatry, 49,* 271–277.

Lieberman JA, Yunis J, Egea E, Canoso RT, Kane JM, Yunis EJ, 1990: HLA-B38, DR4, DQW 3 and clozapine-induced agranulocytosis in Jewish patients with schizophrenia. *Archives of General Psychiatry, 47,* 945–948.

Litvak R, Kaelblin G, 1971: Agranulocytosis, leukopenia and psychotropic drugs. *Archives of General Psychiatry, 24,* 265–267.

Lowy MT, Reder AT, Antel J, Meltzer HY, 1984: Glucocorticoid resistance in depression: The dexamethasone suppression test and lymphocyte sensitivity to dexamethasone. *American Journal of Psychiatry, 141*, 1365–1370.

Lyman GH, Williams CC, Preston D, 1980: The use of lithium carbonate to reduce infection and leukopenia during systemic chemotherapy. *New England Journal of Medicine, 302*, 257–260.

Lyskowski J, Nasrallah HA, 1981: Lithium therapy and the risk for leukaemia. *British Journal of Psychiatry, 139*, 256.

Mandel A, Gross M, 1968: Leukopenia and psychotropic drugs. *Archives of General Psychiatry, 24*, 265–267.

Miller AH, Anis GM, Van Praag HM, 1986: The influence of desmethylimipramine on NK cell activity. *Psychiatry Research, 19*, 12–14.

Morton AR, Yu R, Waldek S, Holmes AM, Mundy K, 1986: Withdrawal of nomifensine. *British Medical Journal, 293*, 452–453.

Myers DH, Carter RA, Burns BH, Armond A, Hussain SB, Chengappa VK, 1985: A prospective study of the effects of lithium on thyroid function and on the prevalence of antithyroid antibodies. *Psychological Medicine, 15*, 55–61.

Neil JF, Himmelhoch JM, Licata SM, 1976: Emergence of myasthenia gravis during treatment with lithium carbonate. *Archives of General Psychiatry, 33*, 1090–1092.

Orr LE, McKernan JF, 1979: Lithium reinduction of acute myeloblastic leukaemia. *Lancet, i*, 449–450.

Paladine WJ, Price LM, Williams HD, 1981: Hairy-cell leukemia treated with lithium. *New England Journal of Medicine, 304*, 1237–1238.

Patel H, Keshavan MS, 1987: Interstitial pneumonitis with nomifensine. *Clinical Neuropharmacology, 10*, 190–191.

Pellock JM, 1987: Carbamazepine side effects in children and adults. *Epilepsia, 28*(suppl), 64–70.

Pisciotta AV, 1969: Agranulocytosis induced by certain phenothiazine derivatives. *Journal of the American Medical Association, 208*, 1862–1868.

Pisciotta AV, 1971: Studies on agranulocytosis: A biochemical defect in chlorpromazine sensitive marrow cells. *Journal of Laboratory and Clinical Medicine, 78*, 435–448.

Pisciotta AV, 1973: Immune and toxic mechanisms in drug-induced agranulocytosis. *Seminars in Hematology, 10*, 279–310.

Pisciotta AV, Westring DW, DePrey C, 1967: Studies on agranulocytosis. VIII. Inhibition of mitosis in phytohemagglutinin-stimulated lymphocytes by chlorpromazine. *Journal of Laboratory and Clinical Medicine, 70*, 229–235.

Pohl RB, Berchou R, Gupta BK, 1979: Lithium-induced hypothyroidism and thyroiditis. *Biological Psychiatry, 14*, 835–836.

Post RM, 1990: Non-lithium treatment for bipolar disorder. *Journal of Clinical Psychiatry, 51*(suppl), 17–19.

Presley AP, Kahn A, Williamson N, 1976: Antinuclear antibodies in patients on lithium carbonate. *British Medical Journal, 2*, 280–281.

Resek G, Olivieri S, 1983: No association between lithium therapy and leukaemia. *Lancet, ii*, 940.

Ross JRY, 1985: Fatal immune haemolysis associated with nomifensine. *British Medical Journal, 291*, 606.

Sakalis G, Curry SH, Mould GP, Lader MH, 1972: Physiological and clinical effects of chlorpromazine and their relationship to plasma level. *Clinical Pharmacology and Therapeutics, 13*, 931–946.

Scanni A, Tomirotti M, Berra S, 1980: Lithium carbonate in the treatment of drug-induced leukopenia in patients with solid tumors. *Tumori, 66*, 729–737.

Schleifer SJ, Keller SE, Myerson A, Stein M, 1984: Lymphocyte function in major depressive disorder. *Archives of General Psychiatry, 41*, 484–486.

Schoonover SC, 1987: Depression. In: *The practitioner's guide to psychoactive drugs*, 2nd edition, edited by EL Bassuk, SC Schoonover and AJ Gelenberg. New York: Plenum.

Shenkman L, Borkowsky W, Holzman RS, 1978: Enhancement of lymphocyte and macrophage function in vitro by lithium chloride. *Clinical Immunology and Immunnopathology, 10*, 187–192.

Shenkman L, Borkowsky W, Shopsin B, 1980: Lithium as an immunologic adjuvant. *Medical Hypotheses, 6*, 1–6.

Shukla VR, Borison RL, 1982: Lithium and lupuslike syndrome. *Journal of the American Medical Association, 248*, 921–922.

Steinherz PG, Rosen G, Ghavini F, 1980: Effect of lithium carbonate on leukopenia after chemotherapy. *Journal of Pediatrics, 36*, 923–927.

Visca U, Mensi F, Spina MP, Bombara R, Giraldi B, Massari A, Rossi F, Santi G, 1979: Prevention of antiblastic neutropenia with lithium carbonate. *Lancet, i,* 779.

Weilburg JF, 1987: Temporal lobe epilepsy. In: *The practitioner's guide to psychoactive drugs,* 2nd edition, edited by EL Bassuk, SC Schoonover and AJ Gelenberg. New York: Plenum.

Whalley LJ, Roberts DF, Wentzel J, 1981: Antinuclear antibodies and histocompatibility antigens in patients on long-term lithium therapy. *Journal of Affective Disorders, 3,* 123–130.

Zarrabi MH, Zucker S, Miller F, Derman RM, Romano GS, Hartnett MS, Varma AO, 1979: Immunologic and coagulation disorders in chlorpromazine-treated patients. *Annals of Internal Medicine, 91,* 194–199.

Zavala F, Lenfant M, 1987: Benzodiazepines and PK11195 exert immunomodulating activities by binding on a specific receptor on macrophages. *Annals of the New York Academy of Sciences, 496,* 240–249.

Concluding Remarks

Adverse Cutaneous Reactions

Adverse skin reactions are commonly seen during psychotherapeutic drug treatment. They may arise from both immunological and nonimmunological mechanisms, and, in many cases, the precise pathophysiological mechanisms may remain unclear. The allergic reactions may range from urticarial rashes to exfoliative dermatitis. Nonimmunologically mediated skin reactions include cutaneous pigmentation and photosensitive reactions commonly seen with antipsychotic drugs. Establishing a cause-effect relationship is often difficult in relation to psychotropic drugs and skin reactions.

Complications of the Eye and Ear

Side effects of psychotropic medications often involve the eye and ear. Complications involving the ear are considerably less common and less severe than those affecting the eye and are usually reversible. Psychotropic drug side effects involving the eye are more common and cause considerably more morbidity. Virtually all classes of psychotropic drugs have been known to be associated with these adverse effects.

Hepatic Side Effects

Psychotropic drugs frequently cause liver dysfunction. Some psychotropic drugs also induce liver enzymes, thus stimulating their own catabolism. Because the liver is the major site of metabolism of many psychotropic drugs, hepatic dysfunction may cause impaired metabolism of drugs, resulting in prolonged activity or toxicity as the drug accumulates. Phenothiazines and monoamine oxidase inhibitors are among the psychotropic drugs more likely to manifest with significant adverse hepatic side effects.

Adverse Cardiovascular Effects

A number of significant adverse cardiovascular effects have been reported with psychotropic drugs, particularly tricyclic antidepressants. A variety of psychotropic drugs cause postural hypotension, a significant clinical problem. Monoamine oxidase inhibitor treatment is associated with a significant risk of hypertensive reactions, especially in relation to certain drug and food interactions. Disturbances of cardiac conduction, which may be severe and occasionally fatal, are often seen during treatment with tricyclic antidepressants and some antipsychotic drugs.

Sexual Dysfunction

Psychotropic drugs may cause unwanted alterations in libido, activity, or sexual performance. The mechanisms of these alterations may involve both central and peripheral pathways. Many psychotropic drugs act through more than one neurotransmitter system and have the potential to produce sexual dysfunction. Dopaminergic, noradrenergic, serotonergic, chlolinergic, and opiate systems may all be involved. An unusual and very serious complication of sexual function is priapism. Priapism is known to occur with several psychotropic agents, including antipsychotics, and among the antidepressants, most commonly with trazodone.

Adverse Hematological Effects

Blood dyscrasias such as leukopenia, agranulocytosis, aplastic anemia, hemolytic anemia, and thrombocytopenia are all known complications of psychotropic drug therapy. All classes of psychotropic drugs may result in these complications, but clozapine and chlorpromazine are among the more significant agents implicated. In general, early detection may prevent hematological disturbances from becoming severe.

Adverse Endocrine Effects

Several clinically significant endocrine side effects are known to occur during psychotropic drug treatment. Notable complications include antipsychotic-induced hyperprolactinemia, lithium-induced hypothyroidism, and diabetes insipidus—the syndrome of inappropriate antidiuretic hormone secretion often seen with diverse psychotropic agents and weight gain seen with a variety of drugs. Early recognition and laboratory monitoring are important in minimizing morbidity and preventing such complications.

Immunological Alterations

Both antibody and cell-mediated immune changes are known to occur with a wide variety of psychotropic drugs; these include skin reactions, hematological reactions, and hepatitis.

Appendix A

Generic and Trade Names, Dosages, and Half-lives of Commonly Used Psychotropic Drugs

Class	Generic name	Trade name	Halflife (hours)	Daily adult oral dosage range
Benzodiazepines	Diazepam	Valium	20–100	2–60 mg
	Chlordiazepoxide	Librium	24–48	15–100 mg
	Clorazepate	Tranxene	2–100	7.5–60 mg
	Halazepam	Paxopam	14–100	60–160 mg
	Prazepam	Centrax	48–78	20–60 mg
	Clonazepam	Clonopin	20–60	1.5–20 mg
	Flurazepam	Dalmane	47–100	15–30 mg
	Oxazepam	Serax	6–24	30–120 mg
	Lorazepam	Ativan	9–24	2–6 mg
	Alprazolam	Xanax	12–15	0.25–6 mg
	Temazepam	Restoril	4–10	15–30 mg
	Triazolam	Halcion	2–3	0.125–0.5 mg
	Midazolam	Versed	2–3	2–4 mg
	Quazepam	Doral	15–35	7.5–15 mg
	Estazolam	Prosom	12–30	0.5–2 mg
Nonbenzodiazepine/ hypnotics/sedatives	Buspirone	Buspar		20–60 mg
	Hydroxyzine	Atarax Vistaril		10–200 mg
	Promethazine	Phenergan		50–200 mg
	Chloralhydrate	Noctec	4–9	0.25–2 g
	Meprobamate[a]	Equanil Miltown	6–17	1.2–1.6 g 400 mg–2.4 g
	Gutethimide[a]	Doriden	5–22	0.5–1 g
	Ethchlorvynol[a]	Placidyl	10–25	0.5–1 g
	Methyprylon[a]	Noludar	4	200–400 mg
	Methaqualolone[a]	Quaalude	10–42	150–400 mg
Antidepressants	Imipramine	Tofranil Janimine	5–30	100–300 mg[b]
	Desipramine	Norpramin Pertofane	10–30	75–300 mg[b]
	Amitriptyline	Elavil	10–50	40–300 mg[b]
	Nortriptyline	Aventyl Pamelor	20–60	10–150 mg[b]
	Protriptyline	Vivactil	50–200	15–60 mg
	Doxepin	Sinequan Adapin	10–25	75–300 mg
	Clomipramine	Anafranil	15–60	75–300 mg
	Trimipramine	Surmontil		150–300 mg

(Foonotes at end of table)

(Table continues on next page)

Generic and Trade Names, Dosages, and Half-lives of Commonly Used Psychotropic Drugs
(*Continued*)

Class	Generic name	Trade name	Halflife (hours)	Daily adult oral dosage range
Antidepressants (*Cont.*)	Amoxapine	Ascendin	30	150–300 mg
	Trazodone	Desyrel	5–15	250–600 mg
	Maprotiline	Ludiomil	30–50	75–225 mg
	Fluoxetine	Prozac	48–216	5–80 mg
	Bupropion	Wellbutrin	8–24	75–450 mg
MAO inhibitors	Isocarboxazid	Marplan		10–20 mg
	Phenelzine	Nardil		45–90 mg
	Tranylcypromine	Parnate		20–30 mg
Mood stabilizers	Lithium	Lithobid	7–20	300–1800 mg^{b,c}
		Lithanate		300–1800 mg^{b,c}
	Carbamazepine	Tegretol	10–21	600–1200 mg^{b}
	Sodium valproate	Depakote	6–16	750–2000 mg^{b}
	Valproic acid	Depakene		15–60 mg/kg^{b}
Phenothiazine antipsychotics				
Aliphatic	Chlorpromazine	Thorazine	16–79	50–400 mg
Piperazine	Prochlorperazine	Compazine		15–60 mg
	Perphenazine	Trilafon	8–12	12–24 mg
	Trifluoperazine	Stelazine		5–20 mg
	Fluphenazine	Prolixin	ca. 14	1–15 mg
	Acetophenazine	Tindal		20–40 mg
	Butaperazine	Repoise		5–50 mg
Piperidine	Thoridazine	Mellaril	16–24	100–300 mg
	Mesoridazine	Serentil		30–150 mg
Nonphenothiazine antipsychotics				
Butyrophenones	Haloperidol	Haldol	14–21	1–15 mg
Thioxanthene	Chlorprothixene	Taractan	10–20	50–400 mg
	Thiothixene	Navane		6–60 mg
Dibenzoxazepines	Loxapine	Loxitane		20–100 mg
Dihydroindolone	Molindone	Moban		5–150 mg
Diphenylbutylepiperidine	Pimozide	Orap	ca. 10–20	0.5–5 mg
Rauwolfia alkaloids	Reserpine	Serpasil	4–200	0.1–1 mg
Dibenzodiazepine	Clozapine	Clozaril		150–400 mg
Antiparkinsonian drugs				
Anticholinergic	Benztropine	Cogentin		2–8 mg
	Biperiden	Akineton		2–6 mg
	Procyclidine	Kemadrin		6–20 mg
	Trihexiphenidyl	Artane		5–15 mg
Antihistamine	Diphenhydramine	Benadryl		25–100 mg
	Orphenadrine	Disipal		50–300 mg
Dopaminergic	Amantadine	Symmetrel	ca. 15	100–300 mg
	Bromocriptine	Parlodel		2.5–10 mg

[a]Not generally recommended for use.
[b]Monitor by blood level.
[c]Daily dose is dependent on phase of illness.

Appendix B

Therapeutic Blood Levels of Selected Psychotropic Drugs

Drug	Therapeutic levels
Imipramine	200–250 ng/ml[a]
Desipramine	> 125 ng/ml
Amitriptyline	120–250 ng/ml[a]
Nortriptyline	50–150 ng/ml
Lithium	0.7–1.2 mEq/L
Carbamazepine	8–12 μg/ml (4–12 for epilepsy)
Valproic acid	50–100 μg/ml
Propranolol	40–85 ng/ml
Phenobarbital	15–30 μg/ml
Haloperidol[b]	3–17 ng/ml
Doxepin	100–250 ng/ml
Primidone	4–12 μg/ml (Primidone)
	10–40 μg/ml (Phenobarbitol)

[a]Sum of parent drug and N-desmethyl metabolite levels.
[b]Clinical values uncertain.

REFERENCES

Guthrie S, Lane EA, Linnoila M, 1987: Monitoring of plasma concentrations in clinical psychophar-macology. In: *Psychopharmacology, the third generation of progress,* edited by HY Meltzer. New York: Raven.

Hyman SE, 1988: Appendix. In: *Manual of psychiatric emergencies,* second edition, edited by SE Hyman. Boston: Little Brown.

Kaplan HI, Saddock BJ, 1990: *Pocket handbook of clinical psychiatry.* Baltimore: Williams and Wilkins.

Index